Validating Preventive Food Safety and Quality Controls

Validating Preventive Food Safety and Quality Controls

An Organizational Approach to System Design and Implementation

John M. Ryan, Ph.D., PCQI
President, Ryan Systems, Inc. Palm Bay, FL, United States

ACADEMIC PRESS
An imprint of Elsevier
elsevier.com

Academic Press is an imprint of Elsevier
125 London Wall, London EC2Y 5AS, United Kingdom
525 B Street, Suite 1800, San Diego, CA 92101-4495, United States
50 Hampshire Street, 5th Floor, Cambridge, MA 02139, United States
The Boulevard, Langford Lane, Kidlington, Oxford OX5 1GB, United Kingdom

British Library Cataloguing-in-Publication Data
A catalogue record for this book is available from the British Library

Library of Congress Cataloging-in-Publication Data
A catalog record for this book is available from the Library of Congress

ISBN: 978-0-12-810994-6

Publisher: Nikki Levy
Acquisition Editor: Patricia Osborn
Editorial Project Manager: Jaclyn Truesdell
Production Project Manager: Caroline Johnson
Designer: Greg Harris

Contents

Preface

This book will introduce you to proven tools and techniques that you can quickly adapt to your organization as you move step-by-step to the point that you, your company, your auditors, and your customers know that you have food safety and quality under your control. Verification of system implementation is no longer satisfactory. Validation is required. The journey is one from wondering why things go out of control to one where you know you are in control.

Validation requirements for the United States food industry are relatively new to the food industry. Validation of food safety systems requires that food safety process controls must be proven to be preventive. This is done using research and statistical methods which are not commonly understood by the vast majority of people in the food supply chain.

While validation strategies have been employed in other industries for quite some time, the food industry is quite unprepared to meet the challenges that will accompany the required cultural shift in thinking and actions. In the European Union, committees worked to develop guidelines for the food supply chain in 2008 and in the United States, the FDA and others published similar guidelines for drug commercial manufacturing processes in 2011.

As of this writing, the FDA continues to waffle around in providing guidance that is primarily HACCP based and inspection dependent. Inspection, tests and audits not preventive activities and HACCP is primarily based on an aging approach to preventive process control.

The bottom line on validation is that it is legally required and must be implemented by people in your company.

The question becomes "How can companies and the people in those companies meet validation requirements without understanding the details of research and statistics requirements?"

The answer is that it can be done the same way hundreds of companies in other industries have done it, by following the trail in this book.

The preventive control rules require that you or someone known as a Preventive Controls Required Individual (PCQI) oversee the preventive controls play. The problem is that in order to become a qualified PCQI by going through FDA training, you will not learn about validation or what to do to validate your system.

The validation information required for you to competently establish a valid preventive food safety system with valid process controls is not included in the FDA certification training. You must hire outside help. But unless your company can afford what amounts to a full-time research department, people within the company must add validation to their daily workload and that is exactly how it should be done.

For instance, do you know how to establish a statistical process control (SPC) system? Can you calculate control limits and process capabilities? Do you know the difference between management or system causes and assignable causes? Does everyone in your company clearly understand cause and effect and do they know how to intentionally move a food process from an "out of control" level to one that is in control and has justifiable process capabilities?

In short, you must know these concepts and be able to prove that your food safety system can isolate and remove both system and assignable causes of potential food safety problems, establish capable processes, and keep them in control.

The difference between system and assignable causes represents a critical basis from which your company needs to start separating work into management controllable issues and those controllable at the supervisor and hourly level. A basic understanding of prevention, appraisal, internal, and external failure costs will help to push you and your company from a state of reaction to one of prevention.

Knowing who is responsible for what changes is critical to success. Knowing how to divide responsibilities between management-level personnel (common cause system level) and hourly employees (assignable causes) and how to organize each group to take charge of what they are clearly responsible for means attacking food safety and quality problems from the appropriate levels of control and eliminates confusion and finger pointing.

After a quick review of international laws and guidance covering different food safety and quality control approaches, you will take a journey through the Food and Drug Administration (FDA) Food Safety Modernization Act (FSMA) requirements for preventive controls and begin to understand the need for harmonization of standards and data requirements among different systems.

The need to take a team approach to the planning and implementation requirements is basic to any dynamic business shift, and the move into preventive food safety and quality controls is no different. Understanding the hazards that can impact both your products and processes is critical. From a basic risk-based hazard analysis, the company implementation plan will slowly grow as processes, and variables that can impact food quality and safety and plan your sampling and control strategy are defined. You will need a solid organizational approach to upgrade sampling plans established by environmental monitoring requirements. With the data from those samples, you will need a tool kit of basic statistical techniques to help you analyze what the sample results mean over time and through the changes you need to make to upgrade your system to meet these new requirements. Your fear of statistics will disappear as you discover that statistical tools including statistical process control are based on addition, subtraction, multiplication, and division and may be learned by anyone in your company. You will learn to use a solution tracking sheet for data and analysis to look at cycle times and to establish baseline and improvement trends, establish team and company priorities, analyze potential causes, set up individual and team action items, report your results to upper management, and provide an outstanding documentation system detailing continuous improvement efforts.

Although today's food safety laws and guidance do not begin to approach the many problems that might impact food safety and quality, you will need to consider a myriad of critical issues that are looming in the dark to cause your company problems. Traceability and recall, poor packaging, cross-contamination, improper supply chain controls, food fraud, cargo theft, and other potential problems are waiting in the wings to upset your strategy. Preventive systems plan for such consequences.

1. With these tools and techniques in your quiver, you will be able to begin taking a leadership position that will enable your company to surpass competitors with less commitment and organization.
2. You will use your new found knowledge to review what happened in a case study of Chipotle, critically analyze what changes to food safety and quality Chipotle has made and continues to make. You will learn from their mistakes and apply a vastly more mature approach to food safety and quality than they have.
3. You will learn a simple planning and implementation scheme that makes sense out of what might seem to be a confusing mass of legal and customer requirements.
4. The numbers will change in your favor.
5. The problems associated with such major system changes will be forgotten.
6. Your company will have a new way of doing things.
7. The old system and approach to food safety and quality will simply fade into the past like they never existed in the first place.
8. And your company and the world will be better off for it.

Introduction

Congratulations on your choice to enter a career long effort to establish preventive food safety and quality controls in the food industry!

New jobs and careers, safer and better quality food, award winning competition, higher corporate profits, less human illness, fewer deaths, reduced recalls, safer processes, and happier consumers wait for you and your company to struggle through the massive challenges facing you.

In the United States, the Food Safety Modernization Act (FSMA) is now law. In a recent article, Shawn Stevens published an article entitled "Criminal Consequences of New Human Standard." In that article, he explores the impact of FSMA's legal impact noting that "Under this new Human Illness Standard, a food company executive, manager or employee can be charged with a crime even if they did not know they were selling product that was contaminated or making sick." If you re-read that sentence carefully, it can be interpreted to mean that quality and food safety managers, the president, vice presidents, directors, and others are now liable for preventing people from getting sick and corporate shields can no longer protect company employees [1].

Obviously, you are not alone. Every person in the food supply chain is impacted and faces the same challenges that you face. Change! Whether you are conservative and comfortable in your niche in the world or are a go getter wanting to learn to build a better world, change is on your door step and staring you in the face. Although there are many in the food industry who deny all this is necessary and many more who will simply go along with the changes, new industry leaders will emerge. And they will emerge to become the new champions of the industry.

FSMA under Food and Drug Administration (FDA) challenges is complex and far reaching. It is designed to change the culture of the food industry. The law covers everything from the producer through all food-handling phases.

You will be challenged to learn things you never learned (or forgot) in school. You will get to dabble in statistics, build teams, improve environmental monitoring, control your suppliers, control sanitation and temperatures, establish a solid and improving food safety base, fight with those who are afraid of and don't want to have to do all this and attend new training that not only helps you learn to stand on your own two feet, but also prepares you to take on more and more responsibility, and to teach those you work with how to get things under control.

You are sitting in the doorway of a skydiving plane getting ready to jump. You have two choices. Do you jump into this new challenge or not?

For 70 or more years, the FDA and other countries have failed to designate or implement preventive food safety controls throughout the food industry. In 2008, a massive tomato salmonella recall inspired members of congress to begin work on new food safety regulations. Three years later, in January 2011, President Obama signed the FSMA into law launching a 5-year effort on the part of the FDA to reorganize in an effort to develop implementation rules.

Confusion regarding how to go about development, implementation, and measurement of the impact of final rules saw the FDA attempt to bring government officials together to address issues such as how to merge and focus disjointed federal, state, and local government efforts into an integrated food safety system.

In September, 2015, the FDA published the first sets of final FSMA preventive control rules. Of critical importance were the final rules for the Preventive Controls for Human and Animal foods.

Under these rules, all food processors, handlers, packers, and distributors are required to submit and maintain adherence to valid preventive control plans. The food side of the FDA is moving from old style visual inspection systems to the more valid, scientific approaches practiced by the drug and medical device side.

The final rules have been published under FSMA mandates require a major cultural shift of food industry participants that will take a generation to implement. The requirements of the new rules are not new to other industries. Preventive controls, supplier qualification and management, quality and safety systems, and other components of normal business operations have previously been implemented in many industries. The strategies employed by drug and medical device industries are not new or any more impossible for the food industry to learn to implement than they were for other industries. The food industry is about to face the learning curve and change requirements that move into a more preventive posture based on more objective scientific and statistical evidence than has been required over the past century.

This dynamic shift requires, at the onset, training, and the ability to translate what has happened in other industries to what has to happen in the food industry. The techniques and tools are not new. They need translation into the food arena.

Although there are books, training, and advices available for you to use, this book is about taking those previously proven tools and enabling you and your team to move positively toward these new preventive control challenges. Many of the currently touted preventive controls training programs provide food industry personnel with what they need to do, but this book gives them step-by-step instructions in how to do it.

Any book written at this stage in the newly evolving history of preventive food safety controls for the food industry cannot possibly foresee the technology that will evolve over the next few decades. Most of the technology needed to help supply-chain players establish preventive systems have not yet been envisioned when other technologies are in the offing. Yet, many of the problems and causes we face in today's food safety arena can be managed almost to extinction with positive commitment, teamwork, and new organizational approaches.

No doubt, there are decades of work, challenge, and change ahead. Hopefully, neither the FDA nor the scientific community will retreat from solving problems that today seem impossible to solve. Michael Taylor who was the FDA food safety czar for the critical years during which the FSMA rules were in development envisioned a cultural shift for the food industry. Cultural shifts take at least a generation and go through different phases.

The long march to prevention will become evident when the FDA is able to report fewer and fewer recalls and food related illness outbreaks. As our measurement and oversight capabilities become more mature, we can expect to see rises in outbreaks because of our improved ability to measure and report them. With a lack of a truer historic recall baseline, we can expect the measurement of food safety issues over the next few years to exhibit decreases in food safety rather than improvement. Many will wonder if all the effort is worth continuing until the time comes when the baseline data is surpassed by the annual measurement data and begins to show the results of the industry's efforts.

As Michael Taylor stated in September 2012, "stated in the simplest terms, the recognized solution to the problem of food borne illness is a comprehensive prevention strategy that involves all participants in the food system, domestic and foreign, doing their part to minimize the likelihood of harmful contamination. And that is the strategy mandated by the FSMA. It is not a strategy that assumes we can achieve a zero-risk food supply, but it is a strategy grounded in the conviction that we can better protect consumers and the economic vigor of the food system if everyone involved implements reasonably available measures to reduce risk.

The FSMA strategy recognizes that the food industry has the primary responsibility and capacity to produce safe food, but it calls for a new definition of public and private roles on food safety and a modern new framework for regulatory oversight, integration of government food safety efforts, and a public–private collaboration." [2]

REFERENCES

[1] S.K. Stevens, 2016. Criminal consequences of new human illness standard. Food Qual. Safety 23(3), 14–16.

[2] Progress on FSMA changes within the FDA Foods Program and on Partnerships, 2012 FDA Science Writers Symposium, Silver Spring, MD (as prepared for delivery by Michael R. Taylor, Deputy Commissioner for Foods, U.S. FDA) <http://www.fda.gov/Food/GuidanceRegulation/FSMA/ucm319053.htm>, March 11, 2016.

CHAPTER

Background: understanding common and assignable causes, laws, and costs

1

PREVENTIVE THINKING

The idea of preventive controls is not new. Seatbelts and airbags are considered preventive controls as they help to prevent injury or death in the event of automobile collisions. Prevention is a word often used in many applications as the forefront of reducing costs, damaged equipment, lost lives, injury, and the like.

Within the scope of food safety and quality, preventive controls as an operational concept is still evolving because of the evolution of many food supply chain adjustments from old world approaches to more modern systems capable of tracking and documenting the impact that applying preventive controls may have on human health. For the most part, food producers, processors, packers, transporters, retailers, restaurants, and others involved in growing and delivering food to the world's millions are, too many degrees, confused about just what preventive controls are, or how they work or whether or not they are effective.

Although many food supply players have worked diligently to define and implement controls that prevent food from losing shelf life or from causing people to get sick and die, many others are left in a state of confusion regarding what, when, or how to do many of the things needed to establish effective preventive controls.

The idea that the food supply chain should implement a system of preventive controls means that a systematic approach to controlling and eliminating those systemic and assignable causes that can define, measure, and control or eliminate pathogenic, chemical, or physical contaminants in food must be taken. As health threatening bacterial, chemical, and physical objects can be introduced into the food supply from any of hundreds of sources and as how to control of many of these hazards is not yet known by the scientific (let along farming) world, confusion reigns.

Regardless, in many industries over the past 20 or so years, highly effective preventive control systems have been developed beginning from similar levels of ignorance, resistance and confusion. Trial-and-error approaches have basically led the charge.

The challenges facing the food industry are not new. The only really new issue is that as the food industry is only the latest industry to have to step up to the plate. Initial resistance may be seen from those who simply don't believe food safety is an issue. Other companies haven't waited for the crowd and have simply moved on implementing those pieces of a food safety and quality system that they know is

Validating Preventive Food Safety and Quality Controls. DOI: http://dx.doi.org/10.1016/B978-0-12-810994-6.00001-8

needed. These companies have also led their suppliers and customers into new ideas and solutions for the problems made public in the daily news.

Wikipedia defines hazard prevention as "the process of risk study, elimination and mitigation in emergency management" [1].

That definitions sort of parallels what is becoming the groundwork for basic requirements in the food industry. Identify what risks are associated with different food types and the processes the food is going through then work to eliminate those risks through better control systems. Of course, truly preventive systems are not based solely on emergency management but are based on determining, controlling, and eliminating causes for the emergencies.

PREVENTIVE ACTIONS VERSUS CORRECTIVE ACTIONS: REQUIREMENTS FOR NEW THINKING

Much of the documentation you will read about the Food Safety Modernization Act (FSMA) uses the words "corrective action" while promoting "prevention." Unfortunately, corrective actions are often conducted in a way that encourages quick fixes to get some operation back up and running after something has gone wrong. Such necessary operational adjustments are not preventive.

Take recalls, for instance. When a food company has produced a product that might be harmful to humans or animals, the company is encouraged or forced to implement a recall. It is unfortunate to hear even Food and Drug Administration (FDA) officials calling recalls "preventive." That type of thinking exhibits a belief that the recall will prevent more people from getting sick or dying. However, recalls, if one is to follow preventive thinking, are in no way preventive. They are a reaction to a problem that is simply a quick fix or attempt to backtrack from what can be called an external escape.

A recall is exactly like trying to get the horse back into the barn after it has escaped. Prevention of the horse escape would imply that the owner had put in place gates or barriers that actually kept the horse in the barn in the first place. Prevention of the horse escape would go much further that having gates in the barn, prevention, in this case, might mean that the horse was tethered to the stall in which the horse resided.

Prevention and the establishment of a preventive control plan (PCP) means to go as far back into the process as possible to understand the causes of a problem. Understanding causes is not the same as looking at a symptom of a problem and circumventing the symptom with some temporary adjustment. Prevention means to establish a formal approach to looking at the symptom or problem and performing a standardized and systematic approach to determining the cause of the symptom. Such a process may be called causal analysis.

Simply, the product that escaped, either to other food chain members or to the public, is the result of the company's system to establish and manage a preventive control system. Recalls are a symptom of the lack of a valid PCP and an indication of a lack of ability or understanding regarding causal analysis.

Most people in the food supply chain, from the farm through to the retail or restaurant operation, are capable of understanding what the FSMA calls bacterial, chemical, or physical adulterants or hazards to food safety. Many bacteriological adulterants come from the farm. Things like salmonella, listeria and *Escherichia coli* are found on farms. They get onto the product and are moved like a contaminated river into and down the food chain. One must assume, therefore, prevention of these hazards must begin on the farm. And while these bacteriological adulterants exist in nature and are virtually everywhere, humans have to date failed to develop an ability to find and eliminate these causes at the farm.

The symptoms that occur from bacterial contamination are usually found at the human level weeks or even months after the product on which the contamination existed was shipped from the farm. With no formal definition or guidance for traceability that could be called "universal" or standardized, back tracking to investigate probable causes is, quite simply, a joke.

How many times has the FDA and the Centers for Disease Control and Prevention (CDC) conducted recall exercises for large-scale food safety outbreaks without finding and reporting the cause? More often than not [2].

CRITICAL CONCEPTS NEEDED FOR EFFECTIVE PREVENTIVE CONTROLS: THE DIFFERENCE BETWEEN COMMON OR SYSTEM AND ASSIGNABLE CAUSES

Common causes of food safety failures result from a lack of system controls or from improper decisions made at the management level. It is estimated that 85% of all food safety failures come from some breakdown in the system processes employed to harvest, handle, process, pack, transport, distribute, and sell food.

Preventive controls must be clearly focused on causes, and those working on preventive systems must not only be able to distinguish between assignable and common causes, but they must be capable, motivated, and allowed to take action to eliminate whichever type of cause is encountered.

Fig. 1.1 breaks causes into those that are called assignable and those that are more of a common system type of cause. Assignable causes are found in specific processes and are regular daily employee responsibilities. They can be analyzed using statistical process control strategies using functional improvement teams.

Common causes are system causes. Regardless of which system or process the company operates under, that system is the result of managerial decisions or lack of decisions and actions. Most food safety issues come from such system insufficiencies. Finding and correcting such causes come under management and corrective action teams comprised of managerial-level personnel. When management refuses to assume responsibility for food safety, for whatever reason, the organization is

Causes

Assignable causes	Common causes
Problems in processes Employee responsibilities	The system management responsibilities
Functional improvement teams	Top management team corrective action teams

FIGURE 1.1

Assignable and common causes.

jeopardized. It is unfortunate that there are so many opportunities for managerial oversights to cause catastrophic food safety problems because with the new changes in the laws, management in most food supply organizations has not had sufficient time to understand and implement preventive control systems.

VALIDATION

If you are planning to take or have taken the Preventive Controls Qualified Individual (PCQI) training, be aware that the training does little to help you understand FDA FSMA validation requirements. Validation of process or preventive control systems must be planned, often involve validation studies and significant reporting requirements.

Prevention means to get control of many potential hazardous causes through the use of analysis, measurement and team involved improvement. Once under control, these hazards must be kept under control. Proving that the hazards are under control and are being kept under control is performed through validation efforts. Validation is a specialized area of preventive controls that requires a specially qualified individual who is capable of conducting related research, experiments, collection of data during operation and may include mathematical modelling or even consumer surveys. Such individuals are qualified in research and statistical methods and may be expert microbiologists.

VERIFICATION IS NOT VALIDATION

Validation provides proof that the process design and verification activities actually control the process and food related biological, chemical and physical hazards identified during hazard analysis.

Validation studies are required at process design, during process operations and after any change to process operational procedures. The validation part of the overall preventive control plan, regardless of the PCQI training omission, requires an integrated team approach, studies throughout the product lifecycle (getting control through team solution tracking sheet (STS) activities), keeping process controls (perhaps through the use of statistical process control (SPC) tools) and continuous protection of the process against new or unknown sources of variability.

Recalls, for example, may be caused by any of a number of issues such as poor process controls, uncaring management, untrained personnel, substandard incoming ingredients, lack of bio-contaminant or chemical testing, poor measurement or even inaccurate labels.

Under preventive controls potential hazards must be identified at each stage of the process, from incoming, through processing and through outgoing stages. All parts of the final product must be considered at every throughput stage. Every product must have its own preventive control plan and each plan must be validated. Validation includes obtaining and evaluating scientific and technical evidence or conducting studies to determine whether preventive controls for hazards when properly implemented will effectively control the hazards.

Current good manufacturing practices (CGMP) require that manufacturing processes be designed and controlled to assure that in-process materials and the finished product meet predetermined quality and food safety requirements in a consistent and reliable manner. Design validation establishes preliminary control over hazards. Small pilot lines, standardization of line controls and equipment, measurement and analysis, process capability studies and teamwork are required during process design stages.

Maintenance of validated processes requires competent control over any changes in materials, manpower and process changes. Such changes represent a significant threat to the validity of established preventive processes. Due to cost issues, management may be unable or unwilling to implement needed process improvements or initial product design qualification and this reluctance may lead to food safety problems. Another example of a threat to a valid process is often found in inadequate specifications. Specifications are often not clearly, accurately or sufficiently established thus leaving people to wonder what to do. Such lack of definition and clarity leads to unanticipated variation. Processes and equipment can usually control hazards if incoming ingredients are controlled, kill steps are adequate, environmental issues are controlled, monitoring is correctly established, teams control start-ups, runs and shut-downs, sanitation controls are in place and causal analysis practices are established as the daily routine.

Often process and product kill steps can be tested using surrogates (non-pathogens) in lab environments. Kill steps can also be validated when process parameters and control measures are in sync and time and temperature controls are firmly established.

Processing parameters may be established using related research or through process variability studies. It is often advisable to test process controls at high volume to eliminate potential out-of-control conditions during high volume production. In such cases calibration and monitoring equipment accuracy are critical to data collection to evaluate important material characteristics.

Once a process validated and proof is established that the hazards are minimized and under control, any changes to materials, equipment or settings should be under team review and approval. Willy-nilly changes or new engineering requirements may not be slipped in during production runs regardless of customer changes demanded in the middle of production runs.

There are a few key validation requirements:

- An understanding of the sources of variation in biological, chemical and physical hazards
- An ability to detect the presence and degree of variation of the hazard
- An understanding of the impact of the variation on the process and product attributes
- An ability to control the variation in a manner commensurate with process and product risks
- Calculation of process capabilities to separate common causes from assignable causes

In short, quality, food safety and efficiency should be designed or built into the product and process. Food safety cannot be adequately assured merely by in-process and finished product inspection or test. The primary goal should be for teams to find ways to eliminate the need for inspection and testing activities because the process is valid an in control.

IMPACT OF THE ORGANIZATIONAL STRUCTURE ON ASSIGNABLE AND COMMON CAUSES

A clearer perspective of the difference between assignable and common causes might be attained if one considers the difference between operational and operational structures.

On the operational side, most personnel are doing their daily jobs, such as scheduling, shipping, inspecting, producing, testing, and involved in those activities primarily focused on getting product out the door on time. These people and activities are more likely to become involved in the analysis of assignable causes.

Organizationally, policies, procedures, staff meetings, hiring, training, marketing, and planning types of work and activities are more likely to provide structure and direction to operational activities and people. It is during organizational activities that are primarily handled by management personnel that often become the source of common causes. Decisions made and directions set by organizational activities generally impact the entire organization, and even minor misdirections can become the source as far as food safety, and quality go are likely to filter downward to embed common causes throughout the entire organization.

Not all management personnel realize that most of their decisions cause system problems that result in food safety failures and recalls. It is much easier to pass the buck or point fingers at another group or person than it is to objectively analyze a situation that has resulted in process or system failures. To avoid having to deal with system-level issues, companies are apt to hire food safety and quality personnel. Food safety and quality organizations are quickly assigned the responsibility of "getting food safety under control." In this manner, management finds it easy to wash their hands of the responsibilities of many of their own actions.

A sample list of departments, vice presidents, and directors that are commonly found in a medium-sized organization would include titles such as operations, engineering, finance, marketing and sales, human resources (HR), and information technology. Other minor functions such as quality, food safety, maintenance, and logistics might fall under operations or engineering. Most often, the function with the most employees is usually called operations. In companies that are strongest in manufacturing or transportation, even those functions are likely to be assigned organizationally to the operations group. Of course, different companies are organized differently, but in general, if we consider assignable causes to be the responsibility of those not in management positions, and most employees fall under operations, the result is that assignable causes are primarily the responsibility of the operations group.

That gives the engineering, finance, marketing and sales, HR, and information technology functions ample opportunity to create a lot of problems that result in product safety and quality. Take a look at the short list below. There is really no limit to the number of problems that are caused at the organizational level.

1. Poor or no preventive planning (Chipotle)

   A company that does not take the time to learn about preventive food safety approaches and develop plans that are focused on causal analysis will find it difficult to establish a competent approach to preventive food safety. Such oversights represent an overall management failure that is likely to result in an outbreak along with accompanying recalls, financial losses, and reorganization.

2. Lack of training

   Training costs money and takes people away from their jobs. In today's preventive controls world, however, training is specifically called out as a mandatory issue. Compliance with the rules demands that training take front stage as a preventive mechanism. Fortunately, a lot of today's training can be delivered via the Internet in an "as needed" manner. Everyone does not have to be herded into a room or travel to Kansas City for training. Great training is available on tablets or computers in an on-demand manner that allows trainees to schedule the training on the basis of their own time constraints.

3. Poor working conditions

   Poor lighting, working in hot or cold areas, and dirt all contribute to poor working conditions making employees less productive or motivated. Unmotivated employees and the poor working conditions they endure simply means that they know management just doesn't care, so, why should they? Poor working conditions can represent a systematic and major contributor to overall food safety and quality problems.

4. Pressure for volume output

   When the end of the month and the end of the quarter approaches, what matters most in your company? What is the real priority at this time if an interviewer were to talk to employees company-wide? In general, everything a company might say it stands for goes out the window at the end of the quarter because the focus is on "making the numbers." When employees see this, they know where management really resides, and they know the slogans and training are a joke.

   Companies that continually improve planning, scheduling, operational capabilities, and shipping environments do not get caught in end-of-the-month or end-of-the-quarter crunches. They meet customer demands a few days ahead of the end of the quarter.

5. Poor incoming ingredients

   Buying cheap is no act of genius, but when buyers are faced with procurement budgets that are not in line with actual market capabilities, the tendency to cut corners by reducing requirements and specifications often becomes the followed path. Presenting trend lines that show how much money is being saved by purchasing during quarterly reviews also makes people look heroic.

   Of course, the ingredients that are cheaper but do not meet food safety or quality requirements might be caught at incoming inspection or test, but, then again, may be they will slip through.

   Unfortunately, under the preventive control rules, a buying company is now responsible for what suppliers do or do not do. Vicarious liability has been established to the extent that suppliers must be both qualified and certified by receivers because receivers are now required to assure the safety of food coming from their suppliers.

6. Poor product design

   Product design can be a tough job in today's world. Food technologists are supposed to understand the impact of the new products they develop. Processes and process controls are all impacted by new products. New product flows, ingredients, scheduling, food safety, and quality requirements must all be upgraded. It is not an easy task to take a product that passes taste tests to a volume production environment. Packaging, shipping, scheduling, design testing, and many other operational functions are all required to adapt. The costs to introduce new products require changes in marketing and sales changes which decreases the profits temporarily. Inappropriate planning and expenditures set the stage for common cause problems.

7. Failure to provide needed information to workers

   It is easy for managers to sit in staff and product meetings and discuss problems or brainstorm new ideas. Communicating the needed changes throughout the organization is another matter. Ignoring needed procedural, process, and training requirements by assuming that information is not needed by operational personnel means that operational personnel cannot begin to successfully, and with food safety and quality in mind meet the operational changes required for successful compliance.

8. Mix-ups in storage or production

Take a walk through your own ingredient and food storage areas. How is the inventory organized? In many cases, the company kind of grew up with a system for storage and production that, at later stages of success, is an outdated burden that makes the right ingredient difficult to find.

9. Corporate panic

A great example of how a corporation can panic and create internal chaos can be found in the way that Chipotle's management handled the 2015–16 outbreaks. Closing all stores and holding industry-wide meetings to announce the new approach to food safety followed by burying the retail outlets with hundreds of audits and inspections is a great example of corporate panic. Corporate execs buried the farms and retail outlets with thousands of inspection items, many of which had nothing to do with preventing bacterial or viral outbreaks. Recall that Chipotle never did find or never did disclose the sources of the outbreaks consumers suffered. Knee–jerk reactions rather than an initial assumption of food safety along with preventive planning throughout the Chipotle supply chain would certainly have been a better approach, but the focus was apparently on growth, stock prices, and other more important business issues.

10. Lack of supplier controls and
11. Purchase based primarily on price

Buying product and ingredients primarily on the basis of price has always been a common business practice. Unfortunately, food ingredients may be cheaper because the supplier has not put in place required preventive controls. Under new supplier preventive controls requirements, such practices are illegal. For most registered food facilities, suppliers must be evaluated and approved as having implemented valid preventive control programs because the buying company now shares liability for what the supplier does or does not do as far as prevention is concerned. Liability shared in this manner means that purchase based primarily on price can jeopardize a company's existence.

12. Refusal to comply with legal requirements

Not all legal requirements are bad. As far as food safety goes in the United States, the FSMA of 2011 was long overdue. Furthermore, the 5 years it took between the signing of the law and the issuance of final rules were partially a result of the lobbying efforts of large companies to kill or weaken the intent of the law so that new requirements met their own needs rather than that of consumer protection.

For many companies, the refusal to comply with the legal requirements continues in the form of food dragging in view of the FDA-imposed compliance deadlines.

13. Not keeping up with new technology

Technology costs money and new technology costs even more money. However, like it or not, as legal, customer and consumer needs and wants change, the technology need to meet those needs and change accordingly. In some cases, companies that cannot or will not expend capital resources on new technology sooner or later become mired in out-of-date processes incapable of meeting the ever evolving demands they face.

14. One up/one back attitude

As far as traceability is concerned, isolationism and isolationistic attitudes and perspectives can become a serious problem. Today's perspectives on food safety and quality demand a supply chain approach that goes far beyond suppliers and customers. Perhaps, the need for greater cooperation among and between supply chain members is the most challenging issue faced by the food industry today. Everyone has their own problems, and they tend to focus on their own problems. Unfortunately, under new preventive control rules, each receiver is required to accept some responsibility for what their suppliers do or do not do.

15. Lack of maintenance spending

Maintenance takes many forms. On one hand, cutting back maintenance support to save money during tight times causes problems downstream that are likely to later cost more money than anticipated.

Take the case of reduction of compressor maintenance during budget cut time. One large company that reduced costs by stretching out compressor maintenance schedules 1 year found 2 years later that failing compressors were causing spoiled shipments, missed deliveries, recalls, and lost customers. Pay the piper now or pay the piper later.

16. Dirty storage (tools, equipment, packaging)

Let's face it, the lowly mop, bucket, and broom don't demand much attention or win awards. They are often tossed in a corner or storage room after use where no one has to look at them. Under new rules, they must not only be designed to be cleanable but must be stored in a manner that keeps them clean.

Packaging on the other hand rarely sees a storage area that has any capability of keeping it clean. Regardless of the fact that packaging comes in direct contact with the food, storage of packaging in areas where one would not eat their lunch contributes to cross contamination from the packaging to the food held within.

17. Overpromising deliveries

If there is a single factor that tends to impact food quality and safety, it is the idea that when a sale is made, all other operations are in some way impacted. Promising to deliver without appropriate scheduling planning is a primary cause of rushing product through an operation by eliminating or overriding necessary controls. The marketing and sales personnel become heroes and are awarded medals and raises, whereas the rest of the organization tries to adjust to the sales department's lack of assumed responsibility.

18. Poor lighting, temperature/humidity controls

Poor lighting, temperature, humidity, and other environmental controls all contribute to poor working as well as poor food safety and quality conditions. Prevention of such potential problems generally becomes one of capital expenditures. Many company owners would much rather pocket the money or show higher profits for investors than spending large amounts of money on capital expenditures.

19. Lack of protective clothing

Lack of protective clothing under Occupational Safety and Health Administration (OSHA) and as required by new food safety requirements has long been an ignored and resisted issue. Managers cannot always see or understand the needs established by new food safety requirements. The "That ain't the way we do it here," "If it ain't broke don't fix it," or "We've never had a recall" attitude often reigns supreme and provides significant delays in terms of a company's ability to meet compliance or food safety requirements.

20. Lack of environmental controls

Environmental controls require significant capital expenditures in the face of new preventive control requirements. More importantly, many food operations do not have the internal expertise required to correctively or competently establish environmental controls that are truly of a preventive nature. A good example is the implementation of laminar flow air-filtering systems designed to reduce airborne contaminants. Such systems require an entirely new approach to temperature and humidity controls as well. Most food supply companies not only have never heard of laminar flow systems but will resist long overdue requirements needs to implement such controls.

21. Poor hiring practices

Competent hiring demands that competent HR approaches are established. An easy way to look at whether or not a company hires competent personnel is to measure and report turnover rates. Employee turnover often means that knowledge and experience are leaving a company and being replaced by a lack of knowledge and a lack of experience.

A company that has process, cost, food safety, and quality stability can be severely impacted by employee turnover. When sales take off, the demand for new and often inexperienced personnel increases the tendency to fill the numbers by using downgraded hiring practices increases thereby increasing the instability of downstream processes.

22. Lack of good process design

When processes are stable, they tend to have the bugs worked out and operate smoothly with fewer problems than when they were newer. Getting a process to the point where is stable and under quality and food safety control, takes time and effort if the original process design could not originally meet requirements. As new products are introduced, new processes are designed. As new processes are designed, they must be debugged thus causing a recycling of the process improvement efforts.

23. Lack of corporate commitment

If there is no policy or financial commitment to support food safety, there is probably a lack of corporate commitment. Lack of corporate commitment can be translated to mean there is a lack of management commitment. The lack of commitment flows downhill to all employees and results in an "I don't care" attitude. What could be more demotivating?

24. Slogans instead of action and support
    Management often likes to plaster slogans on walls. But slogans without the management and financial support to change processes and put preventive controls in place will soon cause operational-level employees to lose faith and ignore them.
25. Slow payment to suppliers
    Withholding supplier payments for 60 or 90 days to make company profit numbers look good, but suppliers and those depending on ingredients may soon find that they are receiving delayed shipments that later cause a rush to meet customer delivery demands. During such rushes, food safety, and quality go out the window as food safety and quality requirements are overridden.
26. Lack of guidance during slowdowns
    Business slowdowns often cause upper management to vocalize the need to save money, but without careful analysis and definition of what processes or procedures need adjustment, operational personnel will take it upon themselves to interpret the meaning of "save money" upon themselves. Does saving money mean to skip process steps or eliminate process controls? Without careful guidance and definition from management, control over processes can quickly become dysfunctional.
27. Overuse of pesticides/herbicides/fungicides
    On farms, it is unlikely that field employees will determine when to use chemicals on crops. Such decisions are management decisions. If applied too close to harvest, chemicals are quick to end up in distribution centers and on supermarket shelves creating potential consumer problems.
28. Lack of or incomplete or confusing procedures
    Without good standards and commitment, incomplete and confusing procedures that do not clearly define step-by-step food adulteration reduction requirements leave operational-level personnel to make up their own process steps. More importantly, when careful definition of food safety and quality are inadequate or nonexistent, operational personnel cannot possible meet real needs. Quality and food safety require that companies meet specific requirements. This is especially true under new preventive control rules.
29. Law suits against the corporation
    Corporate lawyers are always looking for loopholes in laws to save money or for other reasons. When loophole attempts backfire, lawsuits become public and employees become aware of their existence and any of a number of possible rumors begin that can quickly lead to job hopping by key employees. Loss of key employees means that controls over needed processes are lost.

Those 29 issues represent only a very small set of the likely problems that are critical to classify as assignable or system causes. The decisions made to classify food safety and quality problems or issues to each category means that totally different approaches may be taken to establish preventive control over each one. In the case of system causes, management must take responsibility to recognize and fix the problem. This means that management teams, perhaps at the insistence of the CEO or president, must be organized to work, track, and report their progress. They must apply an appropriate approach that validates the success of their efforts.

Assignable causes, on the other hand, are generally delegated to supervisors and hourly workers as the issues raised are considered within their sphere of control. Of course, once an assignable cause team is assigned, both authority and responsibility are delegated to the team.

Regardless of which causal type is attached, basic continuous improvement concepts apply. For many organizations, facing the differences between system and assignable causes can be daunting, and, often resisted. The tools and techniques outlined in this book are designed to help both management and operational teams to overcome food safety and quality hazards they face on a daily basis.

Each of the small set of organizational issues noted above establishes some type of cause–effect relationship that can and often does result in the downfall of quality and food safety preventive controls. Although the decisions made at the organizational levels might often seem to be sound "business decisions," the impact of such decisions is usually far reaching and often damaging.

To begin to stem the tide of organizational caused problems, a different perspective can be taken. Many industries have adopted a different guiding philosophy on the basis of prevention first thinking. Put simply, it is cheaper to prevent a problem in the first place than it is to clean up the mess resulting from bad decisions at a later date.

Adopting a perspective that focuses on spending at the preventive level has been shown to get wasteful costs resulting from fly-by-night decisions under control.

COSTS ASSOCIATED WITH FOOD SAFETY AND QUALITY

Philip B. Crosby published a book entitled "Quality Is Free" in 1979 that greatly impacted the overall quality profession. The concepts are still valid today although the title could be changed to "Food Safety Is Free." The concepts are not difficult to digest. His philosophy was simple, "Do things right the first time." Of course, he was talking about prevention. Another quote from Crosby that relates to the 30 items listed above is important: "Why spend all this time finding, fixing and fighting when you could prevent the incident in the first place?" This type of preventive organizational thinking that needs to permeate the food safety industry. For sure, many people have learned such lessons, but far too many have not [2].

In that book, Crosby began to define what he called quality costs, and on the basis of his preventive approach, he showed how spending money to prevent problems was far cheaper than spending money to recall or fix problems. Here is a brief list of the approach he recommended:

Prevention costs: Costs of all activities specifically designed to prevent poor quality (food safety) in products or services including

- New product reviews
- Planning

- Supplier qualification and certification
- Process capability evaluations
- Quality improvement team meetings
- Quality improvement projects
- Education and training

Preventive costs associated with food safety could include preventive planning, refrigeration, and others.

Appraisal costs: The costs associated with measuring, evaluating, or auditing products or services to assure conformance to quality standards and performance requirements including

- Incoming and source inspection/test of incoming materials (ingredients)
- In-process and final inspection/test
- Product, process or service audits
- Calibration of measuring and test equipment
- Associated supplies and materials

Appraisal costs associated with food safety issues should include those associated with appraisal and food safety audits, culls, sorting, temperature monitoring, and others.

Failure costs: The costs resulting from products or services not conforming to requirements or customer/user needs. Failure costs are further broken down into two categories:

1. *Internal failure costs* that occur prior to delivery or shipment of the product or the furnishing of a service to the customer including
   a. Scrap
   b. Rework
   c. Re-inspection
   d. Re-testing
   e. Material reviews
   f. Downgrading

   Internal failure costs could also include food safety costs associated with re-sanitizing, ingredient failures, and others.
2. *External failure costs* are costs that occur after shipment or delivery including
   a. Processing customer complaints
   b. Customer returns
   c. Warranty claims
   d. Product recalls

External failure costs associated with food safety could also include lost business by guilty and nonguilty companies, stock losses such as those from the Chipotle problems, and others.

In general, the Crosby cost of quality structure can be easily adapted by food safety and quality personnel in the food industry to develop a shift in management thinking away from subjective decision making to one more in line with business goals.

By taking a cost approach to food safety and quality, a different set of priorities quickly emerges that lends itself to the application of other commonly available quality tools including statistical analysis and application of six-Sigma concepts designed to produce what Crosby would call "zero defects." By zero defects, Crosby did not mean perfection. What he meant was that the customer deserves to see no rejectable products because corporate processes have come under such good control that the likelihood of receiving bad product is extremely low.

INTERNATIONAL LAWS

In the United States, the FDA under the FSMA lists some key requirements under the final rule on the Current Good Manufacturing Practice and Hazard Analysis and Risk-Based Preventive Controls for Human Food. The FSMA requirements include hazard analysis, preventive controls, oversight, and management of preventive controls including monitoring, corrective actions and corrections, and verification that includes "effectiveness" or what the FDA calls validation of preventive controls [3].

CANADA

In Canada, the Canadian Food Inspection Agency calls for a Codex-based Hazard Analysis Critical Control Point (HACCP) approach to preventive controls that includes requirements for a PCP and a Food Safety Enhancement Program controlled by a Quality Management Program [4].

EUROPEAN UNION

The European Union (EU) has been working on food laws since the publication of the general principals established by the European Food Safety Authority Regulation (EC) No. 178/2002 in January 2002. In that document, the published general principles of food law include a call for risk assessment and management, protection of consumers' interests, imports and exports, and basic food safety requirements including "(1) Food shall not be placed on the market if it is unsafe. (2) Food shall be deemed to be unsafe if it is considered to be: (a) injurious to health; (b) unfit for human consumption." These 2002 regulations also place a clearly stated emphasis on the identification of risks, traceability, scientific evidence, member state cooperation and authority, open communication with the public, cooperation and networking among member states, implementation of HACCP principles, and many other issues related to compliance with member agreements.

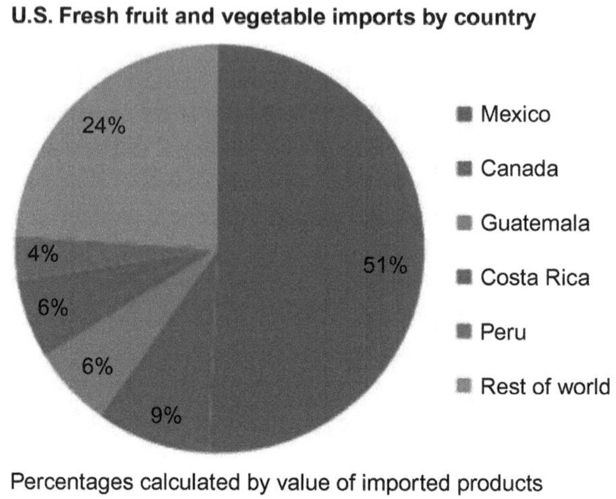

FIGURE 1.2

Integrated food safety system (IFSS)

The EU regulations also cover verification, audit and inspection, monitoring, sampling for analysis, recall planning, and official controls required throughout the supply chain. The EU regulations have been regularly updated by guidance documents through the past several years [5].

MEXICO

Registrar Corp published a pie chart in 2014 showing U.S. Fresh Fruit and Vegetable imports into the United States (Fig. 1.2) [6].

The graphic clearly shows that the United States imported two-thirds of its fresh fruits and vegetables from its border countries of Canada and Mexico with over half of those imports coming from Mexico. Such data moved the United States and Mexico to work on what is called a harmonization agreement intended to collaborate on the practices that prevent contamination through food processes. In the agreement, the United States will establish more FDA offices in Mexico to facilitate facility registration and inspection and to assure that prior notice of shipments is provided at US borders. The two countries agreed to collaborate on laboratory activities, outbreak response, trace-back, training of auditors, developing culturally specific training, and other issues [7].

CHINA

In April 2016, Food Safety Magazine published an article that provided an overview of China's new food safety law. That law became effective in October 2015. The law challenges online food trading websites to assure supplier conformance to avoid liabilities. The law goes further to cover health food ingredients, baby foods and formulae, food producer and processor registering requirements, labeling for genetically modified foods, formula foods used for medical purposes, advertising, increasingly harsh sanctions, and information regarding fines for damages and threats to human health [8].

THE NEED FOR HARMONIZATION BETWEEN BUSINESS AND GOVERNMENT

According to the FDA, there are a number of issues that have driven the implementation of the FSMA.

- The dramatic expansion in the global scale and complexity of the food system
- Reducing the risk of preventable foodborne illness in today's food system
- A focus on improved health outcomes (FDA measurement of the success or failure of the FSMA system)
- Partnerships to establish an integrated world-wide food safety network
- Oversight and enforcement
- New strategies to provide planning, training, operational plans, and capacity building

Of equal importance is the FDA's evolving ability to establish a system that allows them to profile how risky a particular food operation is when it comes to food safety. First, they take a look at the type of food being handled. Some foods present a higher risk to humans (should things not be properly controlled), the manufacturing process involved, the facilities previous food safety record, the facilities history of refusal rates when importing food into the United States, and food safety inspections, foreign and domestic.

The FDA and other federal, state, and local agencies work together to provide information on these and other factors in an effort to develop what they call "integrated food safety systems" (IFSS) capable of calculating the risk level for any food handler, processor, or producer. High risk means that that food operation is more likely to violate food safety standards and, therefore, more likely to gain close attention and FDA audit schedules.

Fig. 1.3 illustrates how the federal, state, and local governmental agencies work together.

On the left are shown the federal, state, and local agencies. The goal of the IFSS is to bring the food operations' various inspection and test data from all involved agencies into a single database rather than the 50–100 databases they currently use. The current databases are basically unable to talk to one another or to extract common data from one to another in any single investigation. The inspection and test data is combined in a single file to allow the IFSS to risk rank different operations and to establish which low scoring operations are most risky and, therefore, most likely

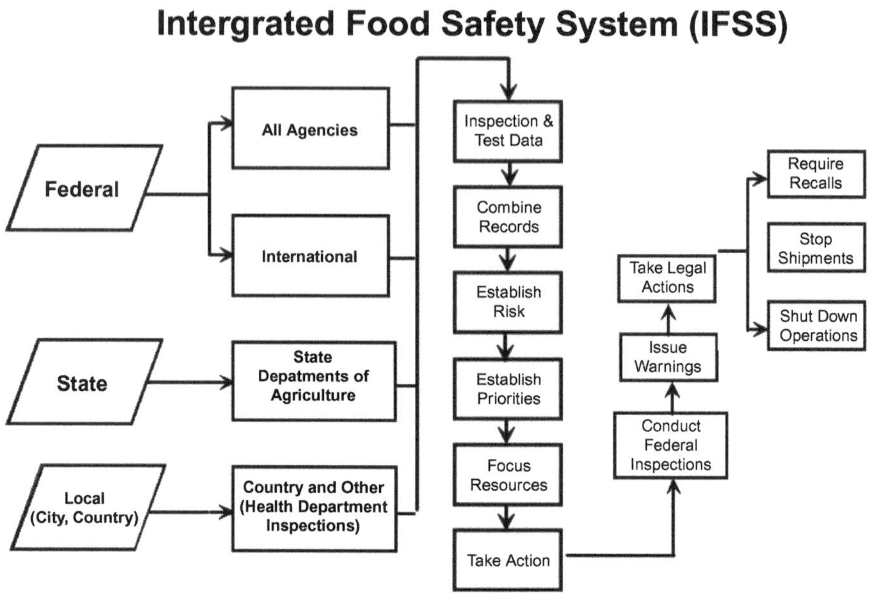

FIGURE 1.3

Integration of governmental food safety systems.

to have caused an outbreak. Governmental resources are then focused on those high risk operations for inspection and test purposes. If the company is found to be problematic in terms of high contaminant levels or lack of compliance to governmental standards, warnings are issued and legal action such as recalls, stopped shipments, or shut down of the operation could occur prior to criminal actions.

A primary downfall of the governmental approach to an IFSS lies in its one sidedness. If an IFSS were to provide insight into the overall food safety system, both government and business data should be included. Of course, that would mean that any governmental efforts to standardize data requirements would need to include standardization of data on both the government and business sides. To some extent, this objective is being worked on as the government requires businesses to register and report recalls.

Interestingly enough, almost all governments lean on CODEX Alimentarius standards.

Of course, the overall rules and the ability of a food facility to successfully plan and implement preventive controls means that all foreign and domestic facilities that manufacture, process, pack, or hold food intended for consumption in the United States must register with the FDA. Failure to register is an illegal act and requires the email address of the legal contact person and an assurance that the FDA will be permitted to inspect the operation at any time chosen without resistance. In other words, if a company wishes to work in the food industry in the United States legally, that operation basically gives up all rights of refusal when, and if the FDA chooses to inspect or investigate the operation for any act, the FDA suspects might be a reason to inspect.

This is right to inspect records is an important part of the FDA's overall desire to disable the legal refusals that denied them the ability to prosecute for the past several decades.

From the business side, food safety and quality data are critical to protect the business, provide visibility into what product is at different locations (inventory) and standardizing data across suppliers and customers.

Other advantages available to businesses when they attempt to harmonize or standardize requirements through the integration of food safety requirements and data lie in locating contaminated foods (traceability and recall), ranking suppliers with regard to their likelihood of failure, reducing recall times, and stopping extended illnesses and deaths, and, most importantly, protecting themselves and innocent partners from involvement in blames associated with recalls.

INTERNATIONAL STANDARDS ORGANIZATION

The International Standards Organization (ISO) has established 22000 "Food safety management systems—Requirements for any organization in the food chain." The ISO organization has also published ISO 22005, "Traceability in the feed and food chain—General principles and basic requirements for system design and implementation." The ISO food safety management system calls for HACCP principles and prerequisite programs (PRPs) calling for hazard analysis and control. The system is CODEX dependent, requires compliance to food safety laws, meeting customer requirements, seeks to establish international standards to protect consumers and requires communication of food safety issues to suppliers, customers and others in the food supply chain [9].

The ISO 22000 standards also call for system management, prerequisite programs, and interactive communication "to ensure that all relevant food safety hazards are identified and adequately controlled at each step within the food chain."

The ISO 22000 system calls for food safety management systems and control through policies, planning, assignment of responsibilities, food safety leaders, emergency preparedness and response, and procedures and extensive documentation. Management responsibilities are clearly defined and challenge management to provide appropriate food safety resources, training, competence, and awareness, an infrastructure in support of all requirements, planning of safe products, clear definitions for ingredients and final products, product and process flow charts, traceability, control of nonconformities, validation of the food safety system, monitoring and measurement, evaluation of improvement results, continual improvement, and controlling ISO system updates [10].

On the ISO 22005 (Traceability) side, ISO provides traceability principles and objectives that include support of food safety and quality through verifiability, consistent application, results orientation, cost effective, practical, compliant, and accuracy of the traceability system. Included in ISO 22005 are issues covering design considerations, regulatory requirements, the need for definition of products and ingredients, competent design, procedures; traceability system planning, responsibilities, training, monitoring, auditing, and system review.

ISO 22000 and 22005 are being updated as of this writing.
ISO 22005 (E), 2007, published in Switzerland.

REVIEW OF THE U.S. FDA FOOD SAFETY MODERNIZATION ACT PREVENTIVE CONTROL RULES

If your business is functioning within the food supply chain, unless you have completely ignored the change going on around you, you are probably somewhat familiar with the overall U.S. FDA FSMA rules recently finalized (September 2015). Basically, rules are the FDA's way of translating the law into some type of set of regulations telling the industry what they have to do to comply with the intent of the written food safety law. In the rules, the FDA will not tell you how to do what you need to do or how to implement compliant solutions, they simply try to put into words what you must do to comply with the law.

In general, the FSMA under the FSMA expects food operations that manufacture, process, pack, or hold food for sale in the United States to define their processes, establish levels of risk for the processes in question and the products, perform a hazard analysis, establish preventive controls, plan to control those hazards, implement, verify and validate the PCP, establish adequate record keeping, and have a tested plan for possible recalls of impacted foods. In short, each food handler was to establish what has become known as a hazard analysis risk-based PCP.

IDENTIFYING HAZARDS RELEVANT TO A FOOD OPERATION

There are a couple of suggested ways to identify hazards that are likely to cause food illness outbreaks if not properly prevented and controlled. For any particular food product or process, common Internet search engines such as Google, Bing, or any of the others, the type of food followed by the word "hazard" can be searched. As an example, a simple search for "spinach hazards" yielded a reference to the World Health Organization's publication on Microbiological hazards in fresh fruits and vegetables. A similar search for "spinach recalls" takes you to the fda.gov website that lists all known FDA recalls [11].

Food suppliers must remember always that the FDA is an enforcement agency. Although the organization may be faced with many of their own internal conflicts

Table 1.1 Primary FSMA Rules

- Final Rule: Accredited Third-Party Certification
- Final Rule: Standards for the Growing, Harvesting, Packing, and Holding of Produce for Human Consumption
- Final Rule: Food Supplier Verification Programs (FSVP) for Importers of Food for Humans and Animals
- Final Rule: Current Good Manufacturing Practice and Hazard Analysis and Risk-Based Preventive Controls for Human Food
- Final Rule: Current Good Manufacturing Practice and Hazard Analysis and Risk-Based Preventive Controls for Food for Animals
- Sanitary Transportation of Human and Animal Food
- Focused Mitigation Strategies to Protect Food Against Intentional Adulteration

and challenges, their job is to enforce industry's willingness and capability to prepare and present safe foods to American consumers.

In 2010, before President Obama signed the FSMA into law, the food side of the FDA had been only modestly supported by congress in their efforts to define and improve food safety. Undoubtedly, there are many members of the FDA who saw no need for any new law and, to this day, are still reluctant to have any part of changes they probably believe will destroy the food industry.

A few months after the new law was signed the established "food safety Czar" was out and was replaced by a new one. That change indicated that new blood was needed in the food side of the FDA to get on with the brutal and hard fought business of establishing the momentum needed for the massive changes yet to come. No doubt many of those employed on the food side of the FDA came to work on Monday wondering what or who would be next.

Table 1.1 is a list of the primary FSMA rules written to establish FDA enforcement capabilities.

One final rule not listed in Table 1.1 is the Final Rule: Record Availability Requirements: Establishment, Maintenance, and Availability of Records, which was finalized in April 2014. The final rule for record availability requirements is an important rule as it basically establishes the right of the FDA to enter facilities and make copies of records they believe may be critical to establishing sources of contaminants, or, even, guilt or innocence in cases where violations of the law are concerned.

At first glance and, indeed at first study, the rules seem to be segmented and anything but directed at the establishment of a synergistic food safety system. If we take a look at the FDA's approach to the development of final rules, there are a few not so simple steps they list as their rules development process.

Step 1: FDA proposes a rule and requests comments
Step 2: FDA considers your comments and issues a final rule
Step 3: Companies comply with the rule based on the "Effective Date"

ADDITIONAL TOOL: FDA ISSUES GUIDANCE DOCUMENTS TO ASSIST INDUSTRY

Of course, the Office of Management and Budget (OMB) is actively trying to estimate cost–benefit tables for each rule. As most of you are aware, this seemingly simple process has taken the FDA over 5 years to complete (2011–16). And that process is just to come up with some "final" version of final rules. When we add on the time required between 1 and 3 years as a full compliance implementation requirement for food supply chain members, the process is, indeed a long one.

On one hand, one of the drawbacks of such a lengthy process is that many food suppliers are on idle meaning that these companies see no reason to change what they have been doing for many years. On the other hand, knowing that these rules will all become law, other food supply chain members succumb to industry pressures to begin establishing improved food safety systems. There are other advantages to a long drawn-out rule-making process. The infrastructure needed to support what the FDA calls a change in the food safety culture simply does not exist to the extent needed for full compliance on the part of all food suppliers, handlers, transporters, processors, distributors, packers, retailers, and restaurants.

The initial proposed rules provided the food industry with enough initial information for many private companies not directly in the food supply chain to begin to develop the services and technology that would be needed over the next generation if food suppliers were to achieve compliance. Following the proposed rules, the comment period and the OMB as well as the Environmental Protection Agency studies all impacted the finalization of rules.

Undoubtedly, the extensive delay also provided the FDA with time to continue its reorganization and improve its focus on concepts that may have previously had less attention than deserved or understood.

Take the concept of prevention for example. The food industry, because of internal rather than external pressures, has worked hard to try to establish some food safety practices. Obviously, no one wants to produce or deliver food that would make people ill or cause death. Well, almost no one (hence the rule on intentional adulteration). The problem with the approach the food industry has taken is that it has followed old, and well established, practices on the basis of subjective observations rather than the more objective and undeniable data that results from taking samples and managing processes on the basis of analysis of that data. I'm taking about food safety audits and certification to certain schemes that rely on external audits.

Although food safety audits drive some level overall system improvement in a business, they increase costs and, in general, are provide little assurance that a supplier knows anything about prevention of food safety problems. Indeed, some food safety audits have failed so miserably that the company that passed the audit was later indicted for transporting foods that killed people.

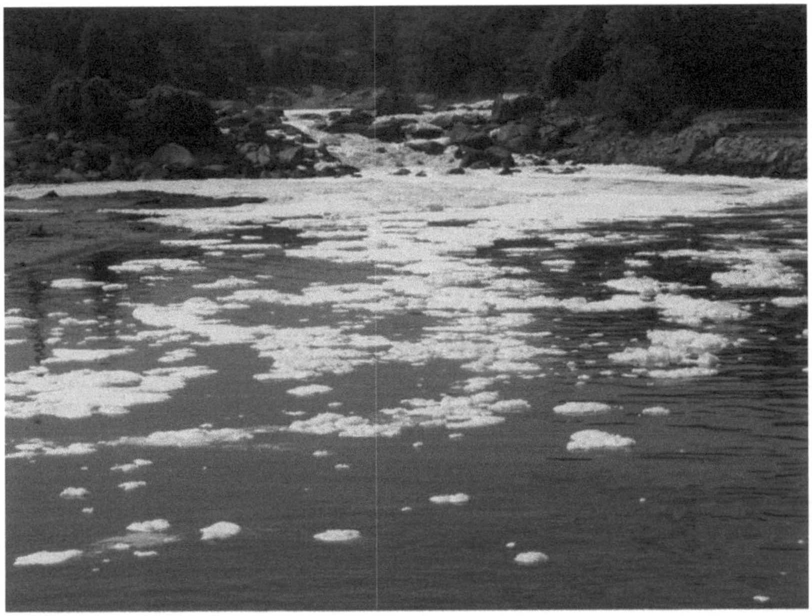

FIGURE 1.4

The river of no return.

THAT'S NOT ACCEPTABLE

If you open your home refrigerator and look at the food inside, on the average, your food has traveled over 2000 mi. to arrive at your home. The world is changing and the ways and distances food travels are also changing. Visual inspection of processes and companies throughout the supply chain cannot keep up with food safety demands. More importantly, as so many companies handle the food as it travels from home to destination, some assumption of the responsibility for food safety must be shared throughout the food chain. Liability for what one company buys from what the company considers a qualified supplier becomes shared. That means that the buying company is responsible for the food safety of the supplier and must be able to quickly identify the source of any contaminant and work with the supplier to prevent such outbreaks, vicarious liability has become a critical issue and everyone in the supply chain is suspect. Unlike the river pollution shown in Fig. 1.4, chemicals, bacteria, and physical hazards are unseen and often undetected by visual inspection. The human eye is simply not capable of seeing such contaminants without some type of laboratory assistance.

All types of contaminants are likely to get into food. In terms of the FSMA, these contaminants may be called hazards, and they have the potential to impact human health and to cause death.

Table 1.2 represents a good sample of these hazards.

Table 1.2 Examples of Food Hazards

- Pests (Bug parts, bird droppings, etc.)
- *Chemicals*
- *Bacteria*
- Food Residues (reuse of package materials)
- Intentional Adulteration (Security)
- Economically Motivated (EMA)
- Objects Such as Foreign Matter/Objects (Glass, wood, etc.)
- Radiation
- *Physical (Paint chips, metal, mold, any other contaminant)*
- Spoilage
- Chemical Extraction and Migration
- Contamination of Food from the Package Materials
- Allergens

PREVENTIVE CONTROLS UNDER FSMA

The FDA's definition of preventive controls states "Risk-based, reasonably appropriate procedures, practices, and processes that a person knowledgeable about the safe manufacturing, processing, packing, or holding of food would employ to significantly minimize or prevent the hazards identified under the hazard analysis that are consistent with the current scientific understanding of safe food manufacturing, processing, packing, or holding at the time of the analysis." [12]

In short, all companies required to be registered with the FDA as food suppliers. You will note that food transporters are not required to bend to preventive control rules; however, by reading the rules on the sanitary transportation of human and animal foods, the emphasis is clearly on prevention. What this means is that companies would be advised to establish some level of environmental sampling and take preventive actions based on that sampling. For instance, adenosine triphosphate or ATP testing of floors and walls after truck trailer wash or sanitation can serve as a basic wash process validation test for food residues. The testing is only used to establish wash procedure validity and, in a manner similar to other environmental monitoring and sampling, establishes a basis for process improvement because it requires causal analysis and preventive action cycles.

The rules entitled "Current Good Manufacturing Practice and Hazard Analysis and Risk-Based Preventive Controls for Human Food" cover requirements for a written food safety plan that includes hazard analysis, preventive controls, oversight, and management of preventive controls that includes monitoring, corrective actions, and corrections and verification.

The FSMA tends to focus on three primary types of hazards: Chemical, biological, and physical, but that list does not really focus attention on other important issues such as the threat of radiation. Radiation became an important issue subsequent to the tsunami that destroyed the nuclear power generation operation after being hit by the tsunami tidal wave.

The FSMA stream of rules from farms impacts the entire food chain from farm to retail, for local and imported foods, with heavy fines for noncompliance, include stoppage of shipments suspected of adulteration, emphasize vicarious liability that is shared from upstream to downstream, and includes new documentation requirements for all impacted entities. Preventive control rules also require a hazard analysis, preventive controls, and oversight and management of preventive controls that cover monitoring, corrective actions, verification, and validation that may include product and environmental testing as well as process monitoring and measurement instrument calibration.

The rules exclude what the FDA calls "primary production farms" but include what is called a "secondary activities farm" if it is not located on a primary production farm, but may harvest, pack or hold raw agricultural commodities (RACs). However, both and secondary activities product farms must comply with the rules.

The rules update Current Good Manufacturing Practices (CGMPs) that include allergen cross-contact.

Under preventive control validation concepts, a trained and certified preventive controls individual is required to oversee a company's ability to establish and manage valid preventive controls. Valid preventive controls represent a significant shift in preventive controls thinking and system implementation. While previous rules and thinking required many companies to verify the implementation of various food safety programs such as HACCP, or Hazard validation requirements now establish team building, causal analysis and statistical analysis as part of an entities overall program. The challenge is for companies to prove that the established preventive controls system actually impacts the results found from environmental and other measurements are actually under control and minimized by the entity in question. Validation requirements established by the rules call for companies to get control over hazards found through environmental and other monitoring activities and to demonstrate such control using more scientific means.

The rules also define a "Primary Production Farm" as a single management operation and a "Secondary Activities Farm" that includes packing and holding of RACs.

Of significance are rules related to the supply-chain (Subpart O) that establish requirements for a risk-based supply chain for ingredients and raw materials that need preventive hazard controls to "ensure that these foods are received only from approved suppliers" whose preventive systems have been reviewed and approved by receiving entities.

Fig. 1.5 illustrates some of the complexity of a single supply chain. Beginning on row 1, food is harvested and goes through chilling and packing prior to being palletized and shipped by reefer to a distributor. At the distributor (row 2), the pallet is loaded into a shipping container and shipped by boat through dock load, ship transport and unload operations prior to being reloaded onto a truck. Row 3 shows the distributor re-palletizing the cases from the original pallets onto trucks delivering to retail outlets or restaurants. Upon arrival, the food is ordinarily placed into a chiller waiting to be moved to retail shelves or the kitchen. Row 4 illustrates the consumer purchase cycle through home cooking operations.

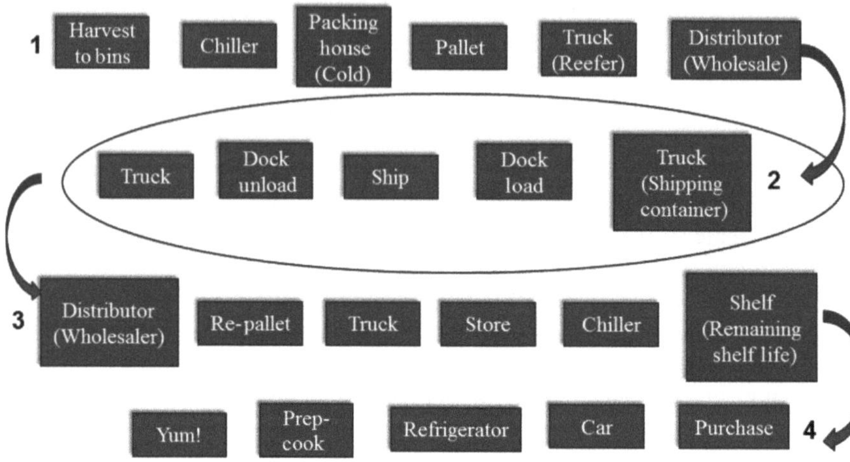

FIGURE 1.5

Supply chain example.

This illustration shows at least four trucking operations with multiple loads and unloads at packing houses, distributors, docks, stores and, at the end, automobiles. The FDA FSMA rules on the sanitary transportation of human and animal foods are established to control this process.

The rules also update CGMPs by requiring employees to be trained to establish competence in the jobs they occupy. The shift to the training requirement is significant to ensure food safety throughout manufacturing practices.

The FDA lists compliance dates based on the September 17, 2015 final rules publication date in the Federal Register.

Compliance dates for businesses are staggered over several years after publication of the final rule.

- *Very small businesses (averaging less than $1 million per year (adjusted for inflation) in both annual sales of human food plus the market value of human food manufactured, processed, packed, or held without sale): Three years, except for records to support its status as a very small business (January 1, 2016).*
- *Businesses subject to the Pasteurized Milk Ordinance (compliance dates extended to allow time for changes to the PMO safety standards that incorporate the requirements of this preventive controls rule): Three years.*
- *Small businesses (a business with fewer than 500 full-time equivalent employees): Two years.*
- *All other businesses: One year.*

Compliance dates after publication of the final rule for the requirements of the supply chain program:

- *Receiving facility is a small business and its supplier will not be subject to the human preventive controls rule or the produce safety rule: Two years.*
- *Receiving facility is a small business and its supplier will be subject to the human preventive controls rule or the produce safety rule: Two years or six months after the supplier is required to comply with the applicable rule, whichever is later.*
- *Receiving facility is not a small or very small business and its supplier will not be subject to the human preventive controls rule or the produce safety rule: 18 months.*
- *Receiving facility is not a small or very small business and its supplier will be subject to the human preventive controls rule or the produce safety rule: Six months after the supplier is required to comply with the applicable rule.*

From Ref. [13].

EXPANDED FDA ENFORCEMENT CAPABILITIES

It is important to note that the FDA does not work alone. The following list contains some of the federal organizations working in conjunction with the FDA to help with enforcement of the rules:

- CDC
- EPA—Activities related to establishing priorities and addressing other issues related to residues of animal drugs and pesticides in food animals, detecting illegal residues, and taking regulatory action against violators.
- U.S. Department of Agriculture, FSIS—Meat, poultry, and processed eggs.
- U.S. Department of Agriculture, Agricultural Marketing Service (AMS) egg shell safety.
- U.S. Department of Agriculture, Foreign Agricultural Service (FAS)—Coordinate future activities and approaches to selected food safety issues facing developing countries and emerging markets.
- U.S. Department of Agriculture, Food and Nutrition Service (FNS)—FDA-regulated products distributed via domestic nutrition assistance programs administered by FNS. Examples of such programs include the National School Lunch Program and Emergency Food Assistance Program.
- U.S. Department of Homeland Security (DHS)—Authority to ensure the safety and security of imported food—DHS personnel formally commissioned and specially trained to conduct cargo and other examinations of FDA-regulated articles. CBP personnel have authority to hold suspect shipments for further examination and sampling.

- U.S. Department of Commerce, National Oceanic and Atmospheric Administration, National Marine Fisheries Service (NMFS)—Seafood—NMFS inspects 20% of seafood consumed in the United States.
- U.S. Department of Defense (DOD)—Information sharing.
- Department of Transportation (DOT).
- U.S. Department of Labor, OSHA—Information sharing.
- Federal Trade Commission (FTC)—Preventing injury and deception to consumers.

By training and coordinating with other agencies, powers of the FDA are extended far beyond the FDA's singular authority and laws as well as the FDA's ability to inspect, seize, hold, reject, or otherwise control food safety. As an example, the DHS has the ability at the borders to stop, inspect and control incoming food shipments. The DOT has transportation rules that go beyond those FDA regulations thus allowing for tighter controls over food transported throughout the supply chain.

EXTENDED PREVENTIVE CONTROL CONSIDERATIONS: BEYOND FSMA

A review of the direction required to establish a company's approach to preventive controls beyond what laws might focus on are several issues that must be addressed.

These include but are not limited to the following:

- Supply chains
- Teams and teamwork
- Statistical requirements and reporting
- Food fraud
- Security and food cargo theft
- Traceability
- Transportation
- Cross contamination
- Integration of food safety systems
- Electronic record keeping
- Technology
- The differences between corrective and preventive actions
- Chipotle as a case study

These topics are covered in different sections of this book.

REFERENCES

[1] August 1, 2016 <https://en.wikipedia.org/wiki/Prevention>.

[2] P.B. Crosby. Quality is Free: The Art of Making Quality Certain, ISBN O-07-014512-1, (1979), published by Mentor, 1980.

[3] August 1, 2016 <http://www.fda.gov/Food/GuidanceRegulation/FSMA/ucm334115.htm>.
[4] August1, 2016 <http://www.inspection.gc.ca/about-the-cfia/acts-and-regulations/regulatory-initiatives/sfca/food-safety-systems/your-business/preparing-a-preventive-control-plan/eng/1427746591578/1427746679297>.
[5] August 1, 2016 <http://eurlex.europa.eu/LexUriServ/LexUriServ.do?uri=OJ:L:2002:031:0001:0024:en:PDF>.
[6] July 1, 2016 <http://fda-news.registrarcorp.com/2014/08/fda-mexico-preventive-food-safety/>.
[7] January 1, 2016 <http://www.fda.gov/NewsEvents/Newsroom/PressAnnouncements/ucm406607.htm>.
[8] June 17, 2016 <http://www.foodsafetymagazine.com/enewsletter/china-an-overview-of-the-new-food-safety-law/>.
[9] August 1, 2016 <https://www.iso.org/obp/ui/#iso:std:iso:22000:ed-1:v1:en>.
[10] ISO 22000: 2005(E), first ed., 2005-09-01, Switzerland.
[11] March 21, 2016 <http://www.who.int/foodsafety/publications/micro/MRA_FruitVeges.pdf>.
[12] May 3, 2016 <http://www.fda.gov/Food/GuidanceRegulation/FSMA/ucm334115.htm>.
[13] May 19, 2016 <http://www.fda.gov/Food/GuidanceRegulation/FSMA/ucm334115.htm>.

CHAPTER 2

Teams and teamwork for validating preventive food safety and quality control

Undoubtedly, the transition by most food supply companies from older approaches that stopped at requiring a company to verify implementation of its food safety system to a new approach requiring validation will be difficult. The presentation of common and assignable causes in Chapter 1, Background: Understanding Common and Assignable Causes, Laws and Costs sets the groundwork for how the assignment of problems must be thought out and delegated to either management or functional hourly worker teams. The organization and the people requiring training and tools needed to successfully make the transition into valid preventive controls must be thought out, properly prioritized and attacked.

This chapter presents a team focused strategy for making the transition smooth and cooperative at all levels. Two primary types of teams are discussed:

1. Common cause (CC) teams whose members consist of management level personnel focused on system or CCs and
2. Functional improvement teams (FITs) whose members are from various company functional personnel with members are primarily nonsalaried personnel with daily operational responsibilities.

CC and FIT teams work on problems for which different levels of responsibility are defined in Chapter 1, Background: Understanding Common and Assignable Causes, Laws and Costs. For both types of teams, a team-level organizational structure is defined. Both types of teams are commonly under the initial training and guidance by a facilitator. All teams have team leaders, secretaries, and members working to define problem areas, collect and analyze data, analyze causes, and establish team-level plans focused on preventing the problem from recurrence.

Leadership and facilitation are critical, especially in the beginning until the system becomes an integrated part of how the company operates. Table 2.1 is a recommended list of the things a team leader should do.

The requirements for validation are significantly different enough for most food suppliers to look for or train a new generation of food safety personnel. In Michael Taylor's terms, this cultural shift is more complex and will take the overall food supply system a long time in spite of implementation dates established by laws such as those enacted by the food safety modernization act (FSMA). The shift to requirements for environmental sampling, supply chain controls, causal analysis, and statistical proof will reverberate through the industry for many years.

Validating Preventive Food Safety and Quality Controls. DOI: http://dx.doi.org/10.1016/B978-0-12-810994-6.00002-X

Table 2.1 What Team Leaders Should Do

1. Let team members set action items, plan, handle decision-making and action items, and present ideas.
2. Listen carefully and accept ideas presented.
3. Be a leader, not a boss.
4. Provide a positive "we can" attitude.
5. Keep the group focused on the issues.
6. Encourage participation from all team members.
7. Provide recognition for good work.
8. Help prioritize.
9. Follow up on activity completion during each meeting.
10. Assign or choose a backup leader.
    a. Meetings should be held even when the leader is absent (which should be never).
    b. Leadership skills should be developed in all team members.
11. Interact with other team leaders and members.
12. Refrain from dominating discussions among team members.

For most companies, a project or team approach will be necessary simply because such culturally dynamic changes cannot be planned or implemented by any single person if the changes are expected to take hold. To begin with, there are attitudes and beliefs regarding the overall changes that will endure for some time. For instance, there are some things heard in many companies that will provide easy insight into those willing to transition from the old to the new versus those of a more conservative nature. Myths endure and walls will be erected that will slow the change process.

Listen around your company for some of these comments and you can quickly establish a theoretical change implementation timeline and a company's ability to move forward.

Team systems take 3 years

"If it ain't broke, don't fix it!"

We don't do it that way here!

That will never work here!

We don't have time for THAT!

You can't do THAT here!

Regardless of foot dragging, there are significant forces afoot that will help to move the change mechanisms along and those forces come in the form of enforcement activities. Such comments that are heard daily help to determine a company's willingness (like it or not) to get on with the required system changes.

Other industries that have undergone such overall changes to their thinking and action and have transitioned more or less quickly depending on their approach to the required changes.

Basically, the idea that upper management must be committed is paramount if a company is to plan and successfully implement preventive controls in a manner that would do if management believed they could successfully increase revenues and secure higher salaries. However, in the case of food safety, many company leaders have and remain against implementing preventive controls as they do not perceive either the danger to consumers, or because of increased costs or because they do not believe that changes required for preventive controls will improve food safety.

Whatever the reason, the lack of commitment will drag required changes into the mud.

Management commitment to needed changes in any industry or country is often countered by others in the organization who go ahead with implementation with or without management support simply because it is their job, and they may be tired of upper management ignoring or refusing to support such changes. In shore, change often starts in the streets. Mid-level managers may choose to work with their personnel to establish procedural changes with or without the approval or knowledge of upper level hoping, perhaps, to wrest leadership control from the foot draggers.

As all companies are legally required to establish preventive controls, new processes will emerge slowly as a result of anticipated lower level revolts.

For companies eager to put all this behind them, many will establish project or other teams to get on with planning implementation. One fact remains. When all departments work the plan together and establish an approach to change implementation, open communication and solution sharing are more likely to flourish, and the pain perceived by the need to change will diminish.

Leadership and involvement among all department heads such as those listed below will serve to move things forward more rapidly until the fears, old way of doing things are far in the rear view mirror, and no one will even remember what the old ways of doing things looked like.

Accounting
Quality
Food safety
Distribution
Engineering
Finance
Human resources
Information technology
Legal
Marketing
Design
Production
Purchasing
Research & development
Sales

In this section, an approach to project and team change management is defined for those companies with less fear of the unknown.

Fig. 2.1 is a simple illustration of the relationship among the key system change components. If leadership and upper management support are established, a guidance policy generally leads planning and the development of procedures as preludes to overall implementation.

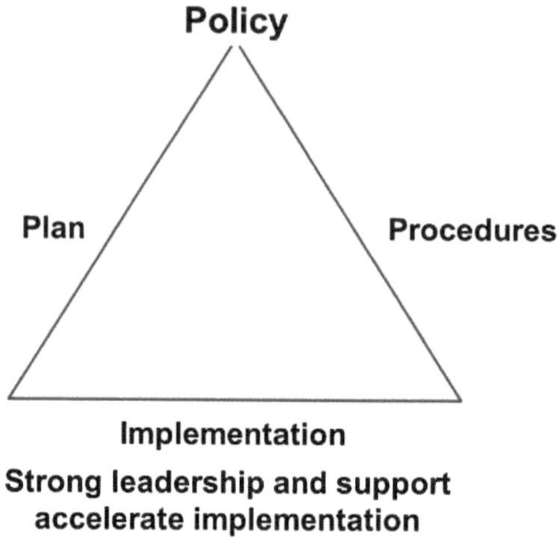

FIGURE 2.1

General system relationships.

A policy that emphasizes and clearly states requirements for validation of preventive controls and causal analysis is clearly different from one that simply states "We are dedicated to food safety."

Implementation can be accelerated through the support of strong leadership or retarded from resistance, the lack of leadership or through strong leadership. Those are three different approaches and the chosen path will dictate the speed with which the organization makes the change and costs associated with the change.

With requirements for preventive control implementation, the dynamics regulating the change process is greatly impacted by several factors. Quite simply, upper management does not do or know the tasks required of subordinates. Rapid change often means that lower-level personnel are given the authority and responsibility to define and make needed changes. In other words, the power to make changes by lower-level personnel opens the door to establishing teams with new authority and responsibilities and challenges all personnel to get on with the job.

Empowering change at lower levels is often against current company operational and management approaches; however, change and system implementation can be accelerated through a team approach. Many companies loosely use the word "team" in an attempt to get people to work together. However, there are vastly different levels of success between "teams" that are assigned to do projects and teams that are teams that win. It is no mystery in the world of sports that a team that is truly functioning as a team takes a winning form, whereas the "team" that does not function truly as a team does not end up in the super bowl.

In short, a group is not a team regardless of what they are called. Overuse of the word "team without the focus," knowledge and effort needed to establish team building can be harmful and leave employees rolling their eyeballs when the word is used.

Group	Team
• Works in the same functional unit	• Works together with focus
• Each person has their own job	• Reports team status
• Individual recognition	• Team recognition
• Rewards are for individuals	• Earns team rewards
• Boss runs the show	• Team runs the show
• Normal Organizational Chart	• Team has authority along with
	• responsibility

FIGURE 2.2

Groups versus teams.

There are differences between groups and teams. Fig. 2.2 illustrates a few.

Generally, groups are not given the authority needed to make changes (without approval) along with authority. Wikipedia defines authority as "the right to exercise power given by the state (in the form of government, judges, police officers, etc.), or by academic knowledge of an area (someone that can be an authority on a subject)" [1].

"Academic knowledge" can be interpreted to emphasize the difference in process knowledge by upper level management versus such knowledge held by individuals actually doing a job.

There are a number of important factors to consider when establishing levels of process knowledge. Put simply, it can be assumed that management, by virtue of their responsibilities and involvement in management issues, has, for some time, been out of lower level functioning for some time. Those who have risen through the ranks may have known how things were done a few years ago, but with or without their knowledge, process changes have slowly been implemented at lower levels without their knowledge. Furthermore, management has often left their concerns over how a specific job was being done during their tenure and moved into new concerns and responsibilities that have shielded them from lower level change dynamics.

Since being promoted, many internal and external forces may have impacted the company requiring lower-level personnel to adjust without telling anyone.

ADOPTING AN ATTITUDE OF CONTINUOUS IMPROVEMENT

Adopting an attitude of continuous improvement implies that such as "If it ain't broke, don't fix it" is antiimprovement. The statement is certainly anticontinuous improvement which is unfortunate since valid preventive controls are because of a continuous improvement approach.

Some factors need to be considered and established to begin to envision a true team system as the company drives toward fulfilling requirements established by preventive systems. These include

- Measurement
- Setting priorities

- Setting goals and objectives
- Forming functional and cross-functional teams
- Establishing authority with responsibility
- Team and individual activities
- Reporting
- Rewards

One of the primary objectives of a team system is to reduce dependence on inspection and test in all operations. Fig. 2.3 illustrates the self-inspection reduction concept. Self-inspection implies that production and other operational steps in any process are not to be backed up by implementing and expanding inspection and test processes, but must be the target of elimination through changes in responsibilities.

The fact that a process has been cropped up by expensive inspection and test steps is a clear indication that poor quality and poor food safety practices are operational, and preventive controls have been put on the back burner in an effort to support inadequate processes and expedite shipments that have continually exhibited poor output.

Inspection and test steps must be analyzed as expensive band aids that have been slapped on a process to crop it up. Inspection and test reduction or elimination should become a primary organizational goal.

In an effort to get beyond reliance on inspection and test, teams can be initially established, trained, and released to work on a goal of inspection and test elimination.

The fact that some rules such as the FSMA have placed great emphasis on environmental testing is somewhat unfortunate. Activities like monitoring, audit, inspection, and test are expenses no one needs and smack of an inability to establish preventive controls.

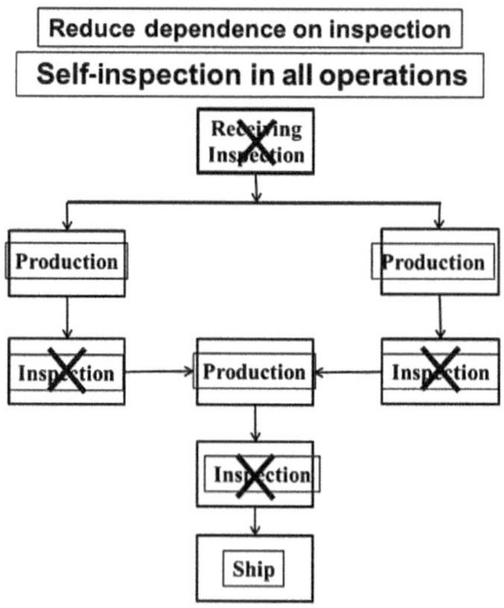

FIGURE 2.3

Self-inspection elimination.

FORMING BASIC TEAMS

Two basic team types can be defined.

1. FIT—A focus on assignable causes
   a. People with the same type of job (e.g., five operators in a single production line, or purchasing folks working on a problem primarily related to purchasing). Functional (I/we can fix our own problems)
2. CC team—A focus on system or common causes—Management controllable
   a. People from different departments working on problems that impact their mutual departments—Problem can't be resolved by a functional team—Team removes barriers. Cross functional means management personnel must work together across company functions to repair interdepartmental processes.

A few basic steps in the formation and implementation of FIT and CC teams can be listed that follow the procedure presented under the solution tracking sheet (STS) presentation.

- Form functional or cross-functional teams (select members)—Empower members to independently make needed changes
- Flow chart the process that has been highlighted as a problem area
- Decide where/how to collect baseline data
- Brainstorm possible causes (Ishikawa diagrams)
- Collect baseline data
- Develop trend data and a Pareto analysis
- Define potential causes
- Establish a recycling plan to continually improve the process
- Establish a final fix level (process goal attainment)
- Allow team members to plan and implement planned change activities
- Upon reaching the process goal, revise procedures
- Retrain involved personnel
- Provide recognition and rewards for successful teams
- Retrigger to identify new problems and new teams as part of the continuous improvement process.

During team activities communication among team members and up the chain of command is important so that everyone understands issues, attempted solutions and needed changes. communication must be

1. Free and open
2. Person to person
   a. Within working functions
   b. Across functions and departments
3. Allows people to talk while working
   a. In the work line
   b. Close location of dependent operations to receive information from previous process steps and to pass information to following process steps

4. Establishment of data systems to support and supply analysis, local understanding and upward reporting
5. Establishment of reporting systems allow for the sharing of findings, information and data with other departments and management

There are a number of team member roles that can be defined. These include

Facilitator,
Leader
Secretary
Member

TEAM ORGANIZATIONS

Fig. 2.4 illustrates a basic team organization with the facilitator taking care of and facilitating both FIT and CC teams. The lines do not create authority levels between the facilitator and team leaders nor between the team leaders, secretaries, and members. This means that each team member gets one vote. The team leader leads but is not "the boss" of the team.

Of course, there can be from one to many CC and FIT teams depending on the organization's current level of expansion. Generally, an organization will start with one of each and facilitate them, whereas team leaders, secretaries, and members come on task and understand the team structure, responsibilities, goals, and operational responsibilities.

TEAM ORGANIZATIONS

Team structures generally work well under normal organizational structures and emphasize the best in employee values that include

- Commitment
- Respect

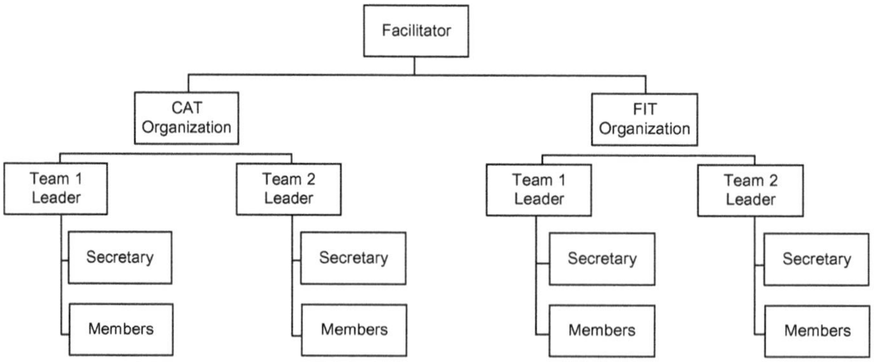

FIGURE 2.4

Basic CC and FIT team organization.

- Leadership
- Integrity
- Patience

Choosing team members implies that selected team members are chosen based on any of a number of personal characteristics. The facilitator is expected to bring any number people together during the team formation process and encourage them to work on the team. Note that membership must be voluntary to eliminate discontented employees from the team.

By bringing potential members into a room and describing team activities, the facilitator can use the list below to discuss team member qualification and requirements.

- Voluntary
- Hard worker
- Want to learn
- Frustrated by "the way things are done"
- Want to improve "things"
- Twinkle in the eye
- May have some specific and important knowledge or specialty
- Respected
- Reliable
- Friendly
- Internally motivated
- Work in connected process to enable cross training

The cross training concept (Fig. 2.5) is important so that each team member can slowly learn the requirements of the process before their own work and the process immediately after their job. The facilitator should introduce prospective team members to this concept to emphasize cooperation and communication between and among members.

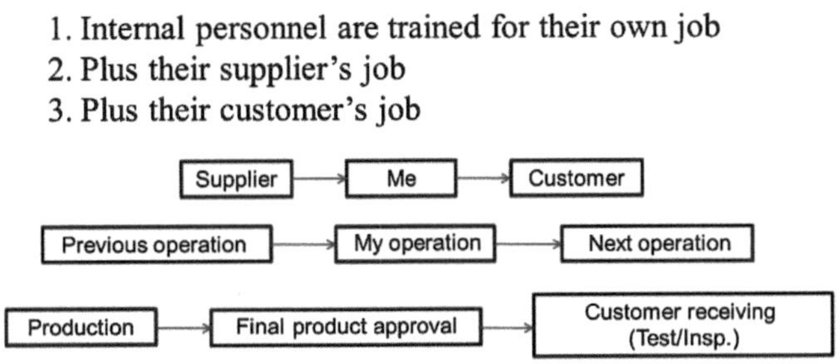

FIGURE 2.5

Cross training concept.

TEAM FACILITATORS AND TEAM FACILITATION

When beginning to establish teams and team objectives, there are some things to keep in mind from a management perspective. Information relative to selecting and training a team organization facilitator is listed below.

- Facilitators are trained to facilitate
- Facilitators do not run the team
- The team leader runs the team, not the facilitator
- Facilitators ask questions—Team members answer the questions
- An individual that is responsible for leading team members to make decisions

Team facilitators must be trained or exhibit competence in the following areas prior to selection. It is management's responsibility to select and assign a facilitator.

1. Facilitation (tested and must go through an observed practicum)
2. Problem selection
3. Causal analysis
4. Food safety and quality principles and practices including
   a. Defect or Pareto analysis
   b. Causal analysis
   c. Data collection and forms
   d. Statistical process control (SPC)
   e. Teams
   f. Planning
5. Training

Facilitators must be comfortable speaking in front of groups. The facilitator is assigned to each team until the team is on task and self-operating.

A team is considered to be "on task" when the team is operating without the need for the facilitator. On task implies that a clear project has been defined, a problem chosen and all members are actively participating in team members.

The facilitator is critical during initial team stages. After proper orientation with a team leader and secretary chosen, the following procedure is followed to help the team select the first problem that needs attention.

PRIORITIZING PROBLEMS

Problem prioritization is a team activity designed to narrow a large list of identified problems into a shortlist and finally to the problem on which the team will focus. The assigned facilitator will guide the team through this process. There are some requirements for the problem selection process including the following brief list of rules to be managed by the facilitator.

1. Teams will choose their own problems on which to work
2. Problems will not be "assigned" or dictated from above
3. Teams will work on only ONE problem at a time.

The following steps should be considered when choosing a team focus:

- Once seated, the facilitator asks team members what problems they experience in their daily work (expect to elicit many issues)
- There should be no discussion of problems during the listing process
- Any and all problems can be considered
- None are too small or too big
- None are too ridiculous
- Team members respond verbally
- Facilitator lists all known problems on board
- Facilitator divides board into two parts
- Problems the team can solve B. Problems the team cannot solve
- Team members tell facilitator which problems go into A and B categories
- Secretary takes notes and keeps record of A and B groups
- Facilitator holds a discussion of "our problems (A)" versus "not our problems (B)" (finger pointing)
- Removal of "not our problems"—"We cannot solve these problems" (assigned to a CC team)
- Cycles of voting take place—Each team member gets three votes (what each member thinks are in the top three problems in their area)
- All problems not in the top 10 (counted votes) are removed from the list
- Rejected problems are filed for later review
- The top 10 problems are voted on—Each member gets only three votes
- All except the top three problems (counted votes) are removed from the list
- Team members get only one vote
- The top problem (counted votes) becomes the prime target for the first team assignment.

TEAM LEADERS

The team is expected to select a team leader under the following set of rules:

1. Any team member can become the team leader
2. It is recommended that team leadership revolves meaning that over time any person may take a turn as the team leader
3. Team selects team leader—Volunteer, assigned or by vote
4. The team leader is not the boss of the team, but a member whose job is to keep the team on task by making sure that the steps outlined in the STS are followed.

TEAM SECRETARY

1. The team secretary can be any member—Volunteer
2. Secretary takes notes during team meetings
3. Maintains team STS with team member help

4. Updates data on STS
5. Distribute weekly agenda and updated STS 1 day after regularly scheduled team meeting to during which the STS is updated
6. Sends out team meeting reminder one work day before regularly scheduled meeting.

TEAM MEMBERS

The following list is used to train and provide guidance for team members:

1. Meeting is at the same time and in the same place every week (calendar control)
2. Meetings are held weekly for 1 hour
3. Membership limited (5–7)
4. Work on team activity outside of team meeting requires 1 hour
5. Members choose the leader
6. Members choose a secretary (sets agenda, records minutes, updates data)
7. For functional teams—No managers are allowed on the team or in any team meeting
8. Every person has one and only one vote
9. Every person must complete their action items on time
10. Voluntary: Motivated employees are selected
11. Members must understand and allow for "lag time" when plotting new data
12. Agenda/team meeting updates are reviewed and acted upon by each member within 1 week
13. Add other rules as you require

GUIDANCE FOR ALL TEAM MEMBERS

1. Be on time to all meetings (100% attendance)
2. Have action items completed and on time
3. Participate in solving the problems
4. Provide solutions and highlight new problems
5. Don't be afraid to ask questions and argue your point
6. Think about becoming the next team leader
7. Volunteer to become the secretary.

All teams need a place to meet. A typical meeting room layout is shown as Fig. 2.6

The team meeting room should be comfortable, well lit, quiet, and neat.

Occasionally and in some operations, a meeting room may not be available due to prior reservations for the room. In such cases, a separate production floor or other area may be established to support team meetings. Fig. 2.7 is an illustration of a suggested team meeting layout.

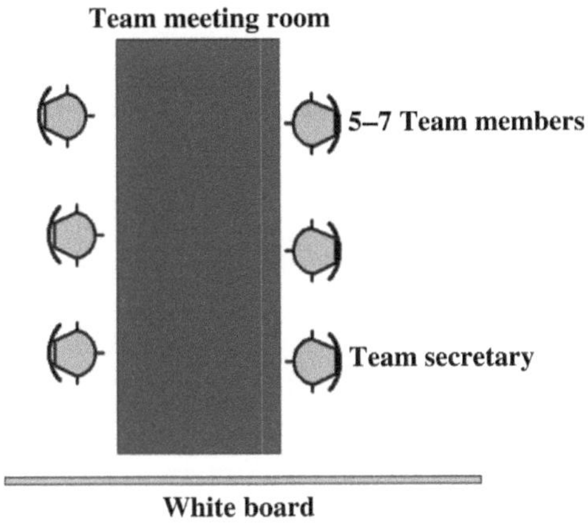

FIGURE 2.6

Standard team meeting room setup.

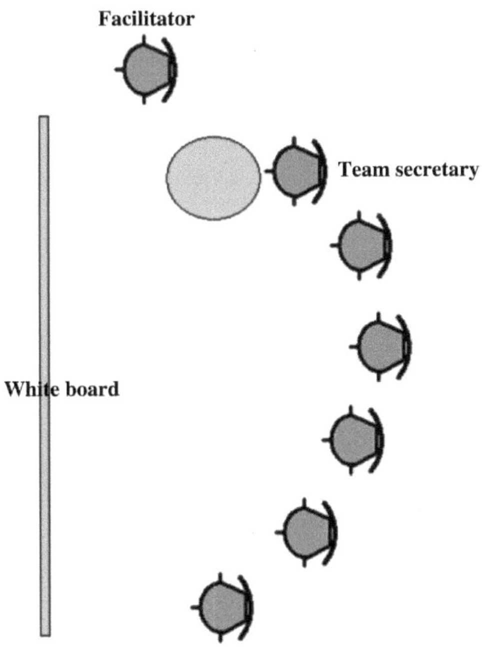

FIGURE 2.7

Production floor team meeting layout.

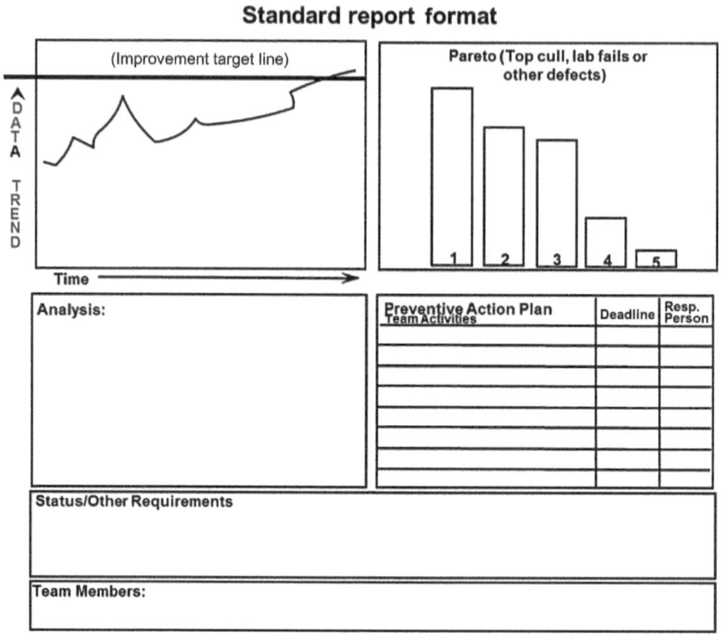

FIGURE 2.8

The solution tracking sheet.

Team meetings should be focused on results and should use the STS to track and record all activities (Fig. 2.8) as outlined in the statistics section of this book.

TEAM REWARD SYSTEMS

Teams that successfully bring a process under control and achieve team goals should receive recognition and rewards as part of the overall team activities. Team reward strategies are designed to motivate and keep teams focused on problem solutions. Teams and individuals may receive impromptu, quarterly or annual rewards. The human resources and other management personnel may design and implement an appropriate team reward system.

Teams and management staff should consider the following when designing reward systems:

- Measure impact of each problem being attacked
- Report outcome costs (prevention, appraisal, internal, and external failures)
- The counting of teams and members is not a hard measure (subjective)
- The facilitator should consolidate team STSs into single page report

Team and operational reports are for hard facility quality and food safety achievements and may include some of the following:

1. Statistical evidence that processes have been brought under control and are preventing food safety and quality problems
2. Zero recalls
3. Reductions in environmental sampling failures
4. Number of suppliers with established preventive control systems
5. Incoming accept rates from suppliers
6. Outgoing customer lot accept rates
7. Return rates
8. Rework rates
9. Scrap/cull rates
10. Test failure rates
11. Inspection and test reductions
12. Bringing vehicle sanitation trends under strict control.

The overall team approach may be evaluated and rewarded by management on some of the following:

- Leadership: Highly visible and active/facilitates/communication
- Information and analysis: Accessible, has depth/breadth, correlated to customer satisfaction
- Strategic planning: Goals and strategies, inputs welcome, resources available, total system
- HR: Internal supplier/customer, employees empowered, low employee turnover, high attendance
- Process management: Preventive, robustness of design, process control, and improvement, cycle time reduced, certified suppliers process assessments/control
- Business results: Continuous improvements (rework, scrap, work in process (WIP), cycle times, recalls, cost structures)
- Customer focus/satisfaction: Company/function focuses customer on what is possible.

Reward systems may be established for monthly, quarterly or annually for best achievement or best team improvement.

FUNCTIONAL IMPROVEMENT TEAMS—ASSIGNABLE CAUSES

The general process for developing and implementing FITs follows the procedures briefly described above. FITs are focused on problems within their own sphere of control and are managed by the facilitator, leader, secretary functions. Within any

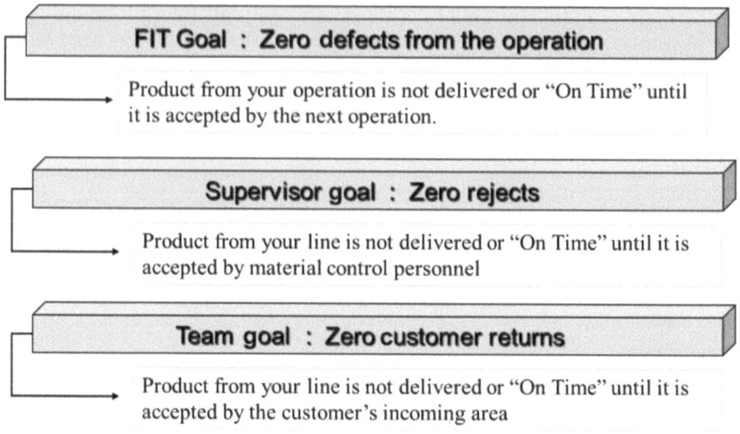

FIGURE 2.9

General FIT goal setting.

single FIT, overall consideration for general goals must be considered in terms of the individual's and team's responsibilities an authority. Fig. 2.9 illustrates goals that might be set at the operational, supervisor, and team levels. Each level of goals is designed to support subsequent and larger goals.

In some cases, more specific rules such as the following are established for operation and FIT members.

1. You are now a member of a rapid response team, and you will remain on the floor during normal production times.
2. Your team is authorized to evaluate performance and to plan and implement changes which will improve food safety, quality or output. Your team and the operators within the operation own the operation and are responsible for product quality, product delivery, the condition of the operation, and everything which happens within the operation.
3. It is your responsibility to respond to RED LIGHT problems within 3 minutes. Any person on the floor (including operators) may turn on a RED or YELLOW LIGHT. The RED LIGHT will NOT be turned off until an acceptable quick fix is in place and agreed to by all team members. The operator at the RED LIGHT station is a member of the team and must approve team fixes.
4. It is your responsibility to perform causal analysis, do a quick fix of problems and put a permanent and preventive fix in place for all RED LIGHT problems. If your team cannot put a preventive fix in place due to a lack of resources or knowledge, one member of your team will attend the daily production meeting, make a brief presentation of the problem and ask management for help.
5. Your team's performance evaluation depends on the following:
   a. The level of operational control as indicated by GREEN LIGHTS and in-control SPC charts

    b. Customer return rates
    c. Scrap costs
    d. Yields
    e. Defective parts per million (DPPM) and lot accept rates
    f. "On time" delivery as measured by the customer's receiving inspection.
6. Your operation is supported by many other people from other functions. Your team has the authority to demand that they assist you when required.

In terms of shared responsibility, the FIT may become a cost center with responsibilities to measure not only food safety and quality, but costs associated with different factors. With a focus on cost controls, the FIT may assume added responsibilities such as these:

1. Each FIT is a cost center
2. Team drives continuous improvement in all operations and may combine or eliminate operations to improve profits
3. Profit measures= ship out value minus cost of rework, scrap, labor and materials, recalls and returns

In the case where FITs may become cost centers, product cost reviews will be conducted monthly using the STS. CCs may be sued to establish FIT cost reduction targets based on product cost reports for each product. The FIT may establish cost reduction plans and work on product cost improvements.

The CC may pick one or two targets from monthly product cost reviews and drivers, work to establish plans and be involved in plan and preventive action reviews that focus on STS trends.

SPECIALIZED TEAMS AND COMMON CAUSE TEAMS

Specialized teams and CCS can be used to focus on many issues not related to the functional improvement efforts of FITs. Recall that far and away more issues are considered common or system causes than assignable causes. CCs and specialized teams are established and function in a manner to that described above, under the same rules, and with similar reward structures.

CCs are generally management level teams and can consider problems under any of the following types of issues:

- Driving company-wide initiatives
- Inventory reduction
- Obsolete and excess inventory
- New projects (bar coding)
- Paperwork reduction
- Implementing international standards organization (ISO), occupational safety and health administration (OSHA), automated processes, or even special issues like establishing a Six-Sigma system

THE COMMON CAUSE SYSTEM IMPROVEMENT TEAMS (REDUCTION OF COMMON CAUSES)

It should be recalled that CCs are comprised of members of management groups, they consist of members from different functions and are assigned to identify and tackle problems that pose barriers, miscommunications and misunderstandings between or among company functions. CCs consist of management members from all functions and are responsible for process maintenance and improvement. CCs may be formed and include members from:

1. Production/operations
2. Food safety
3. Facilities
4. Maintenance
5. Quality
6. Material control
7. Human resources
8. Engineering
9. Maintenance
10. Application Eng.
11. Technicians
12. Tooling

Other departments should be added to the list depending on the organizational structure.

CCs can be focused on problems that are identified in management meetings.

Reviews of daily production or operations status prior to production meeting, determine action items, plans, and establish team actions, plan process improvements, define requirements for support functions.

Summarizes production status and planned actions and reports to and requests support from production meeting attendees using STS format (10:00 am).

Members are considered to be direct report to team leader and indirectly report to functional manager when working on team issues.

CCs may be used to establish and provide immediate in-depth rapid response to manufacturing, distribution, transportation, harvest, or other functions.

RAPID RESPONSE TEAMS

There are critical issues that arise in any company on a daily basis. Such critical issues demand immediate attention and support. Immediate attention and support serves two purposes. First, lower level employees become aware of management commitment to preventive control processes. Second, the support required by daily employees allows them to continue working with the knowledge that the problem that was encountered has a group of professionals focused on providing permanent solutions to problems. Such activities should be carefully recorded because of record keeping demands for evidence of commitment and validation of the preventive control system.

The idea behind management supported rapid response teams is simple. Problems encountered by daily personnel cannot be allowed to languish or be brushed aside. Inaction establishes an attitude of "they don't care" on the part of daily employees.

It is critical to establish an alert system for rapid response team members to get them into the problem area, shipping area, or other function in need of quick help. This can be done by telephone, red lights, or any other means required.

Two levels of response may be required. As a rule, rapid response team members are required to report to the problem area within 3 minutes of notification. Generally, two levels of involvement are required to assure that short (quick corrective actions) and long term (causal analysis and preventive controls) are established and followed up on.

First level team: The floor team leader (supervisor) must be stationed in the line to support the operations at all times and must arrive at the work station within 3 minutes of event notification (red light—Production stop).

The floor team leader must develop a list of team members so that members may be immediately notified.

Second level team: When the assigned team cannot make a corrective action decision, help will be requested from CCs or production meeting attendees or team review attendees.

For rapid response teams, triggering mechanisms, trigger points, and alert systems such the one shown in Fig. 2.10 may be established. Critical control points and information such as SPC charts may trigger the rapid response team and bring it into action. Some of the potential alert issues are listed below:

- Process control plans and trigger system
- ANDON (light systems)
- Customer generated stop ship notices
- Test fails, correlation, calibration, process audits
- Recalls

The key for rapid response, CCs or FITs is simple: Focus on, fix, and control one issue at a time.

A COST FOCUS

Reviewing the cost issues presented in Chapter 1, Background: Understanding Common and Assignable Causes, Laws and Costs means that upper management, team facilitators, team leaders, and members should recall the idea of preventive, internal failure, appraisal, and external failure costs. In a later chapter that presents statistical concepts, Six-Sigma is discussed. Six-Sigma combines the team concept with high cost common or system causes such as those discussed in Chapter 1, Background: Understanding Common and Assignable Causes, Laws and Costs. By

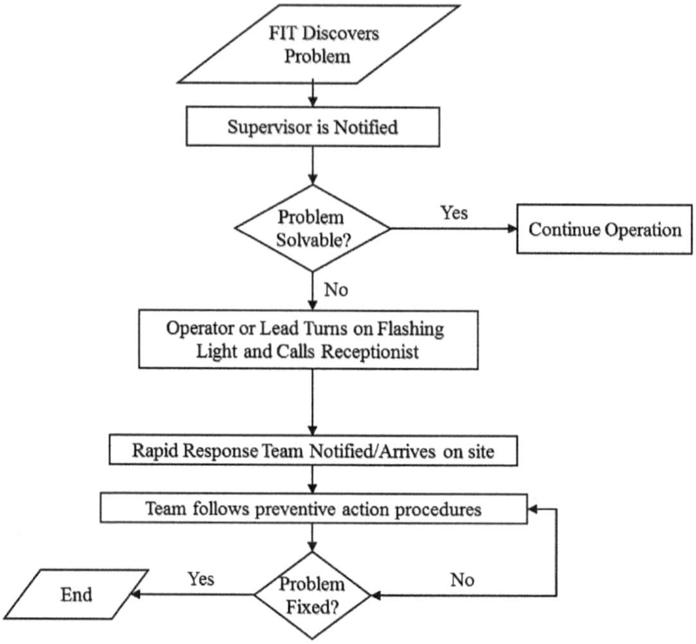

FIGURE 2.10

Rapid response team flow chart.

Table 2.2 Major Company Cost Issues

Response From Group	Estimated Annual Cost
Sale/purchase transactions incomplete	$2+ Million
Incorrect forecasts	2 Million
IT-incorrect decision data	Huge
Engineering design errors	Inestimable
Incorrect or incomplete product specifications	5+ Million
Shipping damage	2.5 Million
Yield losses during manufacturing	4+ Million
Late or missed delivers	1.5 Million
Vendor quality and late delivery	5+ Million
Excess/obsolete inventory	2 Million

implementing a strong team approach that is at least guided somewhat by costs, any company can begin the journey toward implementation of a Six-Sigma program.

Table 2.2 is an example of projects developed by an upper-level management team whose job is to provide financial estimates of costs or losses due to

	Process Step 1	Process Step 2	Process Step 3	Process Step 4	Process Step 5 inspection
Number of rejects	34	11	31	1	44
Cost per unit at each step (Unit cost plus labor/OH cost)	$1	$ 1.5	$2.25	$ 2.75	$3
$ Loss	$34	$15	$69.75	$ 2.75	$132

Total process loss/week = $ 253.50
50 Week annual loss = $ 12,675.00

FIGURE 2.11

CC process cost analysis by operation step.

system problems. Working with upper-level team meetings, annual costs for various problem areas can be established. Teams and cost estimates form the basis of Six-Sigma programs and strategies similar to that presented in Chapter 4, Developing a Preventive Controls Plan: Food Safety and Quality, (analysis) are used to tackle such issues.

In the case illustrated in Table 2.2, a cross-functional CC was assigned by the chief executive officer (CEO) to provide estimated costs. From the CC that provided the estimates, two other CCs were assigned to begin work on a one problem area each.

At the functional team level where causes can be more closely assigned to specific process steps and FITs may become involved, establishing teams for each process can lead to significant cost tracking and improvement. The concept employed for cost focus and analysis for assignable causes is similar to the application of SPC. Each step of the process is monitored for in or out of control conditions (see chapter: Developing a Preventive Controls Plan: Food Safety and Quality, analysis). By developing a tracking sheet that collects the number of rejects at each step in the process, the value of the product at that process step can be calculated by adding together the number of rejects and multiplying the number of rejects by the value-added cost (how much value has been added to the product from all process steps earlier in the process) [2].

Fig. 2.11 illustrates a simplified analysis.

A team review of Fig. 2.11 clearly shows that there is an inadequate acceptance of responsibility or training or supervision throughout the line because there is an overwhelming dependence on process Step 5 to inspect food safety or quality into the product. The solution tracking sheet strategy presented in Chapter 4, Developing a Preventive Controls Plan: Food Safety and Quality can be used by the CC to get control over assignable causes for these losses. The goal of the CC should be focused by the leader on zero dollar and product losses through an elimination of dependence on inspection to catch rejects.

This concept can be further expanded on through supply chains. A supply chain cost analysis is presented in Chapter 8, Cycle Time Analysis in Preventive Food Safety and Quality Control Practices.

REFERENCES

[1] June 28, 2016 <https://en.wikipedia.org/wiki/Authority>.
[2] J.M. Ryan, Guide to Food Safety and Quality During Transportation: Controls Standards and Practices, Elsevier Academic Press, Amsterdam, 2014.

CHAPTER

Environmental monitoring and sampling

3

Regardless of our abilities to detect and control biological, chemical, or physical hazards, the Food and Drug Administration (FDA) and the food safety modernization act (FSMA) have established a new dependence on hard objective data from producers, processors, distributors, packers, and all companies involved in the food supply chain for validation of process and preventive controls. Objective data does not come from visual inspection or observations or reviews of documentation designed to establish conformance to FSMA requirements for detecting hazards. Most commonly, it comes from official laboratory analysis reports of samples taken just about anywhere in the food supply chain. Such samples must now be taken through careful controls and with rigorous reporting on the part of the sample taker and the laboratories hired to analyze the samples.

Chain of custody considerations are now in play. Chain of custody requirements basically means that the sampling, testing, and reporting process has now become a process with legal implications. This sampling, testing, and reporting process may now be used in a court of law to determine innocence or guilt.

The team approach can be applied to planning environmental monitoring and sampling. It is likely that a specialized team consisting of both managers (common cause (CC) teams are assigned to control common cause issues) and nonsalaried functional improvement teams (FIT) teams are assigned to control assignable causes) is the best approach to development of the plan and to reach initial agreements on preventive control requirements. In general, both CC and FIT team members may work together to define sampling plans and the overall environmental monitoring approach.

Environmental monitoring is the key to the establishment of a valid preventive control system. Environmental monitoring is used to establish the objective data used to objectively measure and improve food safety processes throughout the food supply chain. When data is more objective than that supplied through visual inspections, questions regarding the validity of any company's food safety program can be addressed, the samples supplied through a valid environmental sampling and monitoring program provide data that provides much stronger evidence regarding the food safety effort's true ability to control hazardous adulterants.

Environmental monitors are basically established to provide triggers for a company to take action. Taking and analyzing samples as part of an overall environmental monitoring plan is worthless if a company is not appropriately organized to work in a preventive manner designed to either correct for the impact of escaped products or to move into a more cause-and-effect preventive mode.

Validating Preventive Food Safety and Quality Controls. DOI: http://dx.doi.org/10.1016/B978-0-12-810994-6.00003-1

It is important to understand how critical chain of custody concepts is applied with regards to environmental sampling and monitoring. As a means of establishing valid baseline data and showing, the results of process improvement efforts, the chain of custody concept is designed to protect samples from intentional or unintentional dilution or contamination. As mentioned previously, if and when FDA inspectors visit a facility, they will not look at company's food safety certificates; they will immediately begin to take environmental samples for laboratory submission. FDA findings will be based primarily on the results of these samples. While preventive control concepts presented by the FDA are not very clear regarding what a company must, should, or cannot do with regards to environmental sampling, what is very clear are the instructions given to their own investigations personnel with regards to taking samples and controlling those samples through rigorous chain of custody processes.

In short, if the data going in is corrupt in any way, the entire analytic process is considered invalid.

ENVIRONMENTAL PATHOGENS

1. The FDA defines environmental pathogens as
   a. Biological hazards, including microbiological hazards such as parasites, environmental pathogens, and other pathogens;
   b. Chemical hazards, including radiological hazards, substances such as pesticide and drug residues, natural toxins, decomposition, unapproved food or color additives, and food allergens;
   c. Physical hazards (such as stones, glass, and metal fragments); and
2. Known or reasonably foreseeable hazards that may be present in the food for any of the following reasons:
   a. The hazard occurs naturally;
   b. The hazard may be unintentionally introduced; or
   c. The hazard may be intentionally introduced for purposes of economic gain.

Examples of environmental pathogens for the purposes of this part include *Listeria monocytogenes* and *Salmonella* spp. but do not include the spores of pathogenic spore forming bacteria [1].

They further lay out some basic requirements.

(a3) Environmental monitoring for an environmental pathogen or for an appropriate indicator organism, if contamination of a ready-to-eat food with an environmental pathogen is a hazard requiring a preventive control, by collecting and testing environmental samples; and

(4) Review of the following records within the specified timeframes, by (or under the oversight of) a preventive controls qualified individual, to ensure that the records are complete, the activities reflected in the records occurred in accordance with the food safety plan, the preventive controls are effective, and appropriate decisions were made about corrective actions:

(i) Records of monitoring and corrective action records within 7 working days after the records are created or within a reasonable timeframe, provided that the preventive controls qualified individual prepares (or oversees the preparation of) a written justification for a timeframe that exceeds 7 working days; and

(ii) Records of calibration, testing (e.g., product testing, environmental monitoring), supplier and supply chain verification activities, and other verification activities within a reasonable time after the records are created.

Under equipment and utensil requirements, the FDA states "(d) Holding, conveying, and manufacturing systems, including gravimetric, pneumatic, closed, and automated systems, must be of a design and construction that enables them to be maintained in an appropriate clean and sanitary condition."

And "(f) Instruments and controls used for measuring, regulating, or recording temperatures, pH, acidity, water activity, or other conditions that control or prevent the growth of undesirable microorganisms in food must be accurate and precise and adequately maintained, and adequate in number for their designated uses." This last statement means that such instruments must be calibrated by a certified calibration laboratory.

The FDA focus on sanitation controls are clearly focused on prevention of such hazards throughout the food supply chain and cover food-contact surfaces, utensils, and equipment that might be impacted by pathogens due to food handling and cross-contact and cross-contamination. Although the FDA clearly focuses practitioners on allergens, the threat of cross-contact and cross-contamination from people, packaging materials, food-contact surfaces, tools and equipment or from raw product to processed product are also included.

HAZARD EVALUATION

The FDA rules state that a hazard evaluation for environmental pathogens is required through all aspects of the food distribution process including:

1. *The formulation of the food;*
2. *The condition, function, and design of the facility and equipment;*
3. *Raw materials and other ingredients;*
4. *Transportation practices;*
5. *Manufacturing/processing procedures;*
6. *Packaging activities and labeling activities;*
7. *Storage and distribution;*
8. *Intended or reasonably foreseeable use;*
9. *Sanitation, including employee hygiene; and*
10. *Any other relevant factors, such as the temporal (e.g., weather-related) nature of some hazards (e.g., levels of some natural toxins) [2].*

Temperature and weather changes can clearly impact food at any stage throughout the supply chain. Moving food from a cool climate hundreds or thousands of miles by ship and truck, or by truck and air means that the food will go through some degree of extreme external temperature change. Food flying in a cargo hold at 32,000 ft. must be protected from freezing while upon landing, it must be protected from 95°F temperatures with 95% relative humidity. More importantly, the equipment and handling practices required to prevent food from being impacted by potentially extreme temperature changes must be designed to consistently control food temperatures from being impacted by such external changes.

The FDA's Investigative Operations Manual (IOM) 2016 can help food safety and quality personnel to begin to understand the type of controls that need to be established within all food handling processes. The IOM also helps to understand what process FDA investigators will use to evaluate environmentally established threats.

In the FDA's IOM 2016, Chapter 4, Developing a Preventive Control Plan—sampling, the FDA requirements are stated in great detail when the FDA feels a need to do sampling and testing of human and animal feed products. This is an important read because it establishes FDA inspection and audit requirements for their personnel. In other words, this is what and how they will evaluate environmental sampling practices, and from a quality perspective, the information establishes the minimum requirements any operation must meet.

The primary focus is on validation requirements. The document defines a valid sample as follows:

4.1.2—VALID SAMPLE

A valid sample is the starting point and keystone for most administrative and legal actions. As evidence, the sample must support the government's charge there is a violation of the law. Also, it must conform to the rules on admissibility of evidence. A properly collected and prepared sample provides:

1. *A portion of the lot of goods for laboratory analysis and reserve, a 702(b) of the federal food, drug and cosmetic (FD&C) Act [21 U.S.C. 374 (b)] reserve portion if appropriate, and/or an exhibit demonstrating the violation represented by the lot.*
2. *A report of your observations of the lot.*
3. *Labels and labeling, or copies of such, which 'accompany' the goods.*
4. *Documentary evidence of federal jurisdiction over the lot, information about individuals responsible for the violation, where the violation was committed, and similar data.*
5. *Signed statements from persons who may be called upon as witnesses, if there is a subsequent court action.*

Under 4.1.4.1—Definition—Official Sample, the document states:

An Official Sample is one taken from a lot for which Federal jurisdiction can be established. If violative, the Official Sample provides a basis for administrative or legal action. Official Samples generally, but not always, consist of a physical portion of the lot sampled. To be useful, an Official Sample must be:

1. *Accompanied by records establishing Federal jurisdiction, and identifying the persons having knowledge of the lot's movement and custody of the records.*

(Evidence of Interstate movement is not required for medical device samples, but, according to policy, is to be obtained when a seizure, injunction, prosecution or civil penalty is contemplated.) See IOM 4.4.7.

2. *Representative of the lot from which collected.*
3. *If a physical sample, large enough to permit proper laboratory examination and provide a 702(b) reserve portion when necessary.*
4. *Handled, identified, and sealed in such a manner as to maintain its integrity as evidence, with a clear record of its chain of custody. Every physical Official Sample will be fully documented at the time of collection and Collection Reports prepared unless instructed otherwise by the program or assignment.*

In Section 4.1.4.2, the FDA further defines Documentary (DOC) samples

"In a 'DOC' sample, no actual physical sample of the product is taken. Other elements of an official sample described in 4.1.4 and 4.1.4.1 are required—see special official sealing instructions below. This official sample consists of the article's labels (or label tracings, photocopies, or photos), accompanying labeling (leaflets, brochures, promotional materials, including Internet websites, etc.) and documentation of interstate movement (freight bills, bills of lading, affidavits, etc. See IOM 4.4.7) Photos of the product, drawings, sketches or schematics, production records, diagrams, invoices or similar items may also be part of the sample. See IOM Exhibits 4-1 and 4-2. As a rule, no FDA 484, receipt for samples is issued during collection of a DOC Sample. See subparagraph 5.2.4.1 for physical evidence exception.

A DOC sample is collected when an actual physical sample is not practical (e.g., very large, expensive, complex, permanently installed devices), in instances where the article is no longer available, or when there is little need for laboratory examination. A single piece of life support equipment for example, which must remain in emergency service until a replacement is available, may be sampled in this manner.

Another instance where a DOC sample might be collected involves a shipment of product recommended for seizure based on misbranding charges. During availability check, the lot sampled is found to have been distributed; however, a new shipment, identically labeled, is on hand. In this instance, the new shipment may be sampled on a DOC basis since another physical sample and examination is not required. Regulatory action may proceed on the basis of the earlier examination. Thus, only labeling, transportation records, the appropriate dealer affidavits, and an inventory of product on hand need be obtained."

In the IOM 2016, the FDA further defines in-transit, food standards, and investigational samples just to name a few of the investigative sampling conditions. They also note sampling of bills of lading, freight bills, sales re cords, receipts, waybills, labels, and other documents they may sample [3].

ESTIMATION AND SAMPLING BIAS

The primary idea behind any kind of sampling is that samples should provide unbiased estimates of what is going on in the process or product. In other words, it is assumed that unless you test every product, you will not know what the "truth" is. Testing every product is too expensive and time consuming. Sampling reduces both time and cost considerations, but must remain unbiased if an accurate of the overall "truth" is.

The results of any sample that is submitted to a certified laboratory for analysis are numbers that theoretically represent levels of adulterants found in the sample. These numbers become what are commonly called "statistics" and are used to calculate process mean or average or trend estimates of a processes overall "truth". It is therefore critical to control the sampling process so that the resulting statistics do not become biased estimates of the process through mishandling, contamination or improper collection. Samples are taken to estimate true process capabilities but are often impacted by any of a number of erroneous happenings. The goal of sampling procedures and of the person collecting any sample is to reduce any potential for error to a minimum.

Mathematically, this concept can be shown as

$$T = M \pm E$$

where truth (T) is equal to the measure obtained from the lab findings (M) plus or minus some measure of potential error (E). Unfortunately, it is rarely possible to measure error although some statistical procedures can be used to estimate error terms that are not discussed here. This leaves us only with the sample measure or number that results from sampling, handling, and testing procedures. Due to our lack of being able to quantify error, anyone taking samples or handling samples or testing samples must work in careful accordance with sampling procedures to minimize error so that measurement (sample findings) represent the truth as closely as possible.

Of course, it is possible to intentionally bias sampling results. Everyone has heard of how to lie with statistics. False recording of data, taking samples of known clean product, and reporting those results as samples taken from randomly sampled product are just a couple of examples of how data can be falsified if one chose to do that.

Considering the apparent thoroughness that FDA officials will employ based on the brief discussion of IOM 2016, Chapter 4, Developing a Preventive Control Plan, it would not be advisable to doctor locally collected samples or statistics in an effort to appear to be in compliance with preventive control requirements.

SAMPLE SIZES AND SAMPLING PLANS

Samples and sampling plans are designed to allow us to measure and collect data used to estimate what is going on in any process or any part of a process. As noted above, testing every product is expensive and impossible. Therefore, we sample as a means of estimating what kind or level of adulterant is in the product or process. The data resulting from the samples becomes what is called an estimate of the population or an estimate of what is going on in the entire product population or entire population of process steps.

For a company to know that its product or process is under preventive controls, the food safety and quality team must establish a sampling plan that defines who, what, where, and when samples, and tests will be completed.

The questions of "How often do we have to sample?", "How big should our samples be?", and "How many samples do we need?" are difficult to answer due to the complexity of operations throughout the food supply chain. Nonetheless, establishing a sampling plan is a critical part of any preventive control program. Soil, product, water, table tops, processing lines, load, and unload operations for food transporters, conveyors, truck trailer and shipping container walls and floors, packaging, air, blending machines, mixers, trays, pallets, and numerous other types of equipment are now called into the preventive control arena. If any of those listed above or any other piece of equipment is contaminated and has not been properly disinfected or sanitized or is not operating under the correct temperature conditions, adulterants can become a source of cross-contamination that moves chemical, biological, or physical hazards from one piece of equipment to many others.

Preventive control concepts mean that the entire process (whichever process is defined for control) must establish a valid sampling, test, and causal analysis system and become the object of close scrutiny. For this reason, the FDA under FSMA has specified that a "qualified individual" must be included in the development, approval, and modification of any food safety plan. This "qualified individual" is a specialized person who has generally received more than 4 days of training under some training program. In general, like it or not, a statistics professional is required to help determine sample sizes, schedules and the like.

Without a valid sampling plan that defines what, where, when, and how much must be sampled to adequately measure and control any food production or handling operation, the estimates that come from data resulting from sampling might not adequately represent what is going on in the population of products (all the tomatoes in the field, all the bottles in the assembly line, all the water at all points in a field).

But let's face it, even with a good sampling plan, good measurement controls, good testing, and results reporting, problem adulterants can be missed and product may escape into distribution channels. However, the difference between a sampling plan that keeps costs low but also provides excellent unbiased estimates of what is going on in the population or products or process steps and a poor sampling plan is that a poor sampling plan is far less likely to find and prevent illness and death than a poor sampling plan.

The entire game of statistics, preventive controls, and cause-and-effect analyses required to bring food safety and quality control to the food supply chain is simply one of reducing the likelihood that recalls, illness, and death can occur.

The FSMA basically attempts to define a general approach to reducing the probability that such problems reach human populations.

RANDOM SAMPLES EMPLOYED FOR PROCESS AUDIT PURPOSES

To confuse things further, the idea that random sampling should be employed means that occasionally different times and places for samples might be randomly determined to present a higher degree of unbiasedness to the sampling plan.

While establishing a completely random sampling plan might be impossible, from a process audit perspective, a sampling plan that includes occasional samples that might be taken at different times and places can be considered. In short, two sampling plans can be established. First, a standard process control sampling plan, and second, an audit sampling plan that employs randomly selected sites and times for samples to be taken, tested, and included for analysis.

AN EXAMPLE OF SAMPLING AND TESTING ON SMALL FARMS

We would like to believe that there are some governmental oversight activities operative but due to the 2008 recession and government cutbacks, most local departments of health and agriculture have either drastically reduced or completely eliminated random biological and chemical testing as part of their environmental or food safety programs.

Distributors, wholesalers, retailers, and others are left without this "government interference."

This means the cost and responsibility for food safety and testing is now borne by the producer and their customers (the supply chain). Hence, the new FSMA rules for environmental monitoring and the shift for Chipotle to focus and support their suppliers with over $10 million in grants and training.

In June 2008, 2.5 years before FSMA was passed, there was a tomato salmonella outbreak that caused millions of dollars in losses for the tomato industry. At that time, the FDA held what they called "50 State Conference Calls" and invited food officials from all states to attend. As investigations into the cause of the multistate tomato salmonella Saint Paul outbreak were discussed, various FDA personnel reported finding multiple bacterial contaminants on the farms they were investigating. This was not publicly reported as the FDA and the center for disease control (CDC) basically expected to find such contaminants as a result of previous recall investigations. As a result of these 50 state calls, two things became apparent. First, now all listeners knew how highly contaminated farms are. Second, these common contaminants were ignored because of the pursuit of the specific strain that had caused the outbreak, deaths, and illness, and the fact that the contaminants were common, expected, and nothing could be done about them [4].

It was expected by the FDA, CDC, and listeners that no preventive controls could be identified or put in place for all the contaminants being found. Preventive controls were, at that time, not a widely shared concept within the food side of the FDA.

The FDA defines an environmental pathogen as "a pathogen capable of surviving and persisting within the manufacturing, processing, packing, or holding environment such that food may be contaminated and may result in foodborne illness if that food is consumed without treatment to significantly minimize the environmental pathogen.

Examples of environmental pathogens for the purposes of this part include *Listeria monocytogenes* and *Salmonella* spp. but do not include the spores of pathogenic spore forming bacteria [5]."

From the FDA perspective, the pathogens a company is at high risk for and must control are those that might impact products and processes. Generally speaking, detection of such pathogens requires a swab sample submitted properly to a laboratory setting for controlled analysis.

Although there are a number of companies currently working on technologies that will allow testing to take shorter and shorter periods of time, from the time a sample is submitted to a lab to the time results are available is between 24 hours and 72 hours. The time delay between when the sample was taken, and when the results are available, it has serious consequences for companies whose food may lose shelf life and for pathogens to multiply to the point that someone may become ill. If a product company holds freshly picked product for an average of 36 hours, even if chilled, the product is no longer fresh. In the case of Chipotle, not long after the company was hit with multiple outbreaks, centralized receiving, and preparation areas were implemented to test and prepare foods prior to delivery to restaurants. Within a few months, Chipotle discarded these centralized operations due to food quality, although food safety was left, once again, on the back burner.

In Hawaii, funding was provided to determine whether or not state's farms showed similar levels of produce contamination, contamination that seemed to proliferate perhaps in nature or perhaps due to poor farm management. Water and produce samples were tested for biological and chemical (herbicides, pesticides, fungicides) contaminants. Sampling procedures and chains of custody were established, personnel were trained, labs were assigned for analysis and results compiled.

Considering the fact that farms represent the upstream river depicted earlier in this chapter, some study objectives were established that included:

1. Objective 1

   Produce buyers will learn concepts critical to assuring that proper farm water and produce testing are conducted in a manner designed to provide preventive food safety controls.

   Asking the right questions and reviewing the right farm supplied data are critical to protecting consumers at the retail and restaurant levels regardless of food safety certification documents.
2. Objective 2

   Produce suppliers will learn when and where to sample water and food produce to protect their customers and consumers.

The descriptive study aimed to answer some questions:

a. How clean are farms and shipped produce?
b. What levels of contaminants will we find?
c. What is a cheap, effective way for farmers to sample for biological and chemical contaminants?
d. Is there a sampling procedure or device that will put measurement and control in the hands of the farmer as a preventive strategy rather than an enforcement strategy?
e. From the farmer's and farmer's customer's perspectives, what can or should I do or require to protect my business (farm, retail, restaurant)?

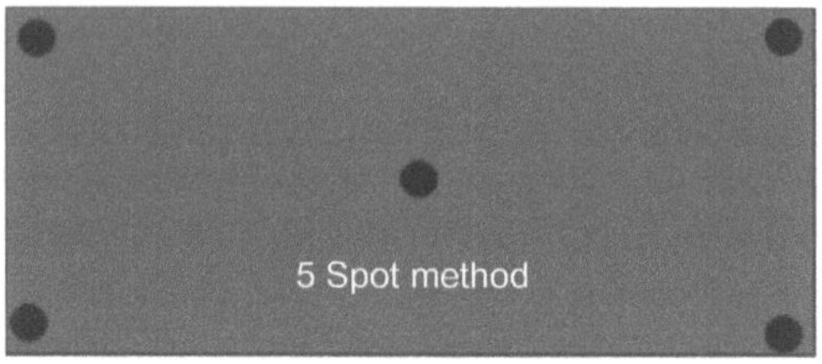

FIGURE 3.1

Sample locations using a five spot method.

At that time, there were other considerations that needed to be noted and cared for:

a. Participating farms were all volunteer farms.
b. Some of these farms were in the process of working towards food safety certification according to GAP, Primus Labs, or some other standards.
c. As such, the data collected as a result of sampling and laboratory analysis was to be kept confidential.
d. The issue of confidentially is one that plagues all food supply chain members and is considered at the state and federal levels to pose a major barrier to more preventive food safety approaches that would be attained if food suppliers had simple, cheap, and rapid contaminant detection devices.

Water was to be tested basic coliform, fecal coliform and *Escherichia coli* at the source and throughout the fields. For most food safety audits at the time annual coliform testing at the source is a basic food safety audit requirement even though if the farm failed contamination levels, the farm could still pass the food safety audit.

As an example environmental sampling for produce followed a basic five-spot method as shown in Fig. 3.1. Samples of produce were taken at each field corner and in the field center. Produce samples were controlled and submitted to the lab for processing. The state lab tested produce samples for biological contaminants and sent samples to a California lab for chemical testing.

Water was samples were taken at the source and at four points along the water distribution system, each point further and further away from the water source.

SAMPLING PROCEDURES

1. Use the "five spot method" sampling procedure, the samples are taken from slightly inside each corner of each field and one sample is taken from the middle of the field (five spots on die).

If the sample crop is located in two or more fields immediately adjacent to one another and have the same crop, treat the two fields as one field and collect your five samples from these fields. If the fields are widely separated, collect 5-1 lb samples from each field. Wipe the pruners with alcohol before using and after taking samples. Also, wipe the pruners with alcohol when taking different crop samples. Label bags correctly.

2. Use sterile gloves provided by the labs kit and wear your long sleeve smocks when taking your samples. It is acceptable according to most labs to simply turn a garbage bag or plastic bag inside out over the hand so that the inside of the bag becomes the sterile outside of the temporary glove to pick up the sample. The garbage bags can be used for the collection of "whole" raw produce samples such as watermelons of heads of lettuce where normal size sterile bags (whirl packs) cannot accommodate the size of the raw produce. Place each subsample in a separate bag.
3. Label bags and place in cooler with blue ice. Do not use wet ice unless the bottles are double bagged in waterproof plastic bags.
4. Complete the chain of custody form. The laboratory must receive the samples within 5 hours. The laboratory hours vary, so make sure you turn in fresh samples as early in the day as possible.

   Pickup sampling kits from lab as well as the chain of custody and analysis request forms.

   a. Make sure the water sampling kit is adequately stocked to take 3–4 water samples per field.
   b. For produce sampling take 5-1 lb samples per field. This may be reduced, but make sure you have enough kits to cover your needs.

A typical kit contains the following items: large nitrile gloves, paper towels, alcohol squirt bottle, pen, sharpie, blue ice, etc.

- Per water microbiological sampling: 1–250 mL plastic bottle (contains a preservative)
- Per water pesticide sampling: 1-L amber glass bottle with no preservative
- Per each plastic tissue sample: one plastic bag.

FINDINGS: REPORT SUMMARY

The final report is summarized here:

Project Title: Development of a Comprehensive Approach to State's Farm-Level Food Safety Risk Assessments

SUMMARY OF RECOMMENDATIONS

1. State farms exhibit a relatively high degree of chemical, fecal, and *E. coli* contamination. This is an indication of farm level mismanagement of chemical and water resources. These preliminary findings appear to be in line with unpublished FDA reports of sampling and analyses of water and produce from mainland farms.
2. Analyses for chemical and sampling of produce and water are currently considered too expensive ($365/sample) for practical application at small farms.

3. Water sampling for biological contaminants ($51/comprehensive test) should be required and should be initiated at the field level rather than at the source due to probable biofilm bacterial buildup in irrigation pipes. (This is an opposite position to most food safety certification recommendations.)
4. All fields should be tested for water contamination due to the high coliform and fecal coliform levels found in this limited study.
5. Water sampling for biological contaminants should be conducted in a manner that provides the farm with measurement and management information. This means that the lowest cost tests (coliform only) should be conducted first to provide the farmer with initial corrective action opportunities. If positive coliform results are found, secondary testing should include analyses for fecal coliform and *E. coli*. However, if the farm can afford slightly increased costs, analysis of water samples should include tests for coliform, fecal coliform, and *E. coli* as a standard due to the relatively low costs for these combined results.

OUTBREAK BACKGROUND

During 2008, *Salmonella* outbreak allegedly reported to be associated with tomatoes, the FDA held a number of 50-state conference calls to keep states appraised of recall and investigation progress. During one of those calls, it was disclosed that during its investigations, the FDA found biologically contaminated samples on many of farms under suspicion, both in the United States and in Mexico. It was also disclosed that the FDA did not want this information to become public as such findings might impact the financial status of all farms producing and selling tomatoes, peppers, and other produce regardless of their association with the outbreak.

It has also been disclosed by XXX Lab's director of quality that the FDA's procedure for investigating possible outbreaks focuses primarily on taking water, produce other samples and testing those samples for biological contaminants. XXX lab personnel report that the FDA ignores food safety certification reports, certificates, and related documentation during such investigations while focusing only on samples.

PROBLEM

On the basis of this information and the potential impact to State's farmers in the event of an outbreak, questions regarding "local" food safety need to be similarly addressed. How clean are state farms? What levels of contaminants will we find? What is a cheap, effective way for state farmers to sample and test for biological and chemical contaminants? Is there a sampling procedure or device that will put measurement and control in the hands of the farmer as a preventive strategy rather than in the hands of the government to be used as an enforcement strategy?

The state has the opportunity grow the world's safest food. Yet, the ongoing inability of numerous state and federal organizations to agree on a standardized set of on-farm food safety protocols, coupled with the outbreak mentioned above and the 2006 deaths and illnesses from organically farmed spinach infected with *E. coli*, highlight an urgent need for new approaches to farm level food safety monitoring. Indeed, the National Association of State Departments of Agriculture clearly indicated a need to develop a "comprehensive integrated approach," perhaps as a precursor to applying Hazard Analysis and Critical Control (HACCP) approaches at the farm level. Furthermore, current laws designed to establish inspection and audit agencies have led to inconsistent and ineffective visual inspection employed by observers of questionable reliability using poorly defined criteria and based on differing approaches to food safety certification. This lack of organization leaves a gap, not only in leadership at the national and state levels, but where leadership is needed most: On the farm.

PROJECT PURPOSE

These issues led to questions that could be best approached through an exploratory study intended to describe the current levels of contamination and to suggest the most cost effective risk assessment sampling and laboratory testing approach suitable for state farms. The study was broken into two phases:

- Phase I: initial overall chemical and biological analyses of water and produce
- Phase II: focus on biological contaminants

STATUS OF OBJECTIVES

Objective 1: Establish a list of most common chemical and biological threats to be used in the screening process.

The project team will use Federal recall data to establish this list based on a ranking of the incidence of recall. This ranking will be analyzed to determine the top five chemical and biological problem areas.

Fig. 3.2 is a breakdown of the most commonly reported foodborne illness causes. The group decided to focus the sampling primarily on water contaminated with fecal matter and produce *E. coli* and *Salmonella* as *Norovirus* was excluded because it is the most common source of gastroenteritis outbreaks of all ages. Noroviruses are transmitted by fecal contamination of food or water and by person-to-person contact, whereas *E. coli* and *Salmonella* are pathogens commonly found on farms.

The results of the study indicate that fecal and *E. coli* water and produce contamination issues are relatively high in the state.

Objective 2: Establish a farm-level sampling strategy.

> *Farm Bureau members and the project team will work to determine appropriate schedules and procedures for sampling produce, water, soil and manure as required. Based on the results of the ranking, the project team and lab teams will determine the appropriate sampling levels and strategies in each of the following areas: harvested produce, ground or irrigation water, manure (found on the property), and soil (as required).*
>
> **Quote from the original proposal.**

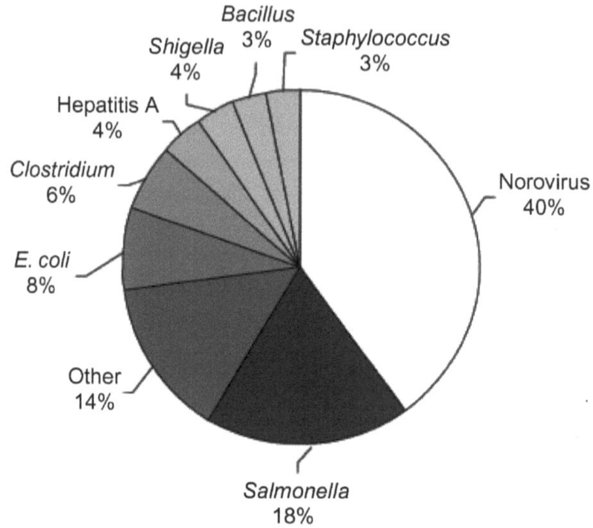

FIGURE 3.2

Common pathogens found in produce [6].

Department of Agriculture, Health and University of XXX, XXX Labs personnel were invited to a number of preliminary meetings to determine a practical scope sampling and sample test strategies for the study. Basic sampling procedures were defined and smocks and other materials designed to protect sample integrity and personnel were ordered from local suppliers.

The proposed study scope included water, soil, and produce. After group discussions, it was decided to eliminate soil as a focus of attention, and this change was approved in a request. Several of the team members thought soil sampling and analysis should be recommended for a subsequent study because analysis is somewhat specialized and expensive.

Food safety and commodities inspectors of Department of Agriculture volunteered to collect samples during farm visits. Farms were not selected on a random basis. Rather, they self-volunteered to have sampling and testing conducted, often as a result of their needs for data prior to food safety certification audits. In this sense, the sampling was biased in favor or farms working on achieving food safety certification.

Objective 3: Identify testing procedures capable of quick turn-around and low cost laboratory strategies and protocols.

Lab personnel will begin work to develop the appropriate procedures to test for the chemicals and biological threats highlighted during activities surrounding Objective 1. Lab personnel will specify parameters for each screening test based on the sampling scheme. Standards for testing will be ordered as required and as funded by this project. Lab personnel will document time and materials required for each test to determine time standards (which will be studied to shorten test times) and costs (which will also be studied to determine how best to reduce costs to the farmer and the Department of Agriculture).

Objective 4: Continue to refine the protocols and preliminary and basic farm review procedures across at least 20 farms throughout the year.

The data collected under Objective 3 will be used to continually look for cheaper and quicker ways to arrive at accurate screening results. All lab initiated iterations in search of cost and time reductions will be documented beginning with documentation.

Objective 5: Establish solutions as part of the State Department of Agriculture Quality Assurance Division preliminary food safety audit system.

Once the lab and project teams have arrived at optimal solutions, protocols and procedures will be prepared at the Version 1.0 level.

See "Recommendations above."

Objective 6: Work with the Farm Bureau to provide outreach to State agricultural community.

Version 1.0 protocols and procedures will be used to describe this new approach to farm associations and economic development councils on each of the major state areas.

CONFIDENTIALITY OF INFORMATION

Participating farms were all volunteer farms. Some of these farms were in the process of working towards food safety certification according to good agricultural practices (GAP), XXX Labs, or some other standards. As such, the data collected as a result of sampling and laboratory analysis was to be kept confidential. This report contains no farm or other identifying information relating to any agricultural business. The issue of confidentially is one that plagues all food supply chain members and is considered at the state and federal levels to pose a major barrier to more preventive food safety approaches that would be attained if food suppliers had simple, cheap, and rapid contaminant detection devices.

ANALYTIC LABS INVOLVED

The State Department of Agriculture and State Department of Health laboratories were contacted for possible inclusion in the study. However, as both labs are supported with Environmental Protection Agency (EPA) funds, both were obligated to report any violations to the EPA. Due to this reporting requirement, both laboratories were excluded from the study.

XXX Labs was the primary contact for the project. This city-based lab specializes in food, water, and environmental testing. XXX Labs offers comprehensive microbiological and chemical testing of food, drinking water, wastewater, sludge, and soil. Examples of food services included quality assurance microbiological and chemical testing, nutrition labeling analyses, and consultation services for sanitation programs, quality assurance (QA) and quality control (QC) programs and food plant inspections. XXX Labs also provides environmental services such as nutrient analyses and metals testing by inductively coupled plasma-mass spectrometry (MS).

The basic water testing assumptions followed for this study are shown in the following paragraph.

Total coliform, fecal coliform, and *E. coli* are all indicators of drinking water quality. The total coliform group is a large collection of different kinds of bacteria. Fecal coliforms are types of total coliform that mostly exist in feces. *E. coli* is a subgroup of fecal coliform. When a water sample is sent to a lab, it is tested for total coliform. If total coliform is present, the sample will also be tested for either fecal coliform or *E. coli*, depending on the lab testing method (Fig. 3.3).

XXX Pesticide Labs located in Oregon is an agricultural and environmental lab specializing in pesticide residue analysis of water, soil, and plant samples providing clients with accurate, defensible data in a reliable timeframe by utilizing the latest methods and technology. XXX Pesticide Lab currently analyzes for over 200 compounds. All analysis is done using a multiresidue screen including insecticides, herbicides, and fungicides that we can do in water, soil, or plant tissue.

XXX Agricultural Laboratory is an analytical laboratory located in Oregon dedicated to the analysis of pesticides, herbicides, and fungicides in a variety of matrices. From low-level water monitoring to food and agricultural commodities screening, Pacific Agricultural Laboratory (PAL) helps with pesticides related analysis in a wide variety of sample matrices offering testing for individual compounds as well as multiresidue screens in water, soil, and plant tissue. The following sections provide PAL references for pesticides screening.

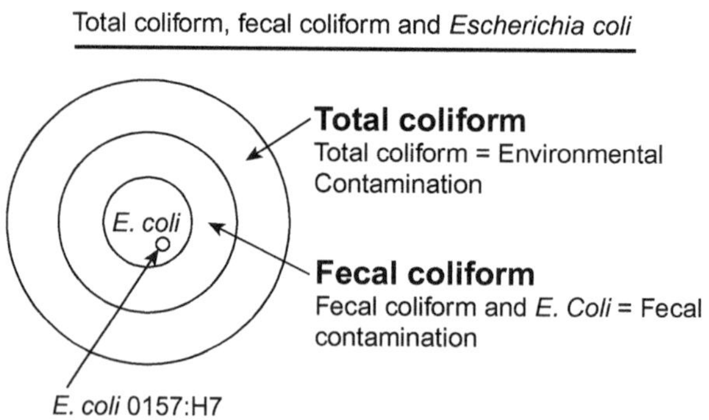

FIGURE 3.3

Total coliform, fecal coliform, and *Escherichia coli.*

FOOD AND AGRICULTURE COMMODITIES

PAL uses the FDA Pesticide Analytical Manual-Volume I as the primary reference for pesticides screening for food products and animal feed. The methodologies are comprised of multiresidue methods. The actual number and identity of determinable residues is dependent on the sample matrix and the number and variety of determinative steps involved. In addition to multiresidue methods listed in the Pesticide Analytical Manual, PAL also provides custom screens based on customer needs. Method reporting limits vary depending on the matrix and may be raised because of interference of coextracted compounds.

MULTIRESIDUE SCREEN IN SOIL AND WATER

These screens are a combination of four Modified EPA methods: EPA 8141B (GC-FPD), EPA 8081B (GC-ECD), EPA 8270D (GC-MS, SIM mode), and EPA 8321B (HPLC-MS). They include over 170 pesticides comprised of organochlorine, organophosphorous, organonitrogen, and *n*-methyl carbamates. It is designed to comply with Oregon department of environmental quality (DEQ) Guidance for Evaluating Residual Pesticides on Lands Formerly Used for Agricultural Production (DEQ-06-LQ-011) and for other environmental screening purposes.

The total number of analytes tested for water and produce from the original water source across all tested fields was approximately 1200 per farm as shown in Table 3.1.

PHASE I RESULTS

Phase I was focused on collecting water from the source across fields and included produce sampling across crops. The initial results water chemical sampling and testing indicated that 10 farms were sampled at the source, through two fields and into the packing house. Samples were collected during the day and submitted to the lab before 4:00 pm daily. The data indicates that four chemical contaminants were found in tested water. This is an indication that fungicides, insecticides and herbicides are somehow migrating into the water supplies at these farms.

Table 3.1 summarizes these data.

Table 3.2 shows the chemicals found in the farm water from the test results.

Table 3.3 shows the number of farms that tested positive for coliform contamination in water. The data shows a low number testing positive at the source but higher positive test results for fields and packing areas. This is an indication of contamination in the field migrating into what were originally clean water sources. The data was collected across five fields and the colony forming unit (CFU) count ranges are shown in the table.

Phase I also included a number of tests for chemicals on produce from different sectors of farms. Table 3.3 is a summary of the data from 14 tested farms. By far, the fungicide Azoxystrobin (molecular formula $C_{22}H_{17}N_3O_5$) was found. Azoxystrobin

Table 3.1 Chemical Testing Screens

Standard Farm Level Chemical Contaminant Test Count		
Source of Sample	**Testing Procedure**	**No. of Tests in Each Screen**
Source water	Organochlorine insecticide screen	27
	Organophosphate insecticide screen	31
	Carbamate insecticide and phenyl urea herbicide screen	43
	Triazine herbicide plus screen	29
	Fungicide screen	36
	Multiresidue screen	34
Postharvest water	Organochlorine insecticide screen	27
	Organophosphate insecticide screen	31
	Carbamate insecticide and phenyl urea herbicide screen	43
	Triazine herbicide plus screen	29
	Fungicide screen	36
	Multiresidue screen	34
Field I sample	Organochlorine insecticide screen	27
	Organophosphate insecticide screen	31
	Carbamate insecticide and phenyl urea herbicide screen	43
	Triazine herbicide plus screen	29
	Fungicide screen	36
	Multiresidue screen	34
Field 2 sample	Organochlorine insecticide screen	27
	Organophosphate insecticide screen	31
	Carbamate insecticide and phenyl urea herbicide screen	43
	Triazine herbicide plus screen	29
	Fungicide screen	36
	Multiresidue screen	34
Produce sample 1	Organochlorine insecticide screen	27
	Organophosphate insecticide screen	31
	Carbamate insecticide and phenyl urea herbicide screen	43
	Triazine herbicide plus screen	29
	Fungicide screen	36
	Multiresidue screen	34
Produce sample 2	Organochlorine insecticide screen	27
	Organophosphate insecticide screen	31
	Carbamate insecticide and phenyl urea herbicide screen	43
	Triazine herbicide plus screen	29
	Fungicide screen	36
	Multiresidue screen	34
	Total tests/farm	*1200*

Table 3.2 Phase I Fungicides, Insecticides, and Herbicides Found in Water Samples

Water Sample Results	
Chemical water sample findings Ten farms were tested at the source and through up two fields and the packing house Water tested positive at three farms for the following:	
Chemical	**Purpose**
Azoxystrobin	Fungicide
Cymoxanil	Fungicide
Imidacloprid	Insecticide
Oxyzalin	Herbicide

Table 3.3 Phase I Coliform Water Sample Findings

Biological Water Sample Findings: Coliform					
10 Farms were tested at the source and through up to two fields and the packing house					
		Source	**Field 1**	**Field 2**	**Packing**
Number	Positive	1	5	3	2
Range	(CFU/100 mL)	2419	200–2419	200–2419	579–2419

Table 3.4 Phase I Produce Chemical Sample Findings

	Produce Results		
	Chemical produce sample findings 14 farms tested: eight farms tested positive		
	Chemical	*Number*	*Purpose*
	Azoxystrobin	8	Fungicide
	Dimethoate	1	Insecticide
	Imadacloprid	1	Insecticide
	Myclobutanil	1	Fungicide
	Spinosad	1	Insecticide
	Triadimefon	1	Pesticide
Produce Impacted	Daikon, onions avodado, basil, kale Lettuce, cucumber, choi sum		

is a fungicide commonly used in agriculture and is considered to be "of low acute and chronic toxicity to humans, birds, mammals, and bees but is highly toxic to freshwater fish, freshwater invertebrates, and estuarine/marine fish, and highly toxic to estuarine/marine invertebrates [7]."

The bottom part of Table 3.4 shows the produce sampled where these chemicals were found.

Table 3.5 Phase I Biological Produce Sample Results

Range of Biological Produce Sample Results		
18 Samples: Two farms showing positive		
	CFU/100 mL	
Coliform range	240–1100	Across five fields
Escherichia coli	3–21	Across five fields
Salmonella	0	Across five fields

Table 3.5 shows the results of coliform tests for the farms 14 farms tested. The data shows that in a total of 18 samples, two farms showed positive results for coliform and low levels of *E. coli*. The data was collected across five fields, and the CFU count ranges are shown in the table. No detection of salmonella was found and lab personnel indicate that they have never seen a positive test for *Salmonella*.

PHASE II RESULTS

The high costs associated with chemical sampling and testing was eliminated in Phase II, and the study was focused more closely on biological contaminants to be found on produce and in water. Unfortunately, due to governmental cutbacks in personnel, only 10 farms were sampled and tested.

Based on the high cost for chemical sampling and the results for Phase I, it could be reasonably assumed that chemicals are finding a way to enter the water supplies, that azoxystrobin is a fungicide in common use (at least for our samples) and that the cost to sample is relatively high. Based on this information, the team decided to eliminate chemical sampling for Phase II and to focus more closely on biological contamination issues.

In phase II, 10 farms were visited and water and plant samples were taken for analysis at the source of water and across up to five fields. Phase II water sampling was consistent with some of the findings in Phase I. Most notably, 9 of the 10 tested farms showed no contamination at the source, but 3 farms showed coliform, fecal coliform, and *E. coli* contamination in the fields.

Table 3.6 shows the number of positive tests for each contaminant and the (above 0) CFU/100 mL findings only for the three farms that tested clean at the source but contaminated throughout the fields. This is an indication that although testing cannot detect contaminants near the source, that biofilms are likely to be developing in irrigation systems. The warmth, moist, and dark conditions within pipes or drip lines provide an environment conducive to bacterial proliferation. This is a substantial argument against testing water at the source as such tests tend to misdirect food safety management attempts.

With water testing clean at the source, the question of whether or not coliform, fecal coliform, or *E. coli* might be actually getting on produce is important any of the

Table 3.6 Phase II Biological Water Sample Results

10 Farms Sampled
Source plus fields 1, 2, 3, 4, and 5
Nine of the ten farms tested clean at the water source
Three of nine farms tested positive in one of the fields

Contaminant	Count	Range CFU/100 mL
Coliform	15	8–1600
Fecal coliform	12	4–1600
E. coli	11	2–17
E. coli 157	0	0

Table 3.7 Phase II Plant Biological Sample Results

Plant Tissue Biological

Ten Farms Tested

Contaminant	Count	Range CFU/100 mL	Found On
Coliform	2	900–1100	Lettuce/Taro
Fecal coliform	2	15–500	Lettuce
Escherichia coli	2	3.6–17	Lettuce
E. coli 157	0	0	N/A

three will cause illness. Table 3.7 shows the number and CFU ranges resulting from testing plant tissues from between one and five fields.

The data shows an unfortunate pattern. Of the three farms that showed negative source water contamination that also showed field water contamination, the coliform, fecal coliform, and *E. coli* contaminants are showing up on fresh produce, most notably lettuce. It appears that pipe biofilms are being created when water is off but when water is again turned on, the bacterial colonies are being blown out onto produce.

SUMMARY

With a relatively small number of farms sampled, but with extensive chemical and biological testing for biological and chemical contaminants conducted, the following observations are made:

1. A high proportion of those farms tested show chemical and biological contamination of water and produce.
2. Chemical testing of water and produce may be cost prohibitive to small farmers.
3. Biological testing of water and produce is not cost prohibitive to small farmers.
4. Water that tests clean of biological contaminants at the source appears to increase in contaminants in the field.

Some basic findings indicated that water that tested clean (CFU/100 mL) at the source tested with increasing levels of coliform, fecal coliform, and *E. coli* found further from the source (in the field).

Of three farms that showed negative source water contamination also showed field water contamination, and the coliform, fecal coliform. and *E. coli* contaminants are showing up on fresh produce, most notably lettuce.

It appears that pipe biofilms are being created when water is off but when water is again turned on, it appeared that bacterial colonies are being blown out onto produce. These findings launched some research into the nature of biofilms that are alive and play host to all types of living organisms.

Bacteria, Viruses, Protozoa, Invertebrates, Algae and algal toxins, Fungi, various *Pseudomonas* species, *E. coli*, Staphylococci, and Microbial toxins are among the most common invading pathogens that can be found in biofilms. Farm irrigation systems contain biofilms. Pipes, hoses, etc. provide warm and moist conditions for biofilm proliferation and biological contaminant growth. Even water tested clean at the source contains some level of contamination which grows in biofilms given the right conditions (warm, moist, dark). Drip irrigation systems lying on the ground may upload chemical contaminants into irrigators. Other irrigation system biofilms play host to bio-contaminants that, while not detected at the source, could proliferate when the water was turned off and the irrigators baked in the sun.

It appears that when systems are turned on after baking in the sun, bio-matter, and bio-contaminants are pressure washed out of the irrigation systems and sprayed on produce when water was turned on after an idle period. This was a disturbing finding that required some further explanation and, perhaps some direction for a solution. A bit of basic research found the following:

What works to destroy biofilms in irrigation systems?

- Continuous ozone treatment
- Continuous chlorine dioxide injection
- Mixed oxidative solutions
- Shock treatments with some forms of acid

None of these options appeared to provide a reasonable solution that could be employed on the farm.

What does not work to destroy biofilms in irrigation systems?

- Heat pasteurization
- UV light
- Chlorine
- Most biocides
- Straight hydrogen peroxide
- High velocity line flushing/scouring
- Copper ionization

There appears to be no known solution for reducing biological contaminants in irrigation systems.

The study had some conclusions:

1. The farms exhibit a relatively high degree of chemical, fecal, and *E. coli* contamination. This is an indication of farm level mismanagement of chemical and water resources. These preliminary findings appear to be in line with unpublished FDA reports of sampling and analyses of water and produce from farms.
2. Analyses for chemical and sampling of produce and water are currently considered too expensive ($365/sample) for practical application at small farms.
3. Water sampling for biological contaminants ($51/comprehensive test) should be required and should be initiated at the field level rather than at the source due to probable biofilm bacterial buildup in irrigation pipes. (This is an opposite position to most food safety certification recommendations.)
4. All fields should be tested for water contamination due to the high coliform and fecal coliform levels found in this limited study.
5. Water sampling for biological contaminants should be conducted in a manner that provides the farm with measurement and management information. This means that the lowest cost tests (coliform only) should be conducted first to provide the farmer with initial corrective action opportunities. If positive coliform results are found, secondary testing should include analyses for fecal coliform and *E. coli*. However, if the farm can afford slightly increased costs, analysis of water samples should include tests for coliform, fecal coliform, and *E. coli* as a standard due to the relatively low costs for these combined results.

It appeared that with a relatively small number of farms sampled, but with extensive chemical and biological testing for biological and chemical contaminants conducted, the following observations are made:

- A high proportion of those farms tested show chemical and biological contamination of water and produce.
- Chemical testing of water and produce is cost prohibitive to small farmers.
- Biological testing of water and produce for coliform is not cost prohibitive to small farmers.
- Water that tests clean of biological contaminants at the source may be associated with an increase of bio-contaminants in the field. There is evidence that biofilms play a role in this issue.
- Better management of water measurement and controls is needed if risk is to be reduced and illness prevented.
- FSMA applies to all domestic and firms importing food to the United States.
- The farm is responsible for developing preventive, risk reducing plans.
- Farms need to upgrade their frequency and type of sampling.
- Sampling procedures for chemical and biological contaminants must be developed and followed as part of the farm's plan. Water and produce sampling are critical—records must be kept that show the farm is following a risk reduction plan.

- No currently known preventive methods for biofilm contamination.
- No known solutions for biofilm contamination until more research time and money are expended.

Although the study was conducted years before the final FSMA preventive control rules there are some farm level suggestions.

- Develop a hazard analysis critical control points (HACCP) or critical control points (CCP) plan based on the potential risk level of the deliverable produce.
- Establish sampling procedures for water and produce.
- Consider both biological and chemical sampling.
- Implement your plan.
- When things are out of control or out of compliance, establish new procedures.
- Establish new data keeping (no data = no work).

There are also some suggestions that are relevant for what a farm's customers should do.

- Determine risk levels for produce purchased.
- Work with suppliers to establish a test plan.
- Qualify suppliers based on their ability to deliver to the plans.
- Certify only qualified suppliers.
- Consider independent produce testing at a facility (costs to be borne by the supplier).
- Establish periodic data and preventive action plan reviews with suppliers.

Regardless of any fear of FDA, United States department of agriculture (USDA), or other enforcement visits, testing on a regular basis shows that a company is working on reducing risk through efforts to find and prevent contaminants.

More importantly, measuring and finding problems gives the management opportunity to improve water supply, irrigation or other processes that might be causing a problem for someone's health and for a company's financial security [8].

MONITORING AND SANITATION TESTING OF FOOD TRANSPORTATION VEHICLES, TRAILERS, AND CONTAINERS

Although the example above focused on farm level environmental testing, food moving through transportation systems now comes under closer scrutiny by the FDA as a result of finalization of the rules on the sanitary transportation of human and animal foods and the FDA's investigative operations manual (IOM) 2016, Chapter 4, Developing a Preventive Control Plan—sampling referenced above [9,10].

Since transportation operations have not previously been a focus of any type of environmental sampling requirements to be imposed by the FDA, the 2016 IOM 2016 becomes an important guidance document to help focus attention on preventive control needs in the food transportation sector. The IOM requirements for all food operations are included earlier in this chapter.

Some important issues highlighted in the IOM related to sampling during transportation processes cover such things as investigation of food fraud (especially for imported foods and raw materials during transportation processes), case and labeling, quantity accuracy, and documentation.

It should be clear that the FDA has the authority to and will sample food ingredients, commodities, documentation, labels, and others through under cover buys, postal seizures, in-line factory sampling, environmental sampling, complaint samples, and reconditioned food samples for domestic and import food shipments at any or all food transportation processes.

Although the final rules on the sanitary transportation of human and animal foods contain no requirements for preventive controls, it should be clear that the FDA can and will sample test for hazardous contaminants throughout food transportation processes. A brief scan of the final rules, however, clearly shows the use of the word "prevention" throughout the final rules document. This can be seriously misleading to shippers, carriers, and receivers since few tests for container, vehicle or truck trailer contaminants. Furthermore, the final rules call for no shipping container, vehicle, or truck trailer testing under normal preventive control practices requiring identification of hazards, cross-contamination and the like. Nor do the rules call for documentation supporting transportation efforts to control contamination. This rule conflict situation is terribly misleading. Some larger shippers and carriers have moved forward and are now becoming certified to standards requiring the development of procedures and practices calling for testing for hazards to be controlled as part of their preventive practices.

To establish preventive controls for containers, truck trailers, and containers used to move food by road or rail in the United States, environmental (container) testing is highly recommended to determine whether or not food carrying containers contain hazardous biological food residues capable of cross-contaminating clean loads.

SAMPLE SHIPPING CONTAINER INSPECTION AND VERIFICATION PROCEDURE

A complete inspection of the trailer or container is performed after completion of the cleaning and sanitation operations. It is done to make sure there are no signs of bad smells, visible dirt, or traces of organic matter. Odors are a sign that additional cleaning is needed as bad smells can be an indication of microbiological contamination and poor cleaning practices.

Final verification and validation of the cleaning and sanitation of the shipping unit is always performed with an adenosine triphosphate (ATP) swab and analyzer. The readings from the ATP-swabbing equipment immediately show if the cleaning and sanitation process passes or fails and helps with the decision of what corrective actions to take.

RECORD KEEPING

A report will be generated from the initial inspection of the truck and from the cleaning and sanitation process and the final readings from the ATP-swabbing machine. This report should be documented and kept on file as a proof that the shipping unit has been cleaned and sanitized properly. Copy of the cleaning and sanitation certification will also be kept in file for reference.

RESPONSIBILITY

All personnel are required to carry out cleaning procedures as instructed and maintain a clean and tidy work environment. The manager or supervisor is responsible for supervising cleaning procedures across the company and ensuring that cleaning records are completed and signed off. The manager is also responsible for monitoring the effectiveness of cleaning and specifying the use of cleaning chemicals. The manager is responsible for approving all cleaning procedures, work instruction, records and certifications.

References

- Cleaning Work Instructions
- Cleaning Checklists
- Chemical Inventory
- PRP Sanitation Programs
- ATP-Swabbing Machine Manual
- Material Safety Data Sheets

INTRODUCTION

The company has established and implemented Standard Operating Procedures (SOPs) for the use of equipment at the facility. These procedures are maintained as part of the operational programs to keep the proper functioning and to meet customer requirements and expectations.

SCOPE

The protocols outlined in this SOP are applicable to guarantee the food safety of the shipping/transportation container, vehicle, or truck trailer. All employees involved with the cleaning and sanitation of truck containers are required to be familiar with and follow these SOPs. This activity covers the procedure to assess the ATP Swab methodology used by the Manager.

PURPOSE

This procedure is established to ensure that the cleanliness and sanitation of the truck container interior has been performed appropriately for the safety of transported food products. An effective microbiological monitoring program ensures that cleaning and sanitation procedures are followed properly and are effective.

FREQUENCY

ATP swabbing will be conducted according to established procedures after completing the cleaning and sanitation of a truck container. This will help collect data and assess the effectiveness of the sanitation process and make appropriate determination where to pass or fail a cleaned container. If container fails, cleaning and sanitation will be done again and ATP swabs will be re-conducted and analyzed.

EQUIPMENT

- ATP Swabs
- Handheld ATP Swabbing Machine

PROCEDURE

Wait until the truck shipping container has been cleaned and sanitized. Select two different areas of the container where the swabbing will be performed (wall and floor are recommended).

SOP FOR ATP SWABBING TO ASSESS THE CLEANLINESS OF SHIPPING CONTAINERS

Test tube

1. Remove from test tube and swab surface. Swabbing motion should be in a $4 \times 4\,in^2$ while rotating swab or a random motion that ensures a good sample collection.
2. Place swab back in test tube.
3. Break plastic Snap Valve at top of swab by bending bulb. Squeeze bulb twice, pushing liquid reagent down swab shaft.
4. Shake test for 5 seconds.
5. Place test in System SURE Plus and close lid.
6. Press "OK" and reading will appear in 15 seconds.
7. The cleaning process is rejected or accepted based on company established upper ATP control limits.

RESPONSIBILITY

The transportation manager is responsible for updating and training company's personnel in the ATP Swabbing methodology. Fig. 3.4 illustrates the ATP luminator and swab and swabbing pattern.

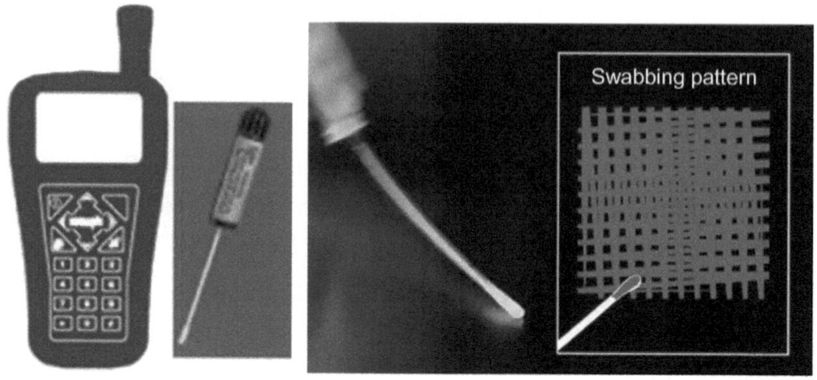

FIGURE 3.4

ATP luminator, swab, and swabbing pattern.

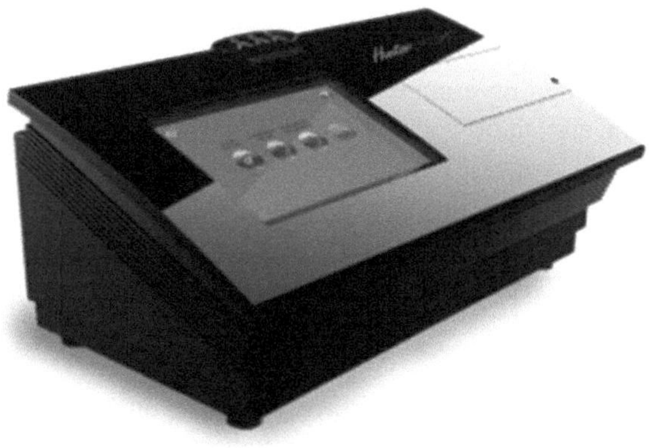

FIGURE 3.5

Polymerase chain reaction test station.

The price for each swab is around $2 while the luminator is priced at about $1200. The luminator provides readings in 15 seconds, is rechargeable and lasts a very long time. ATP products provide a quick 1-minute test for an energy molecule found in living cells.

If sanitation or cleaning process does not remove enough of these cells, the process probably needs to be upgraded with hot water, higher water pressures, or even through the use of sanitizers such as QUAT.

In some cases, carrier and shipper companies would be advised to provide audit level testing for specific types of bacterial contaminants including salmonella, monocytogenes, Vibrio, *E. coli*, and listeria. In such cases, portable and local polymerase chain reaction (PCR) testing stations are available (Fig. 3.5).

Pricing for the PCR test station (excluding supplies) is around $10,000.

MANDATORY CARRIER TRAINING FOR ALL FOOD TRANSPORTATION OPERATIONS PERSONNEL

The final rules on the sanitary transportation of human animal foods also include some serious training requirements for carriers responsible for the sanitation of their containers, truck trailers, and vehicles. These training requirements are shown below and are clearly established to help carriers prevent hazardous practices:

1. Responsibilities of the carrier
   a. Understand US FDA FSMA Law for the Sanitary Transportation of Human and Animal Foods
   b. Understand changes from the proposed FDA FSMA rules
   c. Know the different requirements for shippers, carriers, and receivers
   d. Know who is exempted
   e. Understand the FDA waiver requirements
2. Awareness of potential food safety problems that may occur during food transportation
   a. Understand basic bacterial, chemical, and physical hazards
   b. Know what prevention means
   c. Know how tools and equipment, pallets, trays, bins, gaskets, hoses, load and unload systems, vehicles, containers, and trailers can contaminate foods
   d. Understand the impact of temperature variation on food safety and food quality
   e. Know what conditions occur in transportation operations that may cause bacterial growth
   f. Be able to prevent cross-contamination
   g. Know what missing records can mean
   h. Know what action to take if a reefer fails or a container is out of acceptable maintenance condition
   i. Understand accident protocols
3. Basic sanitary transportation practices to address those potential problems
   a. Develop a contract of carriage and other agreements required between carriers and shippers
   b. Understand basic management, preventive control, sanitation, temperature monitoring and traceability, and training standards
   c. Help to write and implement appropriate container procedures (truck, trailer, sanitation, testing, container traceability, and temperature monitoring)
   d. Learn to keep appropriate records
   e. Understand the transportation food safety audit and certification process
   f. Help to establish preventive controls
   g. Understand how to collect, analyze, and take preventive action using statistical data

MONITORING TEMPERATURES DURING TRANSPORTATION PROCESSES

Environmental sampling and monitoring must go beyond sampling for hazardous contaminants. As all food enters the food supply bloodstream and is transported through multiple handling, load, unload and truck trailer, rail car, or vehicle movement processes, the FDA rules on the sanitary transportation of human and animal foods call for shippers, carriers, and receivers of perishable and frozen foods to maintain bacterial growth temperature limits throughout all handling, load/unload and transportation processes.

If you open your home refrigerator and look at the food inside, on the average, your food has traveled over 2000 mi. to arrive at your home.

Vicarious liability demands that your company is responsible for your suppliers (transporters) ability to deliver temperature controlled, safe, and sanitary food.

These vicarious liability issues imply that companies must consider and establish supply chain visibility and supply chain visibility means that the product type and the temperature and humidity conditions under which the product is being shipped as well as the shipment's location at any date and time should be known in what might be called real-time. "Real-time" simply means that the shipper, carrier, and receiver all have access to data as shipment conditions (temperature, etc.) are sampled with monitoring equipment and transmitted using Internet or cell phone technology to a database and to users. Such systems are commonly referred to as ILC or identification (I), location (L), and condition (C) systems. ILC systems commonly allow for remote configuration of such things as the upper and lower temperature control limits, frequency of read and transmit requirements, and sending of alerts to managers when temperatures and other measured variables go out-of-specification limits.

Preventive control concepts would also imply that such temperature monitoring equipment be adequately calibrated to assure measurement accuracy and that managers collect, analyze, and use available data to take corrective actions to protect consumers against overheated, melted, or otherwise spoiled food. In such cases, causal analysis under preventive control requirements would also require managers or teams to establish projects that can be documented using the STS or statistical process control (SPC) as the teams work through process improvements.

Throughout time there has been an evolution of food transportation models. Some time in history and in countries or regions that lack refrigeration, the warm chain was the primary way to deliver foods. Countries with limited or no refrigeration generally harvested, transported, cooked, and ate fresh food within a single day. Food traveled less than 50 mi. and distribution from harvest to market to preparation and consumption was a relatively simple process.

Today, the cold chain tends to dominate on a world-wide basis increasing the need for temperature monitoring and control. In the cold chain, the length of time from harvest depends on the temperature and conditions under which the food is kept. If things comply with best practice implementation to control humidity and temperature, food is considered fresh if delivered to supermarket shelves within what

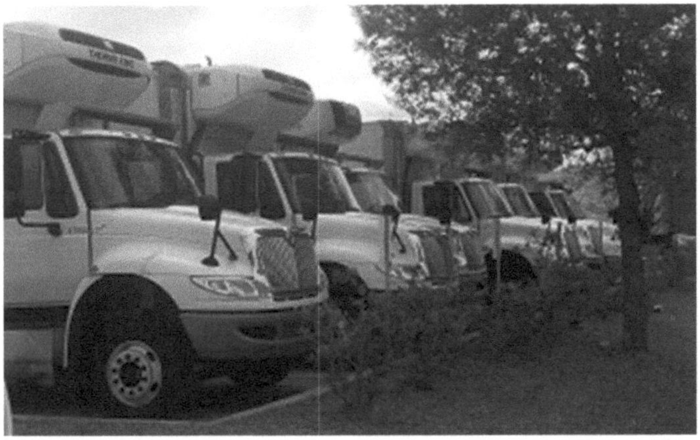

FIGURE 3.6

Delivery truck refrigeration units.

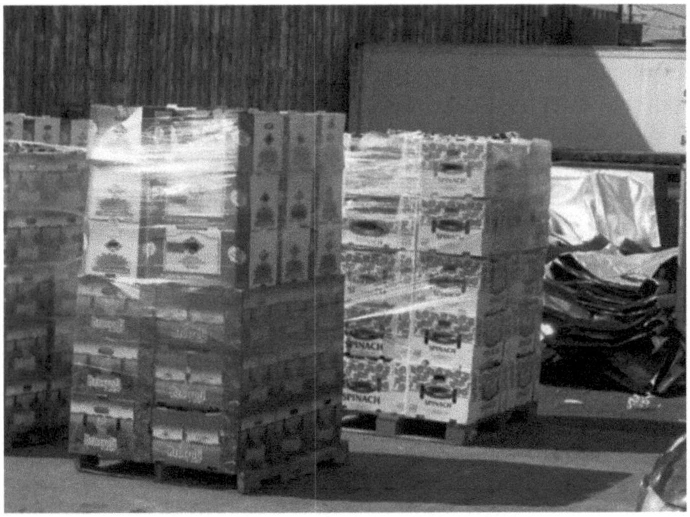

FIGURE 3.7

Pallets of produce baking in the Hawaiian sun.

is called the shelf life of the product even though it has traveled thousands of miles through a complex distribution process.

Generally, reefer or refrigerated transportation is required. Fig. 3.6 shows the large protruding reefer units on the top front of these produce delivery trucks.

Unfortunately, there are many points throughout transportation processes that can result in high bacterial growth probabilities when food is mishandled. Fig. 3.7

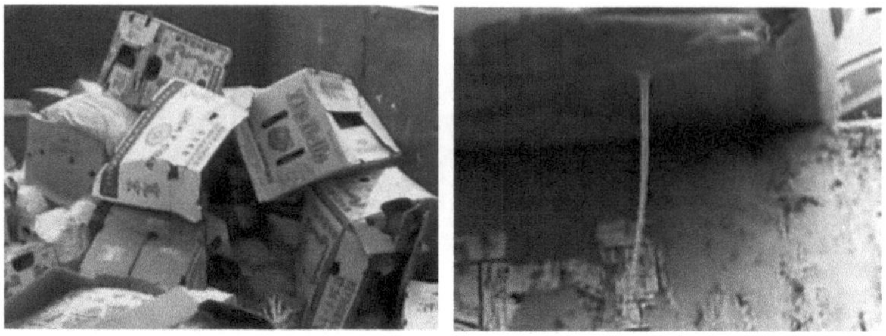

FIGURE 3.8

Cross-contamination during reefer shutdown [11].

illustrates pallets of freshly packaged broccoli and spinach that had been air transported from California to Hawaii. The cost to air freight each pallet was in excess of $800 (that's just for the airfare). After being carefully cleaned, processed, packaged, and protected from freezing during flight and being delivered by reefer transport from the airport to a warehouse, the pallets were left in the 91°F sun for over 2 hours. Such mishandling greatly reduces shelf life and promotes bacterial growth. The inability of the shipping company to sample and monitor temperatures is considered as a lack of ability to establish preventive controls during transportation processes and exhibits the shipper's lack of supply chain qualification requirements.

Some states are known to supply highway patrol or state troopers with temperature measurement devices they can use on the road to enforce food safety regulations. NBC News reporter Tom Rossen had the opportunity to ride along with Indiana state troopers as they stopped reefer enabled trucks, opened the rear doors, and measured temperatures of the food inside. Rosen reported that "Some trucks carry unsafe food, authorities say. Bacteria can breed when temperatures are too high; feds provide little oversight." The report included videos of their findings. Fig. 3.8 shows that frozen chicken was defrosted and the chicken juice was leaking out onto fresh vegetables being shipped below the chicken. Although this is a good example of economically motivated adulteration (the truck driver turned off the reefer to save gas), cross-contamination also became an issue because chicken is known to carry salmonella. When cooked, the salmonella on the chicken may be killed by excessive heat, but the cross-contamination of the vegetables with potentially laden salmonella juice from the chicken will not be cooked and could result in illness or death when the raw and contaminated vegetables are eaten.

Under the FDA FSMA final rules on the sanitary transportation of human and animal foods, some of the FSMA definitions and requirements for shippers and carriers should be reviewed.

> *Carrier: A person who owns, leases, or is otherwise ultimately responsible for the use of a motor vehicle or rail vehicle to transport food (private truck fleets, private fleet truck drivers, contracted drivers, distributors, leased vehicles).*

According to the rules, "Carriers must supply a vehicle and transportation equipment that meets any requirements specified by the shipper and is otherwise appropriate to prevent the food from becoming filthy, putrid, decomposed or otherwise unfit for food, or being rendered injurious to health from any source during the transportation operation.

Must, once the transportation operation is complete, demonstrate to the shipper and if requested, to the receiver, that it has maintained temperature conditions during the transportation operation consistent with those specified by the shipper."

Further, a carrier must develop and implement written procedures subject to the records requirements that

1. *"specify practices for cleaning, sanitizing if necessary, and inspecting vehicles and transportation equipment that the carrier provides for use in the transportation of food to maintain the vehicles and the transportation equipment in appropriate sanitary condition as required (brooms, mops, hoses, etc.)*
2. *describe how it will comply with the provisions for temperature control in paragraph (2) of this section, and*
3. *describe how it will comply with the provisions for the use of bulk vehicles."*

"Food not completely enclosed by a container means any food that is placed into a container in such a manner that it is partially open to the surrounding environment. Examples of such containers include an open wooden basket or crate, an open cardboard box, a vented cardboard box with a top, or a vented plastic bag. This term does not include food transported in a bulk vehicle as defined in this subpart.

Shelf stable food means a food that can be stored under ambient temperature and humidity conditions and, if the package integrity is maintained will not spoil or become unsafe throughout its storage life.

Time/temperature control for safety (TCS) Food means a food that requires time/TCS to limit pathogenic microorganism growth or toxin formation.

Transportation means any movement of food in commerce by motor vehicle or rail vehicle.

Transportation equipment means equipment used in food transportation operations, other than vehicles, e.g., bulk and nonbulk containers, bins, totes, pallets, pumps, fittings, hoses, gaskets, and loading and unloading systems. Transportation equipment also includes a rail car not attached to a locomotive or a trailer not attached to a tractor.

Transportation operations means all activities associated with food transportation that may affect the sanitary condition of food including cleaning, inspection, maintenance, loading and unloading, and operation of vehicles and transportation equipment.

Transportation operations do not include any activities associated with the transportation solely of shelf stable food that is completely enclosed by a container, compressed food gases, or live food animals. In addition, transportation operations do not include any transportation activities for raw agricultural commodities that are performed by a farm.

Vehicle means a land conveyance that is motorized, e.g., a motor vehicle, or that moves on rails, e.g., a railcar, which is used in transportation operations.

Shipper: A person who initiates a shipment of food by motor vehicle or rail vehicle.

Under the rules, a shipper must "Carry out loading and unloading operations under conditions that will prevent the food from supporting such microbial growth

Maintain written agreements as part of the records requirements

Report equipment failures (temperature or other), take "appropriate" action, communicate with other parties to prevent sale or distribution unless qualified person approves the use of the food.

1. And must specify in writing to the carrier "sanitary requirements for the carrier's vehicle and transportation equipment (vehicles, trailers, containers, bins, trays, pallets, load and unload equipment, hoses, gaskets, etc.)
2. specific design requirements
3. cleaning procedures
4. temperature conditions necessary during the transportation operation, including the pre-cooling phase
5. must verify that each freezer and mechanically refrigerated cold storage compartment or container has been precooled in accordance with information submitted by the shipper
6. Assumption of temperature records required of the carrier"

However, if the "shipper assumes the requirements applicable to the carrier with respect to providing a demonstration to the receiver if the shipper and carrier have agreed in writing that the shipper is responsible for ensuring that the food was held under acceptable temperature conditions during transportation operations.

When the shipper and carrier have established such an agreement, the shipper also assumes the corresponding records requirements." Such agreements may take the form of a contract of carriage and all documentation must be maintained for a minimum of 12 months for both shippers and carriers, be kept as original records and must be made available to FDA auditors.

Receiver: Any person who receives food after transportation, whether or not that person represents the final point of receipt for the food.

Transportation: Any movement of food in commerce by motor vehicle or rail vehicle.

Transportation equipment to mean equipment used in transportation operations, other than vehicles.

As an example of what temperature controls might be applied to some produce, the Cornell Cooperative Extension program provides "Storage Guidelines for Fruits & Vegetables shown in Table 3.8. Cornell recommends temperatures, relative humidity, and shelf live or length of storage suggestions for fruits and vegetables listed in the table. Other temperature control tables are available through a simple Google search using the words "product temperature chart."

Table 3.8 Partial Cornell Temperature Relative Humidity Control Suggestions [12]

Vegetable	Temperature (°F)	Relative Humidity (%)	Length of Storage
Beans, snap	40–50	95	7–10 days
Cucumbers	45–50	95	10–14 days
Egg plant	45–50	90	1 week
Cantaloupe	40	90	15 days
Watermelon	40–50	80–85	2–3 weeks
Peppers, sweet	45–50	95	2–3 weeks
Potatoes, early	50	90	1–3 weeks
Potatoes, late	40	90	4–9 months
Tomatoes, green	50–70	90	1–3 weeks
Tomatoes, ripe	45–50	90	4–7 days

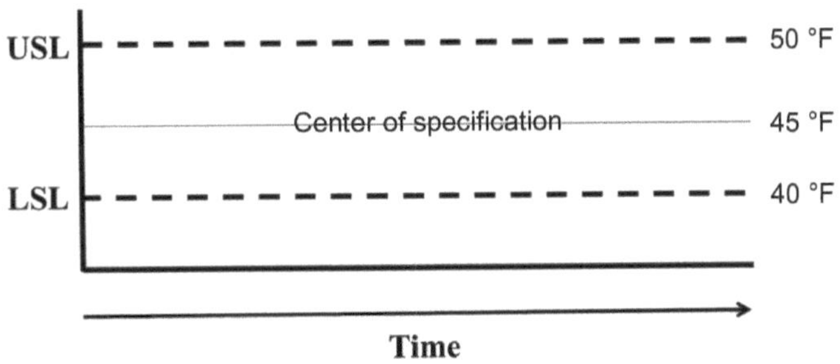

FIGURE 3.9

Temperature monitoring control chart.

If we look at the suggested upper and lower limits set for watermelon (Fig. 3.9), it should be obvious that those limits (45–50°F) can be used for temperature control monitoring for that product. By using the solution tracking sheet or statistical process control chart examples provided elsewhere in this book, the upper specification limit (USL) and lower specification limits (LCL) can be transferred to temperature monitoring trends to determine in or out-of-control conditions. By subtracting the LCL from the USL (50 − 40 = 10), we can determine a middle-of-the-specification line (10/2 + 40 = 45) to determine a center line for ideal temperature storage and transportation conditions for watermelon as shown in Fig. 3.9.

Although temperature monitoring devices generally record temperatures at set periods of time (e.g., 15 minutes or 30 minutes), the recorded temperature can be plotted on the control chart to provide a strong visual depiction of how well a company is able to control temperatures for food products.

Plotted points that show up as out-of-specification or even out-of-control if normal control charts are used, can be used to determine when temperature limits were exceeded. Such charts are often combined with global positioning data thus providing the time, place and temperature for out-of-control conditions. This strategy provides management information that can be used to correct irregularities in temperature control processes.

Considering what seem to be onerous record keeping and documentation requirements for temperature and sanitation monitoring as preventive controls, new systems are evolving in the marketplace to simplify data collection, storage and analysis in a low cost supply chain enabled manner. One must assume that transportation process monitoring and record keeping needs to focus on the FSMA rule requirements noted above and other rule requirements not listed. Although preventive controls are not specified under the FSMA rules on the sanitary transportation of human and animal foods, the rules frequently refer to prevention. This can be interpreted to mean that any FDA audits will include questions such as "How do you know your sanitation and temperature monitoring work?" Companies choosing to ignore the need to prepare to answer such questions will most likely find themselves undergoing increased scrutiny.

PREVENTIVE TEMPERATURE CONTROLS

Some of the examples from the beginning of this section were used to illustrate potential cross-contaminants and their prevention through various supply chain processes. Sanitation is generally considered critical to controlling the spread of bacterial and chemical contaminants from one product to another or from one operational step to another, but food processing often requires temperature controls in packing houses, distribution centers, processing operations, transportation, retail outlets and restaurants. Although bacterial contaminants may not be detected early in the supply chain flow, if processing, storage, handling, and transportation temperatures are not properly maintained to prevent bacterial growth and spread, even initially undetectable bacteria gains the ability to grow and spread thereby contaminating everything and everyone it touches.

For most perishables and frozen foods, it is generally accepted that any temperature above 140°F (60°C) or below 41°F (5°C) are in a temperature range that is conducive to temperature growth.

For this reason, most food processes have established temperature control requirements between 41°F and 140°F for controlling environments through which the food must pass on its way to consumers.

While establishing and maintaining temperature limits might seem to be a rather simple process, today's equipment and operational procedures, especially during transportation operations, are inadequate. Consider a few examples.

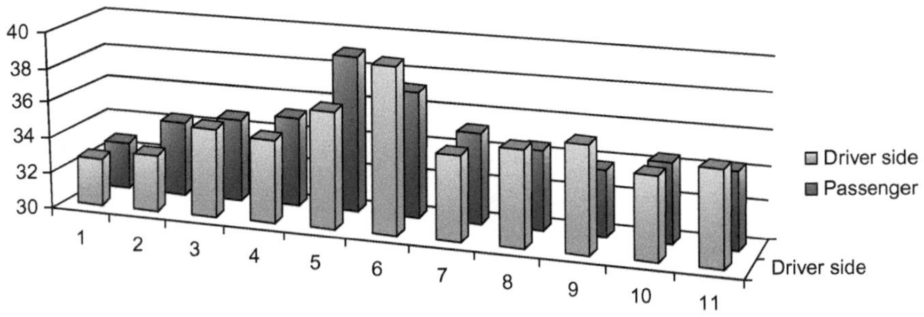

FIGURE 3.10

Pallet temperature recording.

With permission from Intelleflex Corporation.

Fig. 3.10 uses vertical bars to illustrate temperatures measured on pallets from the front of the truck trailer on both the left and right sides. Temperatures at the front and rear of the trailer are considerably lower than temperatures recorded during transportation than those recorded in the middle of the trailer.

A second example is illustrated as Fig. 3.11. The figure shows the recorded reefer record line in the middle of the temperature range at about 37°F. The other lines are temperatures recorded with special temperature monitoring tags placed on different pallets. Some tag recorded temperatures are clearly recorded below the temperature monitoring records from the reefer monitoring system, but other tag temperatures indicate that there is a rise in temperatures throughout the 4-day trip required for delivery. It is likely that the higher temperatures show the emission of stored heat from improperly precooled product. In other words, some pallets of product were not adequately precooled and the heat stored in the middle of the pallets was released into the truck trailer during transportation.

Pre-cooling is considered a preventive control that was long ago established to prevent shortened shelf life but has significant impact on the need for preventive practices on the food safety side as well.

Generally, the idea that temperature controls established to prevent bacterial growth and prolong shelf life should be monitored throughout the entire transportation process to determine if, where, and when temperatures might have gone out of control. Knowing the product (identity), where it is (location) and condition (temperature) along transportation routes provides management with preventive control information that allows them to take preventive action. Fig. 3.12 shows a temperature and route tracking map of the type commonly available with today's wireless monitoring systems.

The map and temperature data recording and delivery show temperatures throughout the route. Each square indicates a temperature recording and data transmission

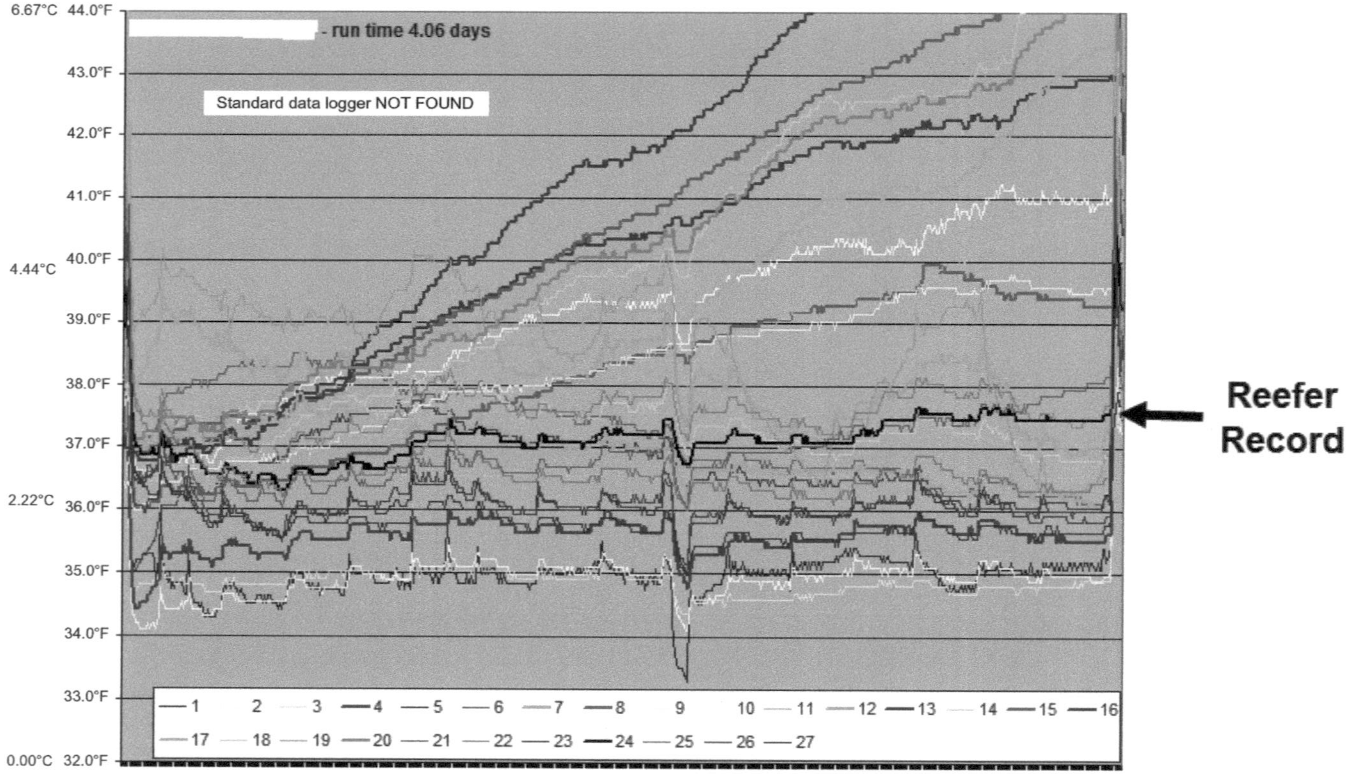

FIGURE 3.11

Effects of improper product precool processes.

With permission from Intelleflex Corporation.

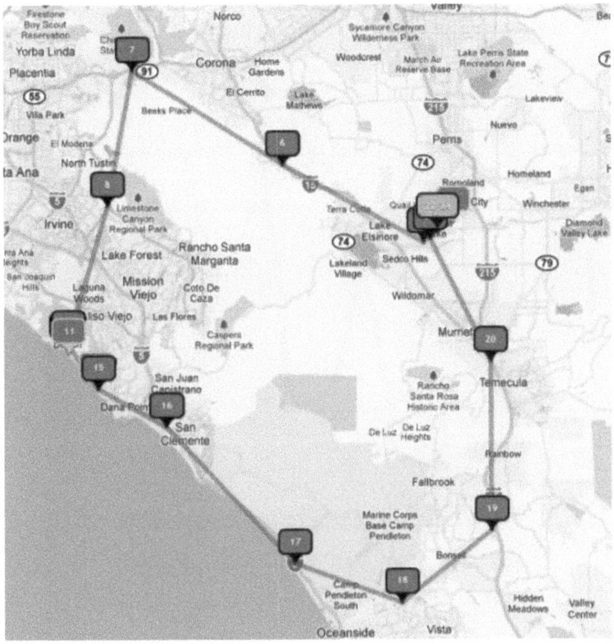

FIGURE 3.12

Delivery temperature recording map.

location. The data are transmitted through cell phone technology to a cloud database where a manager can look at the details for each record. By sitting at a desk with a computer and logging into the system's database, the manager can stop the computer mouse on any of the squares and look at detailed information recorded by a tag from the truck trailer. Further, the system provides a temperature plot (Fig. 3.13) that allows the manager to highlight any particular place where temperatures might have gone out of control.

The data plot shows that the internal temperature exceeded 32°F at about 4:00 pm in the afternoon. Between the plot and the map, the manager can pinpoint exactly where the temperature began to rise and can discuss the situation with the driver to determine likely causes and take preventive action.

There are many other advantages to using wireless temperature monitoring systems including those listed below:

- Monitoring tags are quickly installed
- Technical IT personnel are not required
- Cell phone, tablet, and computer access to the data
- Driver can exercise improved controls
- Information is shared (shipper, carrier, receiver)

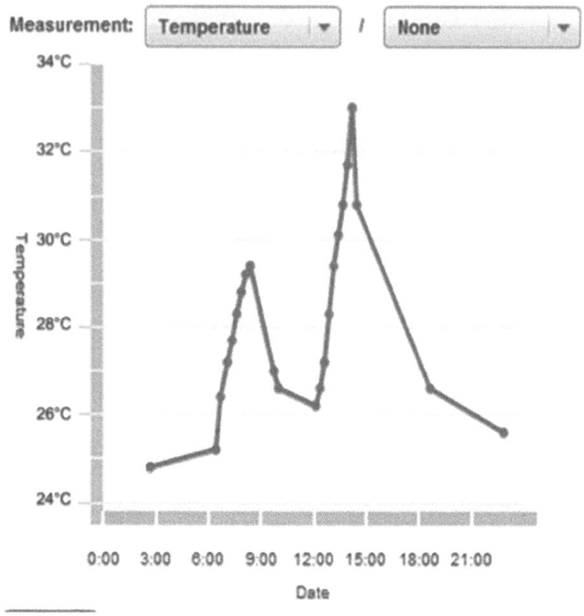

FIGURE 3.13

Route temperature data plot.

- Temperature monitoring devices in the trailer may be remotely configured
- System provides email and phone alerts for out-of-control conditions
- Local or standard zone time recording information is available
- Some products are rechargeable or may allow for battery replacement increasing longevity.

In some cases, such temperature recording systems can be used through the entire supply chain, from the product supplier, through distribution, transportation, and into final store or restaurant destinations. Fig. 3.14 shows tag, reader, and computer layouts for data collection, analysis and transmission to the cloud.

Using special temperature monitoring tags at the supplier, distributor, store and in reefers used for deliveries, tags send data to readers and onto computers hooked up to the internet. This is a supply chain control system that can, with cooperation among players, be expanded into a regional data network such as shown in Fig. 3.15. The figure shows how data flows from suppliers, reefers, distribution centers, and stores and into a centralized database.

All members can view temperature recordings from and to their operations to collectively work to prevent any temperature breakdowns in the food distribution system.

If expanded to any number of regions (Fig. 3.16), the system can supply corporate headquarters with overall management analysis information.

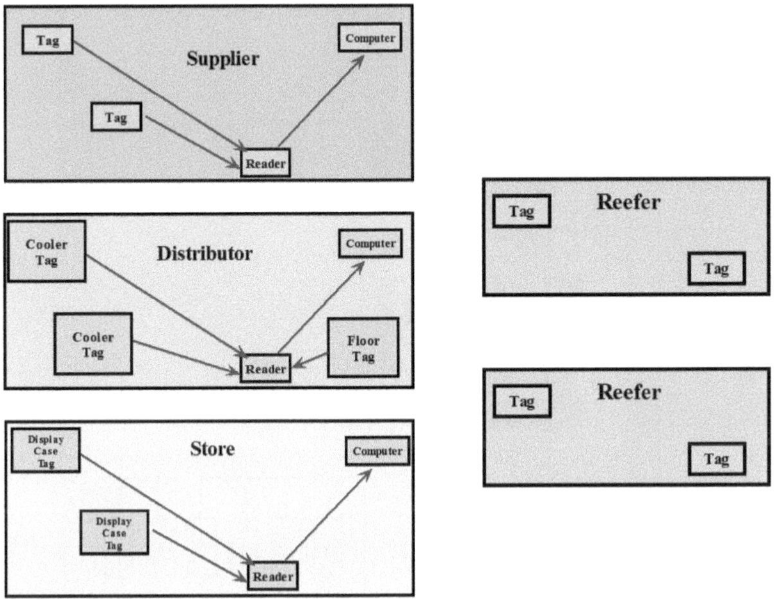

FIGURE 3.14

Temperature monitoring system communications.

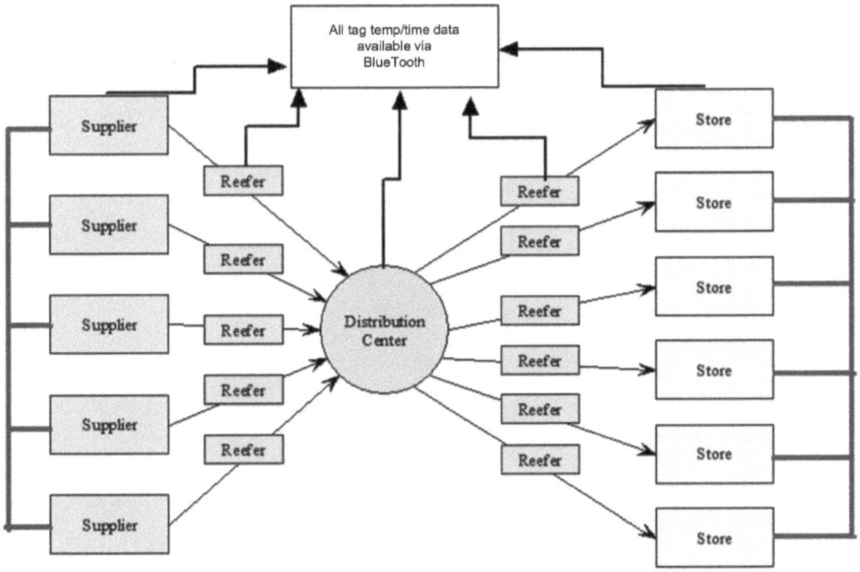

FIGURE 3.15

Regional supply chain temperature monitoring network.

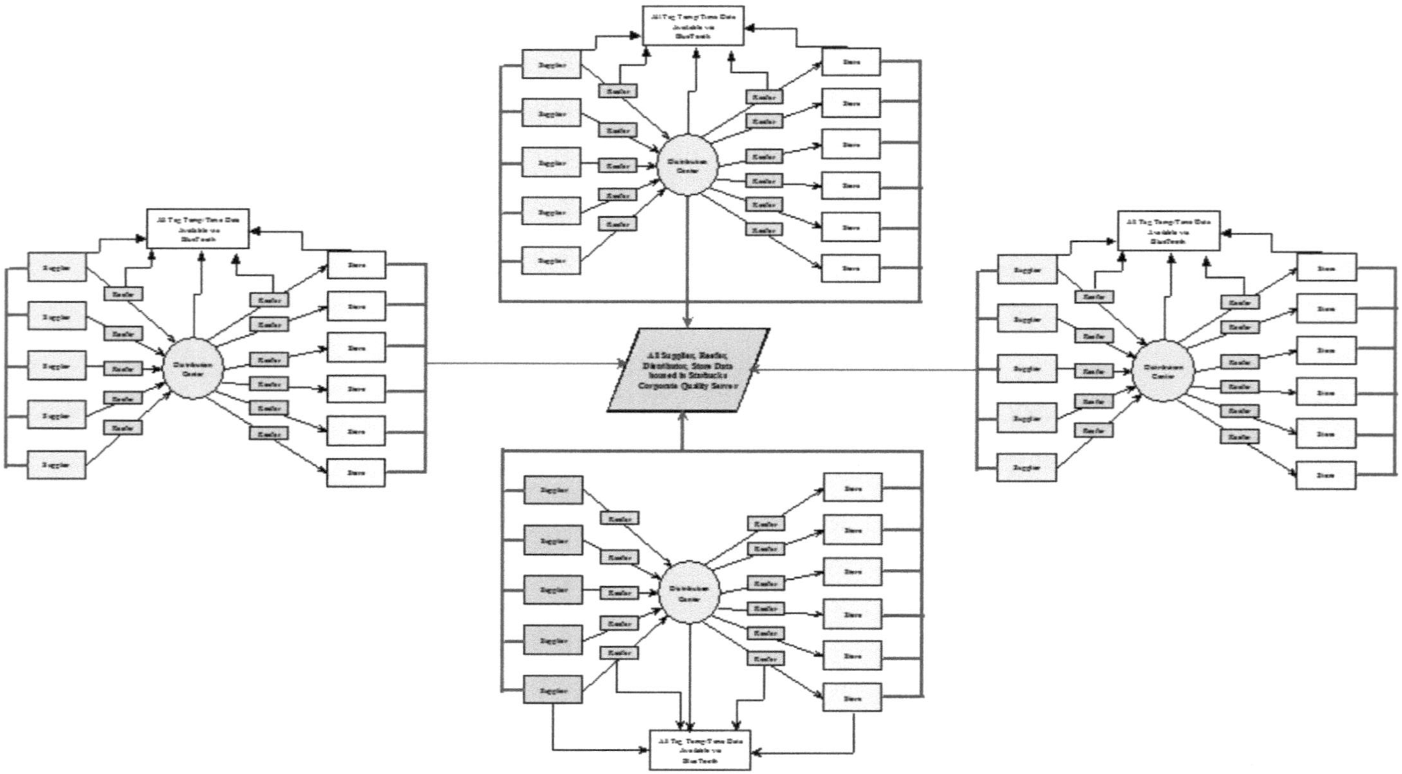

FIGURE 3.16

Corporate management over several regions.

SOME BASIC SANITATION CONCEPTS

Regardless of which food handling process is involved, where the processes is located or who runs the process, some sanitation basics can be covered to help guide an analysis of what should be done to prevent contaminants from impacting human health or from issues like cross-contamination.

There is a difference between disinfectants that destroy or inactivate infectious fungi and bacteria and sanitizers that do not kill microorganisms and there is a cleaning, rinsing, disinfection, rinse, and sanitizing flow that can be basically defined for establishing systems designed as preventive controls. These issues are further discussed in the section on cross-contamination.

ADDITIONAL ENVIRONMENTAL MONITORING ISSUES

From a producer's perspective and since many food quality and food safety issues originate at the production level, new technologies are evolving that might be considered to further help understand and measure variables such as field and food storage temperatures. Many of these technologies have been established to include solar power or battery powered monitors capable of transmitting field and other data directly to a producer's computer or into cloud maintained databases for later analysis.

For instance, drawing a map of a farm operation, mounting tags at specific locations, and recording each tag number on the map is just about as complex as installation might get. Both Zigbee and Smartphone enabled systems can send data to the "cloud" if needed where it can be stored and analyzed for seasonal, annual, or location variations.

In some cases, the supplier of the Smartphone or ZigBee system provides free software that provides trends and other screen shots for user analysis and system management.

Both require batteries that can be changed. Battery use depends on how often the data is sent by the system to the receiver rather than how often measurements are taken. The lithium batteries in each type of device usually last for between 1 year and 2 years.

For relatively flat fields, Fig. 3.17 shows how monitors might be laid out. Each small circle represents a potential monitor location.

Similar systems can be set up for fields that are much hillier such as those used as vineyards (Fig. 3.18).

In the wine cellar, upper, and lower temperatures vary meaning that wine cellars can be monitories using monitor setups such as those shown in Fig. 3.19.

In distribution centers, Zigbee, and cell phone monitors can be set up in a manner such as that shown in Fig. 3.20.

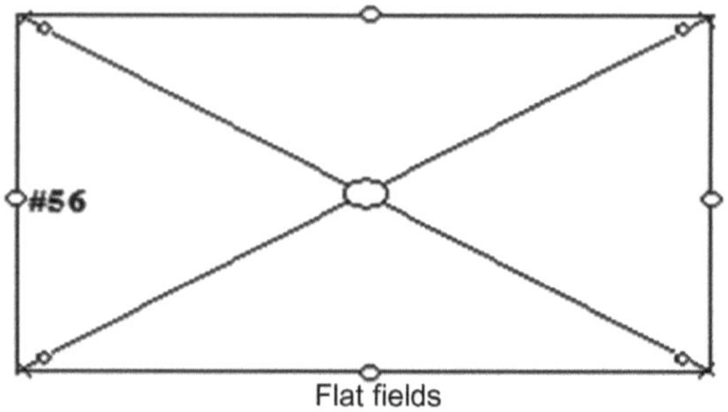

FIGURE 3.17

Flat temperature/humidity temperature monitoring device distribution.

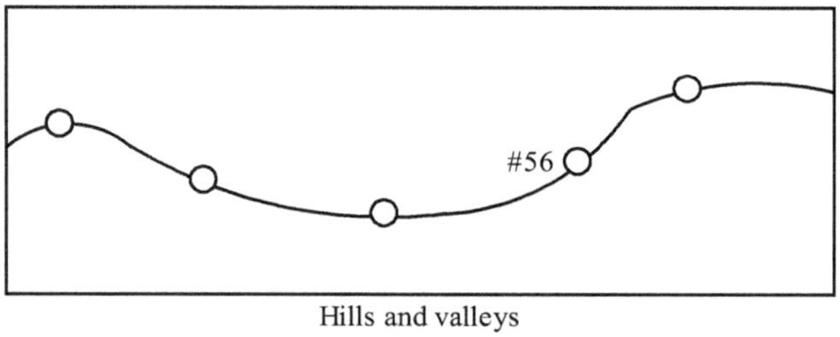

FIGURE 3.18

Monitor layouts for hills and valleys.

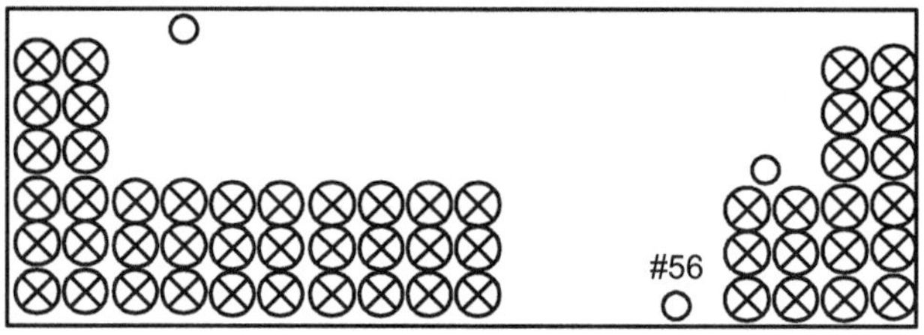

FIGURE 3.19

Wine cellar temperature/humidity monitoring setup.

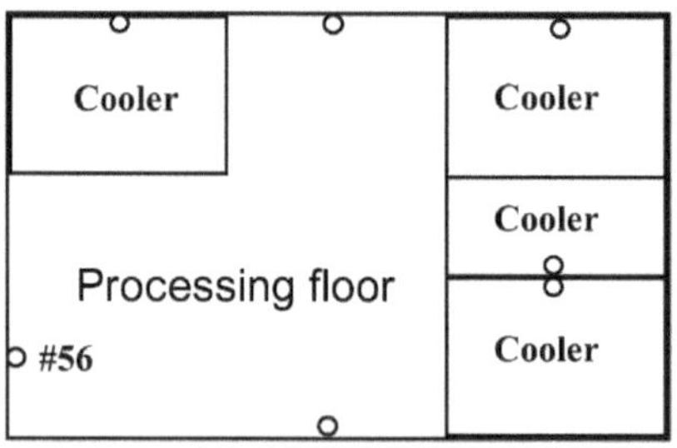

FIGURE 3.20

Packing house or distribution center temperature/humidity monitoring.

REFERENCES

[1] Current Good Manufacturing Practice, Hazard Analysis, and Risk-Based Preventive Controls for Human Food. https://www.federalregister.gov/documents/2015/09/17/2015-21920/current-good-manufacturing-practice-hazard-analysis-and-risk-based-preventive-controls-for-human; August, 2016.

[2] FSMA Final Rule for Preventive Controls for Human Food. http://www.fda.gov/Food/GuidanceRegulation/FSMA/ucm334115.htm; August, 2016.

[3] Investigative Operations Manual 2016, Chapter 4 – Sampling. http://www.fda.gov/downloads/ICECI/Inspections/IOM/UCM123507.pdf; July, 2016.

[4] Multistate Outbreak of Sallmonella Saintpaul Infections Linked to Raw Produce. http://www.cdc.gov/salmonella/2008/raw-produce-8-28-2008.html; March, 2016.

[5] Current Good Manufacturing Practice, Hazard Analysis, and Risk-Based Preventive Controls for Human Food. http://www.regulations.gov/document?D=FDA-2011-N-0920-1979; July, 2019.

[6] Center for Science in the Public Interest. http://www.cspinet.org/foodsafety/Produce%20Outbreaks%20%28IAFP%20Poster%2007%29.pdf; April, 2009.

[7] Pesticide Fact Sheet: Azoxystrobin. https://www3.epa.gov/pesticides/chem_search/reg_actions/registration/fs_PC-128810_07-Feb-97.pdf; October, 2016.

[8] J.M. Ryan (unpublished), Hawaii Farm Bureau Federation, January, 2010.

[9] FSMA Final Rules on the Transportation of Human and Animal Foods. http://www.fda.gov/Food/GuidanceRegulation/FSMA/ucm383763.htm; July, 2016.

[10] Investigations Operations Manual 2016. http://www.fda.gov/downloads/ICECI/Inspections/IOM/UCM123507.pdf; July, 2016.

[11] Rossen Reports: Some trucks carry unsafe food, authorities say. http://today.msnbc.msn.com/id/48691046/ns/today-today_rossen_reports/t/rossen-reports-some-trucks-carry-unsafe-food-authorities-say/#.UEY8yJaaJ8E; July, 2016.

[12] Storage Guidelines for Fruits & Vegetables. http://www.gardening.cornell.edu/factsheets/vegetables/storage.pdf; July 2016.

CHAPTER

Developing a preventive controls plan: Food safety and quality

4

The food safety profession and the FDA are still in need of some simplification that combines concepts into standard approaches. For instance, hazard analysis critical control point (HACCP) has been around for some time and has recently been somewhat translated into hazard analysis risk-based preventive controls (HARPC). Now, we have preventive control planning. In truth, all three are process control strategies and are normal approaches to basic the path from getting control over process problems by defining and eliminating problem causes.

It doesn't matter what industry you are in. Food, electronics, construction, transportation, and others all benefit from establishing and implementing team approaches that recognize the difference between system and assignable causes and implement continuous improvement efforts.

Call the strategy whatever you want. Prevention is the name of the game.

In this chapter, a relatively simple aquaponics process example used to illustrate a strategy for using spreadsheets and flowcharts to help planners and food safety teams to analyze, visualize, and develop the detailed planning that impact food safety throughout their own processes. The planning strategy provides example guidance from analysis of incoming materials through process steps into transportation and into customers.

In the later chapters, more detailed information covering a basic team approach to tackling food safety threats using statistical applications for common cause (CC) teams and assignable cause functional improvement team (FIT) teams are covered. In some cases, a specialized team made of those CC and FIT team members that are most qualified and aware of what goes on in company processes can be established to review common and assignable causes. Other companies have left this phase of the planning to a FIT, and later required a careful review and update by a CC team. Theoretically, any and all team members will be trained in preventive controls and causal analysis before tackling the planning effort. Recall that under the U.S. approach to preventive controls, a "qualified individual" should be involved in all planning and plan reviews, and that, this involvement must be documented. The plan must provide an approach to validate the fact that the plan actually has impact and works in a continuous improvement manner to minimize and eliminate hazards.

If one has to walk around some schools nowadays, they would notice that a significant and growing number of them are getting involved in gardening. Some of

Validating Preventive Food Safety and Quality Controls. DOI: http://dx.doi.org/10.1016/B978-0-12-810994-6.00004-3

them are actually putting shovel to earth, some are organic, some have greenhouses, and some are into hydroponics or even aquaponics. There are a lot of lessons to be learned by gardening, and many teachers and parents are happily getting kids involved in those lessons.

More importantly, many of those gardens are supplying produce and may be even fish from those gardens to cafeterias or local farmer's markets. This is all done joyously and with great feeling of accomplishment. Some of us succeed in gardening before we go into farming. Something about making things grow starts from a people on the agricultural path.

It's one thing to have a garden in your backyard and quite another thing to take your locally grown produce and introduce it into distribution channels as part of a supply chain where you must assume responsibility and liability. The newly passed food safety modernization act allows "small" suppliers to escape food safety responsibility by providing loopholes big enough for a football player to run through. Unfortunately, those loopholes will eventually eliminate the opportunity for small producers to sell into any food supply chain. Buyers will simply not be allowed to purchase from operations that are not food safety certified.

Although compliance organizations have each developed sets of food safety audit standards and paid their fees to provide certification services, the question of just what makes for safe and quality food still haunts us all. It is well known that bacteria and chemicals can harm humans, but there are few, if any, standards that require post-harvest chemical and bacterial testing at the farm level. The farm, by the way, is a primary source of contaminants. These contaminants are usually found further down the chain in restaurants (and blamed on cross contamination) or processing operations. It all becomes a blame game with food origins relatively protected because of a lack of oversight.

Aquaponics systems are particularly interesting because this method of production provides both a source of protein and produce to the marketplace, perhaps making it doubly dangerous. On the other hand, aquaponics provides us with an opportunity to establish both food quality and food safety controls in a preventive manner—at the source. Aquaponics saves water and land, seems cleaner for the environment and allows for the use of solar energy to run pumps. If you talk to aquaponics fanatics, they are after a truly sustainable operation that functions completely off the grid (well, almost completely).

The aquaponics process offers a perspective that provides us with clearly defined inputs, processing and outputs. The inputs, process, and output stream must be defined in detail and completely considered. If the process and system controls are balanced just right, food emerges; food, we assume, that is nutritious, contaminant free, has fresh flavor and can even be sold because it has market appeal. This is a perfect set up for a school yard and a great learning experience.

But, what about food quality and food safety? How are they controlled in any farming or aquaponics operation? We begin with a basic understanding of aquaponics. Aquaponics intends to produce protein and produce in a single system in as sustainable and green manner as possible. Fig. 4.1 shows a fish tank, a bio-filter, and three grow

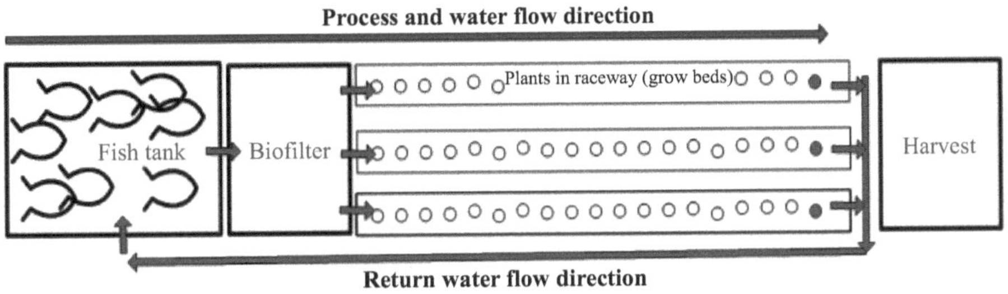

Potential food quality process concerns

- Fish
- Fish food
- Fish treatments
- Water contamination
- Water level
- Pump (flow rate)
- Back flow preventer
- Aerator
- Water hardness
- Water alkalinity
- Fish food storage
- Fish food quality
- Fish food source

- Bell siphons
- Water exchange
- Water level
- Cinder/media
- Fish manure
- Ammonia
- Cinders (media)
- Water
- Worms
- Worm castings
- Bacterial seed
- Exit water contamination

- Cinder/media
- Water levels
- Bell siphon
- Fertilizer
- Pesticides
- pH
- Dissolved oxygen
- Carbon dioxide
- Ammonia
- Nitrites
- Nitrates
- Seed source
- Lime/calcium

- Water exchange
- Waste water disposal
- Harvested fish
- Harvested produce

Potential food safety hazards

- Biological contaminants
- Chemcial contaminants
- Metal contaminants
- Air and water flow rates
- Fish pathogens
- Antibiotics in fish food
- Invasive species introduced in locally grown azolla
- Human illness
- Water source
- Fish treatments (illness)
- Plant grow height
- Local animals (airborne contaminants)

Potential test requirements

- Water sampling & test (contaminants)
- Fish sampling & test
- Produce sampling & test
- Fish food sampling & test
- Aerator and pump maintenance
- Traceability
- Recall

FIGURE 4.1

One version of an aquaponics operation with food quality and food safety options.

beds or raceways. Basically, water, air, and fish work together in the fish tank, the fish are fed, they respire and defecate adding ammonia and other materials to the fish tank water. The fish tank water is pumped into the bio-filter, where, through the miracle of nitrification, ammonia is turned into nitrites and nitrites into nitrates. The water is now rich with nutrients needed by the produce and is pumped from the bio-filter into the grow beds. Lettuce, onion, or other seedlings may be placed in the grow beds in cinder or some other media or might simply float in Styrofoam floats with their roots in the nutrient rich water. The plants grow and the produce is harvested, inspected, and packaged for the market. The fish are also harvested at an acceptable market weight and are usually sold live to restaurants, markets, or through distribution.

That's how the basic process is often setup, but many simpler or more complex setups are currently in existence. Numerous items are added to the basic system to produce and maintain a balanced state.

The figure also shows a significant number of potential food quality process concerns, food safety hazards, and potential test requirements. Not shown are the critical control points for each hazard. Control points are included in the flowcharts presented below.

In the box entitled, potential food quality process concerns note that the team has brainstormed as many process quality issues that they could visualize at planning time. From the fish food, fish, water, pH, water hardness, and alkalinity issues, the team expanded the list to include quite a number of variables needing consideration. Although that box considers food quality process concerns, a similar team exercise is held to list food safety concerns. The result is that both food safety and food quality process concerns must be addressed in the overall plan.

FOOD SAFETY AND FOOD QUALITY PLANNING

There is a significant movement toward establishing strong management systems over both food safety and food quality. The Safe Quality Food (SQF) Institute, for example, has established a level three opportunity for food suppliers to significantly increase food quality. SQF 1000 Level 3 focuses on producer food safety and food quality. Process controls will become increasingly important as the new Food Safety Enhancement Act is clarified and administrative rules established. I anticipate that over the next few years SQF, the global food safety initiative (GFSI), and ISO requirements will evolve as more important standards. These changes will result in food supplier consolidation as many operations will not be able to compete at increasingly maturing food safety and food quality levels.

There are literally hundreds of different setups for aquaponics systems. This article depicts a generic approach to food safety and food quality planning that might be brought to focus on a typical aquaponics operation. Although there has been quite a bit of peripheral research involving various aspects of aquaponics, the opportunity to integrate some of the research findings into food quality and food safety plans is just beginning to emerge. Aquaponics also provides a unique opportunity to begin to apply HACCP concepts at the producer level. Applying HACCP to the farm is generally avoided as it seems to be rather commonly accepted that farms must continue to be dirty and relatively uncontrollable.

The approach to food safety and quality planning requires the development of a flowchart for each that match requirements researched and outlined on two spreadsheets; one for food safety and one for food quality. In addition, certain management, worker, and facility controls that might not fit conveniently on either flowchart or on the spreadsheets can be summarized as shown in Fig. 4.2. The three boxes serve to summarize criteria that are often found on audit checklists.

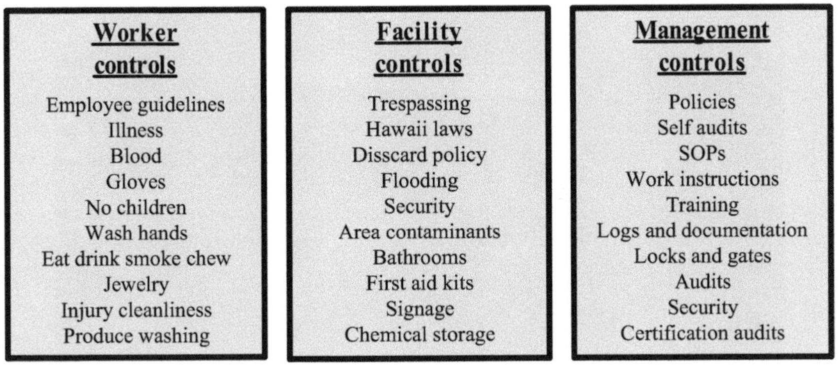

FIGURE 4.2

Worker, facility, and management control considerations.

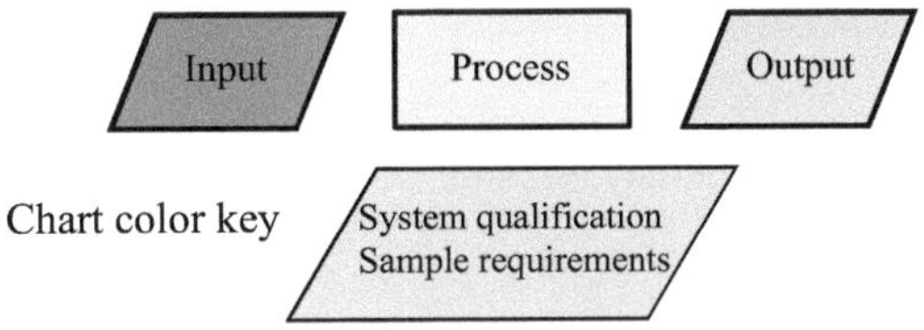

FIGURE 4.3

Plan color coding scheme.

For purposes of clarification, the planning flowcharts and spreadsheets are developed with the intent to show inputs to the system, processes and controls, sample and test requirements, and system outputs. These are color coded in both the flowcharts and spreadsheets so that they might be easily recognized in each document. The color coding is shown as Fig. 4.3.

INPUTS TO AN AQUAPONICS SYSTEM

Fish are an input item to an aquaponics system. Depending on the system design, other inputs include water, fish food, and locally grown *Azolla* (Fig. 4.4) cinders or media that may be used in the biofilter, the plants grown in the raceway, worms (and castings) occasionally used, bacterial seed cultures used to speed up biofilter development. The requirements for physical structures and water flow systems are excluded from this paper but can be added to more extensive food safety and food quality plans. Often aquaponics farms establish their own germination beds to provide plants for the grow beds (Fig. 4.5).

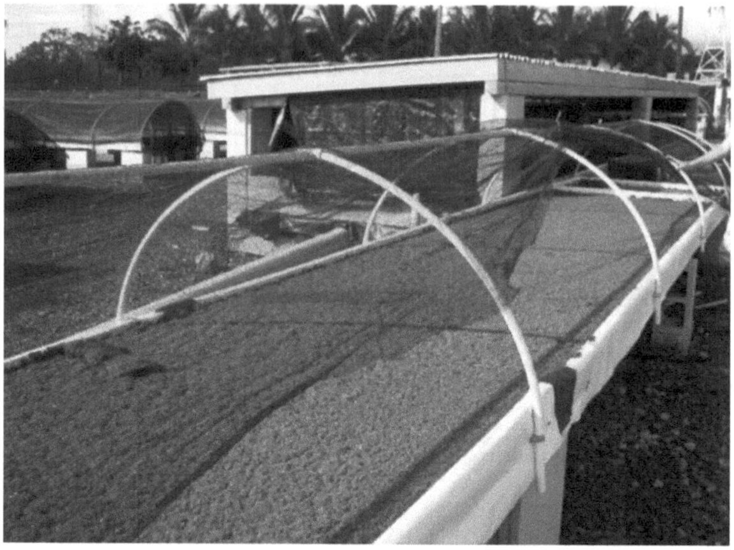

FIGURE 4.4

Inputs: growing *Azolla* as a secondary fish food.

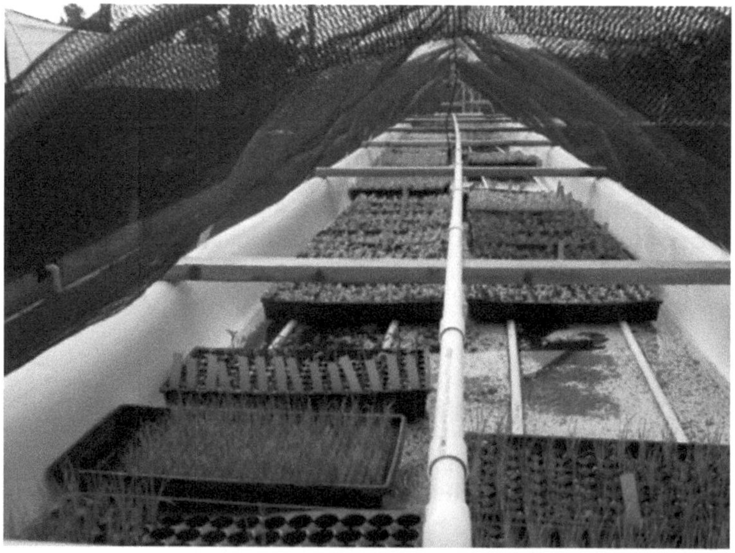

FIGURE 4.5

Inputs: aquaponic seed germination beds.

Fig. 4.6 includes four parts and is a partial spreadsheet showing each input variable, the potential risk, hazard and an example of the procedures to be followed. For instance, the incoming water could be potentially contaminated with metal, chemicals, or biological agents and should be sampled annually at the source (A). The spreadsheet continues through (B), (C), and (D) and if you were to align the sections

(A)

Variable	Risk	HA	Incoming Procedures
Water 1	Contamination	Metal - TBD	1 annual Sample at Source
Water 2	Contamination	Chemical	1 annual Sample at Source
Water 3	Contamination	Biological	1 annual Sample at Source
Backflow Preventer	Contamination	Illness/Death	Obtain city test results
Fish	Pathogens	Multiple	Certify source of fingerlings
Fish Food 1	Contamination	Metal	Certs/Label/Test
Fish Food 2	Contamination	Chemical	Certs/Label/Test
Fish Food 3	Contamination	Biological	Certs/Label/Test
Fish Food 4	Contamination	Dioxin	Sample and Test Feed

(B)

	Critical	Control Point	
Where to Measure	Measurement Equipment	Measurement Frequency	Spec
At source	Lab Kit/Lab System	Monthly	EPA Limits
At source	Lab Kit/Lab System	Monthly	EPA Limits
At source	Lab Kit/Lab System	Monthly	< 100 MPN/g
At Location	Visual Verification	Annual	N/A
At Source	Lab Kit/Lab System	when supplier changes	Per pathogen limits
Sample	Lab Kit/ Lab System	Annual	Per lab suggestions
Sample	Lab Kit/ Lab System	Annual	Per lab suggestions
Sample	Lab Kit/ Lab System	Annual	Per lab suggestions

(C)

Treatment Under Spec	Treatment Over Spec	Corrective Action	Reassessment	Traceability System	Recall Procedures	Complaint Management
N/A	Stop Production	Automatic Failure	After new source	Electronic Preferred	Per Recall SOP	N/A
N/A	Stop Production	Automatic Failure	After new source	Electronic Preferred	Per Recall SOP	N/A
N/A	Stop Production	Automatic Failure	After new source	Electronic Preferred	Per Recall SOP	N/A
N/A	Stop Production	Repair BF System	After Repair	N/A	Per Recall SOP	N/A
N/A	Reject at incoming	Qualify new supplier	Retest new vendor	N/A	N/A	N/A
Terminate vendor	Terminate vendor	Qualify new supplier	Retest new vendor	Traceability required	Inventory Control	N/A
Terminate vendor	Terminate vendor	Qualify new supplier	Retest new vendor	Traceability required	Inventory Control	N/A
Terminate vendor	Terminate vendor	Qualify new supplier	Retest new vendor	Traceability required	Inventory Control	N/A

(D)

			Documentation	
SOP	SOP #	SOP #	WI	Logs/etc.
Water Test and Recall SOPs	1.00	2.00	WI 1.0 & 2.0	Test data/logs
Water Test and Recall SOPs	1.00	2.00	WI 1.0 & 2.0	Test data/logs
Water Test and Recall SOPs	1.00	2.00	WI 1.0 & 2.0	Test data/logs
Building Codes	1.00	2.00	City Test WI	Maintenance Log
Incoming Certification SOP	2.00		WI 3.0 (FISH)	Records on File

FIGURE 4.6

Food safety planning example for input controls (A) Input variables; (B) critical control points and specifications; (C) specification limits, corrective action, traceability and recall requirements; and (D) standard operating procedures (SOP), work instructions (WI) and documentation logs.

left to right, you would have the top few lines of the spreadsheet. In the interests of space for this article, the remainder of the Food Safety Planning spreadsheet and the entire Food Quality Planning spreadsheet are eliminated.

In the spreadsheets and the flowcharts that follow, the system is flowing from left-to-right, from water input, through the fish tanks and biofilters across grow beds and then recycled back to the fish tank.

Notice that in Fig. 4.6B, critical control points are defined somewhat. Quality professionals commonly divide defect types into three categories: critical, major, and minor. The primary idea for such definitions is to help establish priorities for product process controls. Assuming that, a product can have a critical defect of some type, it makes sense to focus on fully preventing critical defects first and once the potential for such critical defects is near zero then focus on major defect types. To quality control professionals, defects are the results of hazards but to a great extent are usually visible or measurable making them easy to count and analyze using statistical techniques.

Fig. 4.7 shows the accompanying flowcharts for water input controls for both food safety and food quality control plans. The plan shows concern over maintenance of the back flow preventer, a divergence of approaches are based on various sources of water, sample points, pass/fail decision points along with logging of data, disqualification of water sources, and potential corrective action loops. As the flowcharts presented below are somewhat lengthy, they have been truncated in an attempt to show side-by-side comparisons between the food safety plan and the food quality plan.

Complete food safety and food quality process control flowcharts are included in the appendix.

As with the spreadsheet planning phase, the flowcharts are sectioned and presented on the basis of the process flow components including water input, fish tank and biofilter controls, grow bed controls and harvest, and shipping controls.

Incoming controls such as the fish tank and biofilter controls become increasingly complicated. Fish food is an input and must be certified or sampled and tested for various contaminants as noted in the spreadsheet. There are also significant concerns on the food quality process controls side with the storage of the feed. The delivery of feed on the basis of the growth rate and size of fish becomes increasingly important as a process and product quality control. In some aquaponics operations, bacterial seed mechanisms are used to start the biofilter and these too must be strictly controlled (some aquaculture systems use cattle manure and urine to seed biofilters). Water, fish manure, vermicast, and cinders (grow media) are all sampled for testing in the food safety chart. Data are logged, corrective action cycles are established for both the fish tank and the biofilter. Water pumps and aerators are important food quality controls (Fig. 4.8).

The system continues flowing into the produce grow beds (Figure 4.10) which are often called raceways. If pesticides and fertilizers are used, the water may be

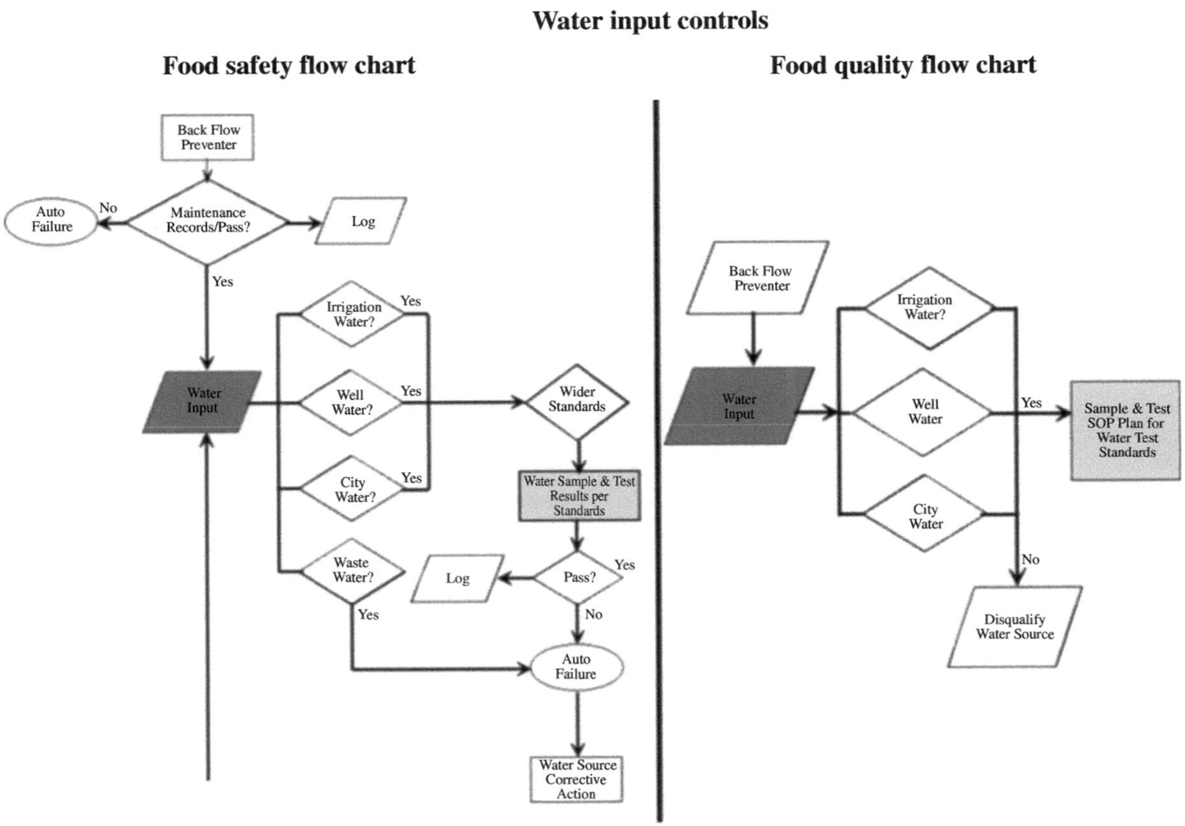

FIGURE 4.7

Food safety and food quality input controls.

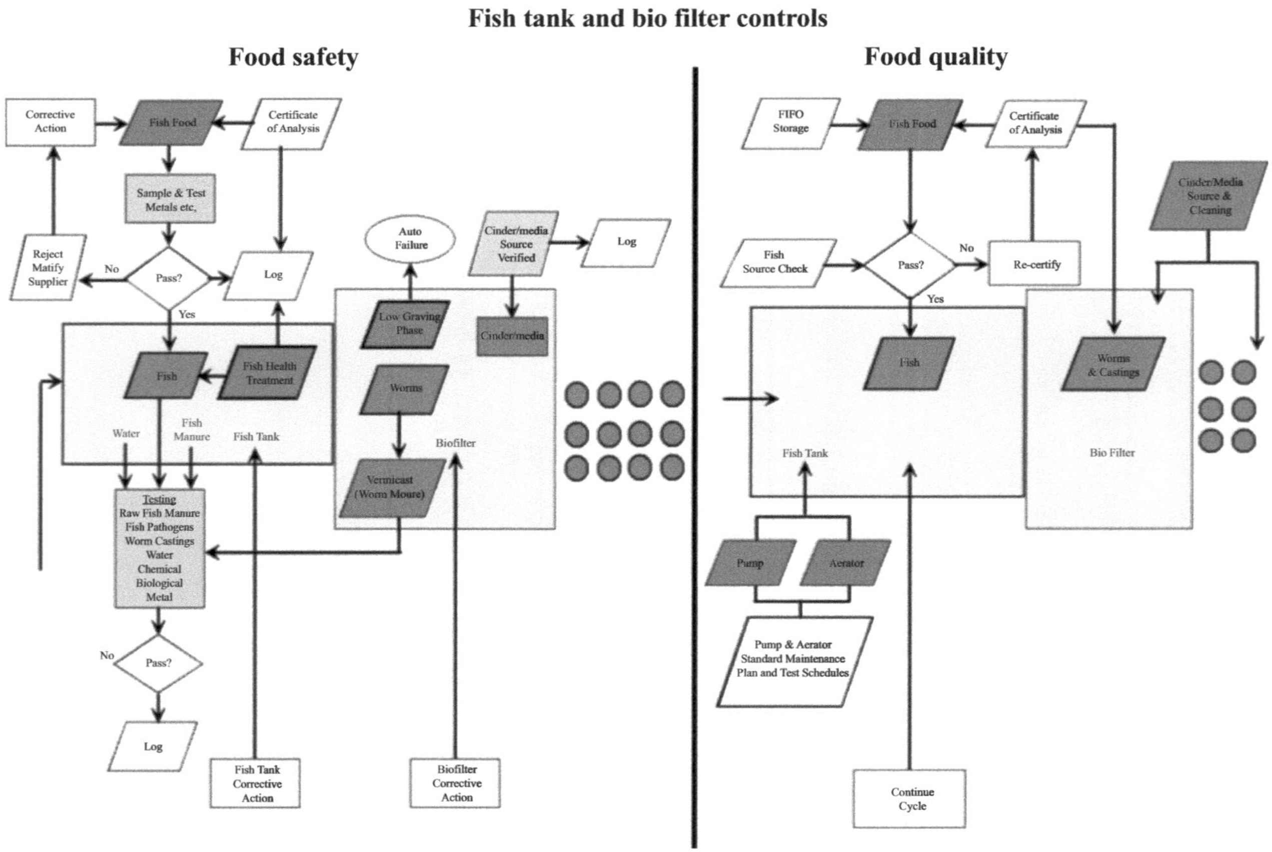

FIGURE 4.8

Incoming controls.

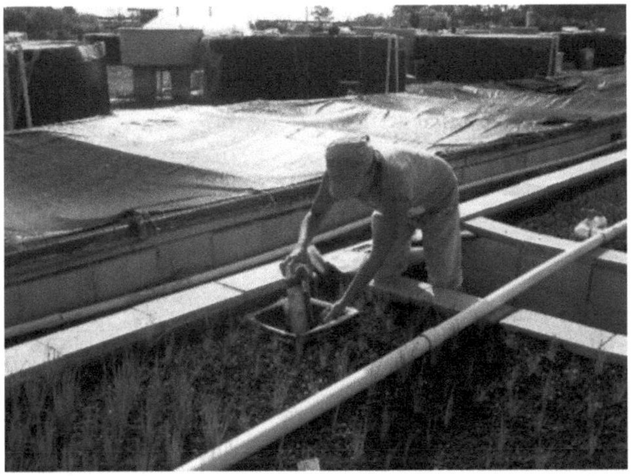

FIGURE 4.9

Checking siphon valve functionality.

sampled and tested on the food safety side, whereas on the food quality side, they may be adjusted to attain maximum produce growth and yield based on visual inspection. Obviously, samples are taken and, when needed, other inputs are added to bring the pH up or down, adjust for nitrate and nitrite levels that are too high or too low, adjust for dissolved oxygen. Other fertilizers may be added. Pesticides may be used. These are all input items that impact the quality and safety of both fish and produce.

Fig. 4.9 shows an employee checking a siphon valve in one of the grow beds.

The final section of the flowcharts and spreadsheets are dedicated to the harvest, inspection, test, and shipping operations (Fig. 4.12). On the food safety side, traceability components come into play to facilitate any need for recall. Data recording and corrective action loops are defined and feedback is established to all preceding operations. Fig. 4.11 shows a typical cucumber harvest.

Figs. 4.14 and 4.15 are difficult to read within the publication space restrictions but are shown here to illustrate what the entire food safety and food quality flowcharts would look like when completed.

The evolution of such plans depends on the attention to detail and the farm manager's willingness to do all possible to protect consumers. There are still a lot of "old farm" attitudes. Resistance to change is a predominant player. But for those farmers that seek to take a leadership role to assure the success and protection for their operations, food safety and food quality planning is a must.

The final food safety flowchart and the food quality flowchart both provide a quick and easy visual representation of the overall final plan. Keeping this initial plan

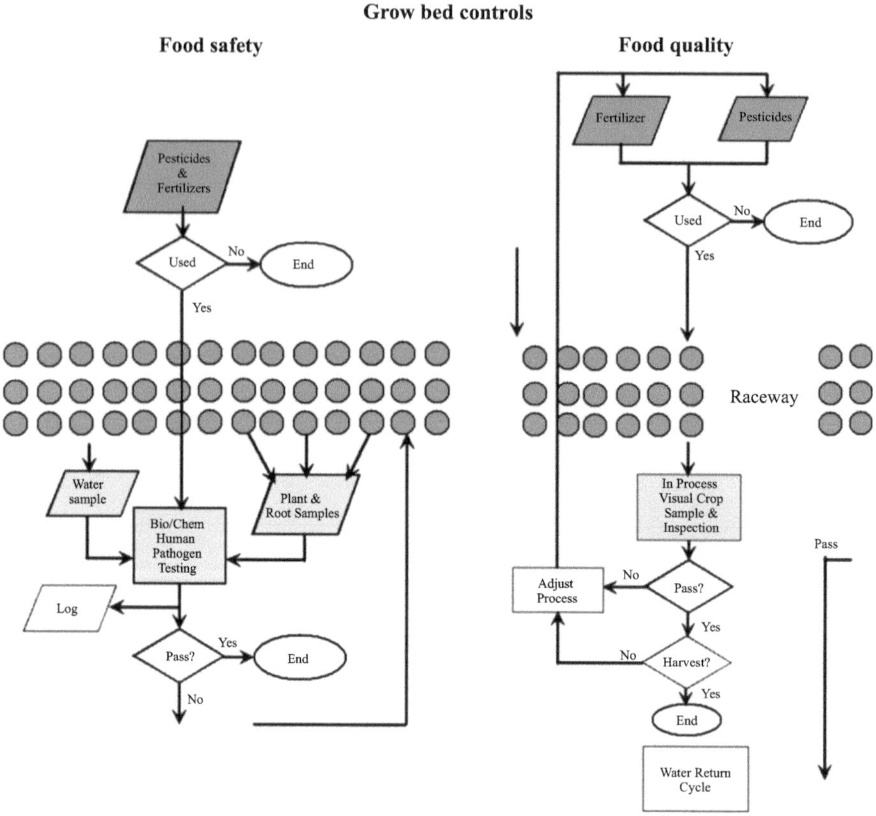

FIGURE 4.10

Food safety and food quality grow bed controls.

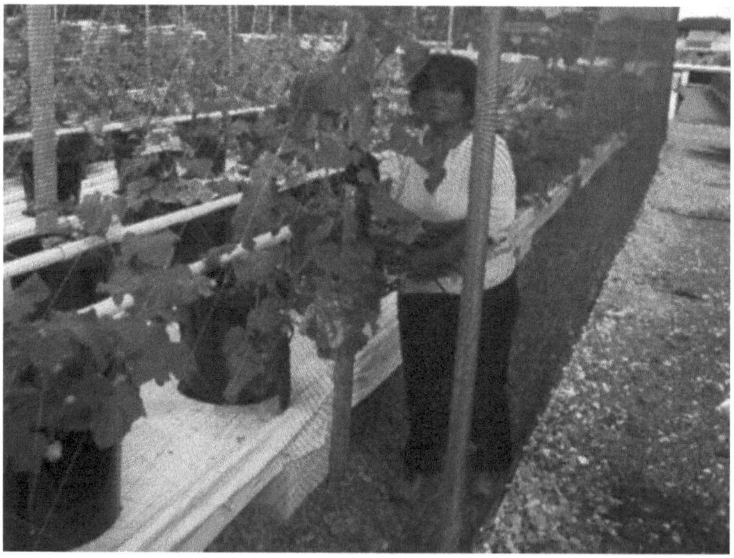

FIGURE 4.11

Harvest.

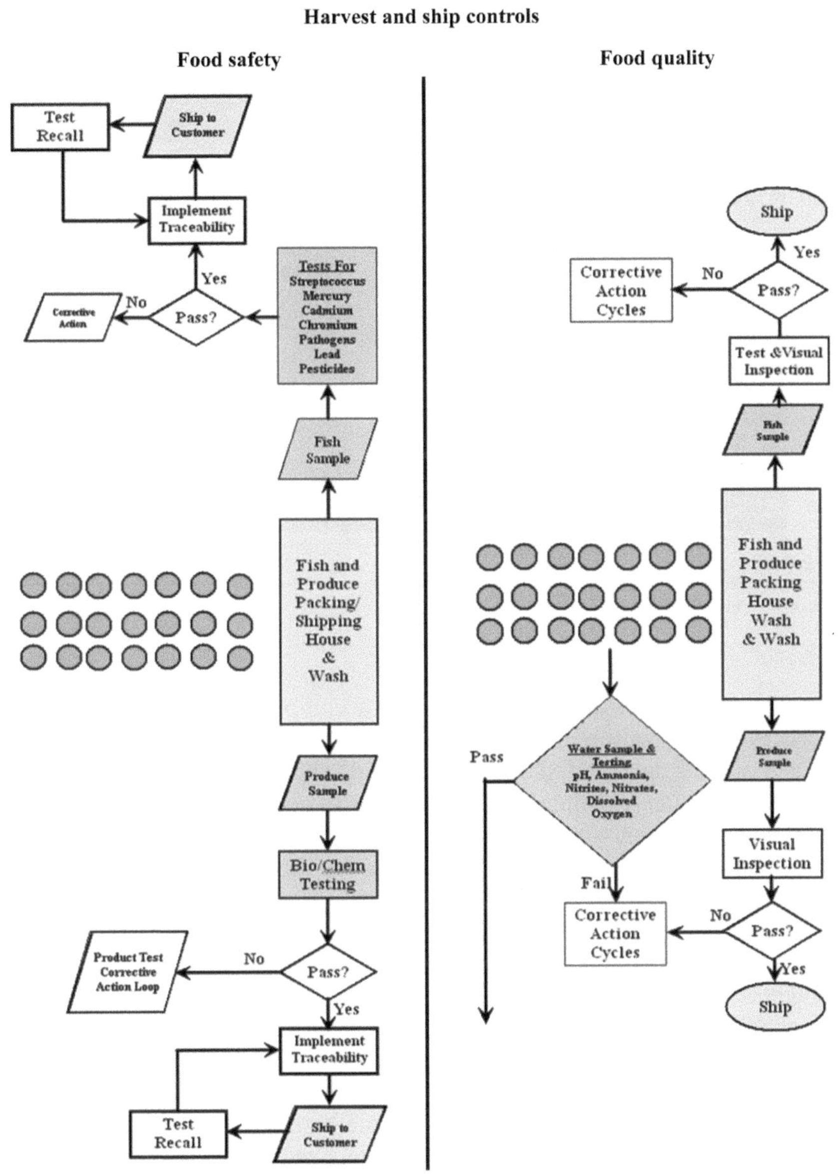

FIGURE 4.12

Food safety and food quality harvest and ship controls.

visual, a flowchart display allows for any individual to quickly review and work on any specific part of the process and provides complete a complete and easily updatable document for any internal or external auditor or preventive controls individual to review and check its adequacy.

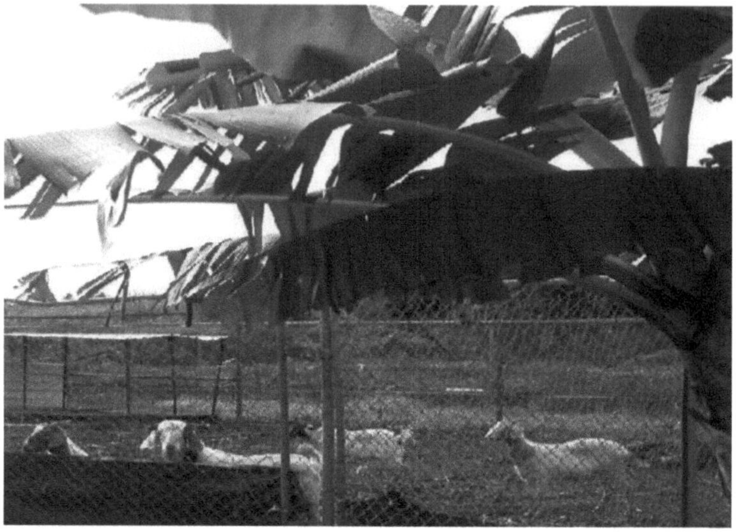

FIGURE 4.13

The unknown contaminant.

The sample plan presented above isn't quite complete but is intended to stimulate process visualization and definition. There are many other inputs, process steps, and outputs that need to be considered in addition to those illustrated in the sample above. As an example, preventive control practices require that verification of plan implementation, and validation practices are followed. By expanding the sample flowcharts and spreadsheets a bit, those strategies can be further detailed.

Although HARPC and HACCP requirements still loom out there, the information from the flowcharts and excel spreadsheets are easily transferrable to other forms that might be required. For instance, take a look at Fig. 4.16. The form calls for definition of the process step, critical limits, and monitoring procedures. Details from the flowchart and the excel sheets can be easily transferred onto the HACCP planning sheets.

Taking that a step further, Fig. 4.17 asks for a bit of detail for each process step, the hazard that could impact the product or process and preventive measures. Again, the information from the flowchart and the excel spreadsheet can be easily transferred to this HACCP form.

Fig. 4.18 is an example of how the hazard analysis details can be transferred from the flowcharts onto a HACCP sheet for a ground pork sausage hazard analysis.

The aquaponics example illustrated in this chapter is only used to serve the need to take a visual and detailed approach to planning. Obviously, any process can be

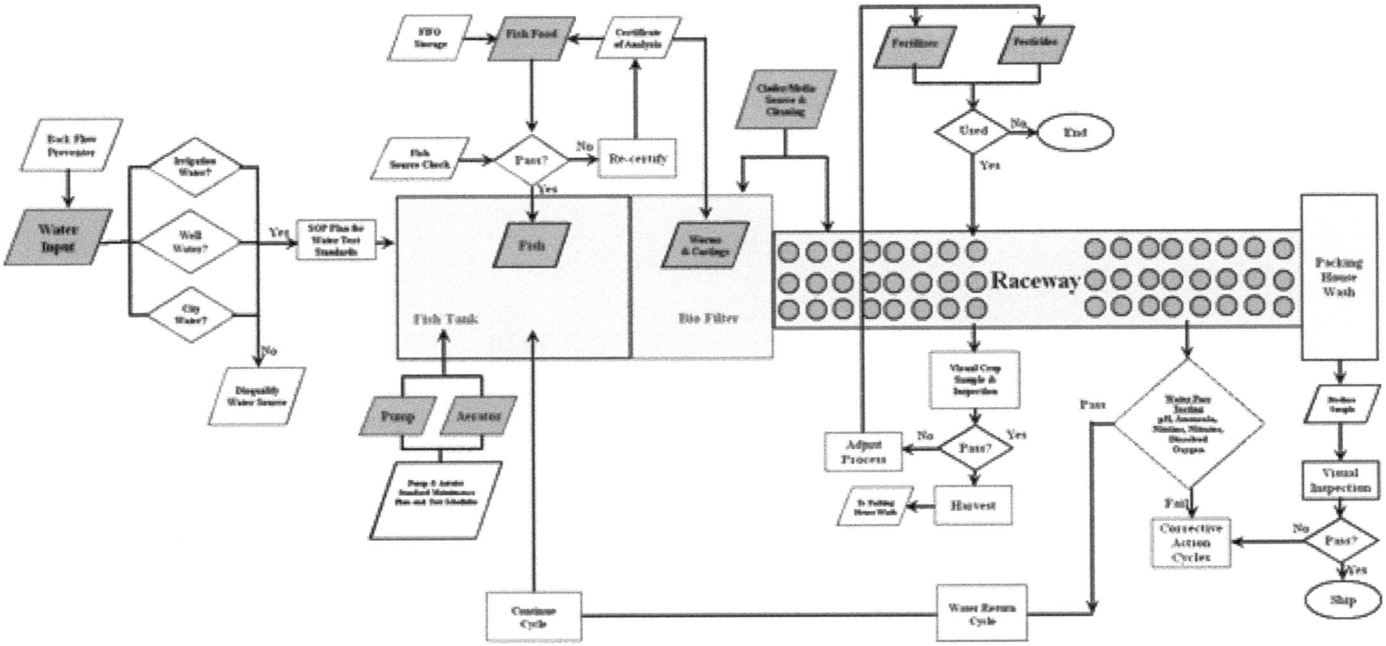

FIGURE 4.14

Aquaponics food safety system qualification flowchart.

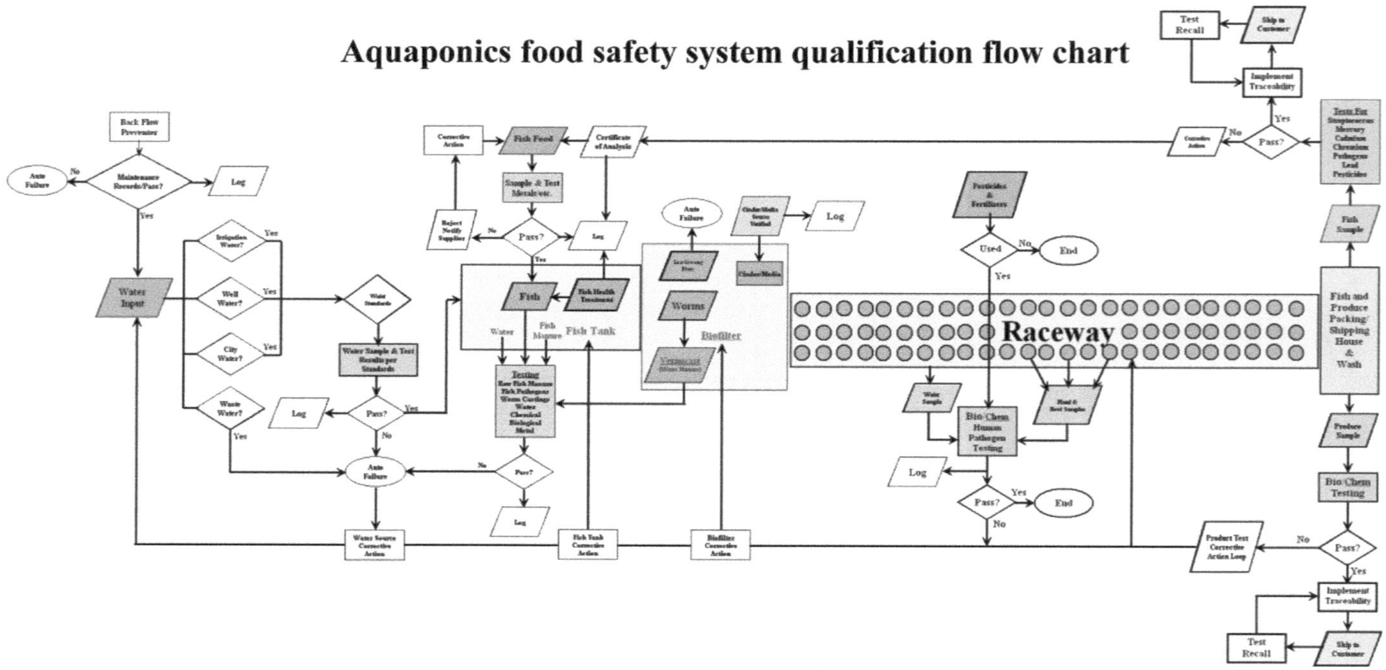

FIGURE 4.15

Aquaponics food quality system qualification flowchart.

HACCP PLAN DEVELOPMENT FORM: MONITORING PROCEDURES AND FREQUENCY		
PROCESS CATEGORY:		
PRODUCT:		
PROCESS STEP/CCP	CRITICAL LIMITS	MONITORING PROCEDURES *(WHO/WHAT/WHEN/HOW)

FIGURE 4.16

Standard HACCP monitoring procedures form.

HAZARD IDENTIFICATION/PREVENTIVE MEASURES		
PROCESS CATEGORY:		
PRODUCT:		
PROCESS STEP	FOOD SAFETY HAZARD	PREVENTIVE MEASURE(S)

FIGURE 4.17

Hazard identification/preventive measures form.

HAZARD ANALYSIS – RAW PRODUCT, GROUND – Fresh Pork Sausage

Attachment 6

Process Step	Food Safety Hazard	Reasonably Likely to Occur?	Basis	If Yes in Column 3, What Measures Could be Applied to Prevent, Eliminate, or Reduce the Hazard to an Acceptable Level?	Critical Control Point
Receiving - Meat	Biological: Pathogens - microbial (*Salmonella, Escherichia coli 0157:H7)*	Yes	Either pathogen may be present on incoming raw product.	Letters of guaranty that supplier meets base line criteria or in process control of room temperature or storage temperature to prevent growth	1B
	Chemical – None				
	Physical – Foreign materials	No	Plant records show that there has been no incidence of foreign materials in products received into the plant.		
Receiving – Nonmeat Ingredients/Packaging Materials	Biological – None				
	Chemical – Not acceptable for intended use	No	Letters of guaranty are received from all suppliers of nonmeat ingredients and packaging materials.		
	Physical – Foreign materials	No	Plant records demonstrate that foreign material contamination has not occurred during the past several years.		

HACCP PLAN

PROCESS CATEGORY: ______________________________

PRODUCT EXAMPLE: ______________________________

CCP# and Location	Critical Limits	Monitoring Procedures and Frequency	HACCP Records	Verification Procedures and Frequency	Corrective Actions

Signature: ___________________________ Date: ____________________

FIGURE 4.18

HACCP hazard analysis sample sheet.

diagramed and flowcharted and the details for preventive controls established using excel or some other simple planning form. Every process is different and every process can follow the same planning strategy. The strategy presented above can be adapted to any process needing preventive controls.

REFERENCE

[1] J.M. Ryan, Developing food safety and quality plans: an aquaponics process control example, Food Safety Magazine, September 18, 2012.

CHAPTER

Preventive system data analysis strategies for common and assignable causes

5

This chapter includes some statistical and mathematical approaches to analysis of data resulting from various data collection points that tend to evolve and change throughout continuous improvement cycles. Three basic types of data analysis that can be easily applied by common cause teams (CC teams) working on common causes and FIT teams working on assignable causes. These include:

- Solution tracking sheets (STSs) (used by both CC and FIT teams)
- Statistical process control (SPC) (primarily used by FIT teams)
- Cycle time analysis (used by both CC and FIT teams)

USING SOLUTION TRACKING SHEETS

Prevention requires a strategy that can be used to statistically determine the impact of changes made in pursuit of causes. The idea is that if one can show that a potential cause for a problem can be modified or eliminated, the problem should also be eliminated. To do this, a causal relationship has to be theorized, changes made and the impact of the changes should show up in terms of the disappearance of the problem.

Causal relationships exist everywhere and aren't too difficult to understand. In an ordinary course in statistical analysis, the idea of correlation is explored. As a matter of fact, correlation is central to many statistical or scientific studies. However, if a general approach to determining causal relationships can be taught to people afraid of statistics or with basic math skills, the ability to solve complex problems can be placed under the control of the people that actually do the job rather than trying to bring in a consultant or some other person more experienced in validation practices.

The team approach lends itself to applying group thinking in pursuit of the ever elusive causes that are related to many problems. When the planning, reporting, environmental sampling, statistical analysis, and other requirements related to preventive controls are all influencing an operation's control over its processes, a clear and standardized approach to getting control is needed.

Fig. 5.1 is a standard report format for what is called the STS. The STS is a team form and serves multiple functions. It is a record of measured environmental factors,

Validating Preventive Food Safety and Quality Controls. DOI: http://dx.doi.org/10.1016/B978-0-12-810994-6.00005-5

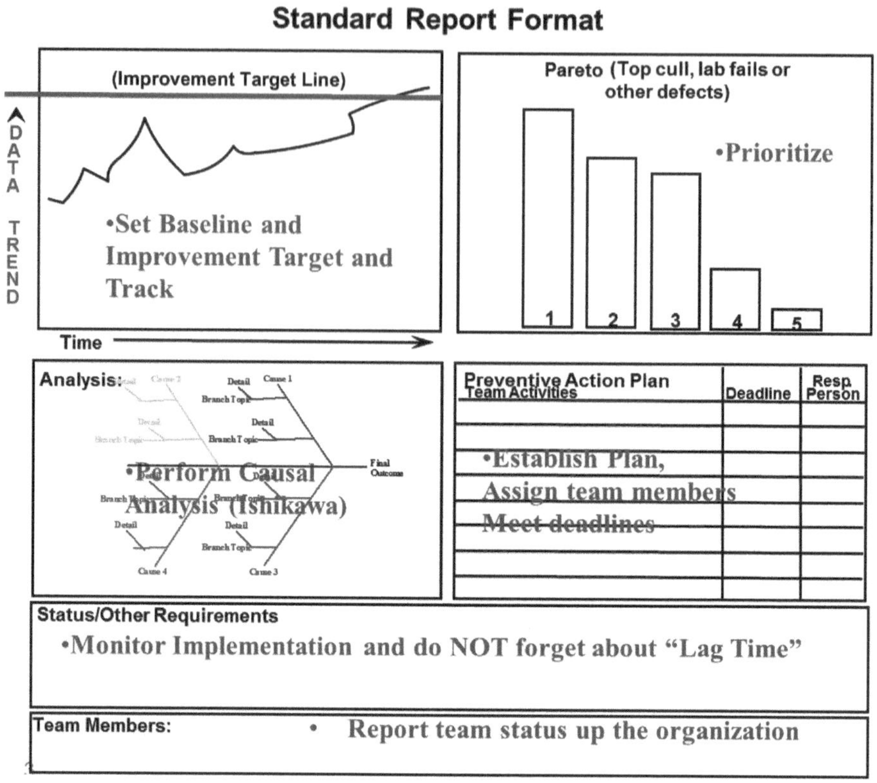

FIGURE 5.1

Solution tracking sheet (STS).

causal analyses, defect analyses, team member involvement, process improvement trends, process baselines, and team successes and failures. The strategy presented by the STS and associated statistical strategies has a single goal: To gain control over errant processes that threaten food safety.

Put simply, when food safety issues arise and are found through measurement or recall, those issues are a clear indication of a company's inability to control processes that threaten human health. Efforts focused on preventive control mean that a company and its employees are actively working on gaining control over errant processes. The STS strategy presented here is intended to allow those people most knowledgeable about a process to understand that they can and must get in control of the process rather than just tending the process. Being in control of a process means that the team members can manipulate it to do whatever they choose to make it do. Being in control of a process is not something employees are normally capable of. Most often, employees are simply a part of the process with little or no control over either the process or their own activities.

The STS provides team members with both control responsibility and control authority.

The STS is a single page form consisting of six sections. The upper left hand quadrant is reserved for plotting three things:

1. The process baseline capability at the start of the improvement project.
2. A trend line depicting weekly or daily process measurements.
3. A team established goal or target line. When the process data exceeds the target line in some way, the team has reached the improvement goal.

The upper right quadrant is reserved for showing the type of defects that are to be considered for control. In our example, three types of bacteria are found in six lines that process raw chicken parts. The team goal is to bring the levels of bacteria to minimum and safe levels. This quadrant is used for what is called a Pareto analysis. The Pareto analysis is nothing more than a bar chart that visually shows the defects in the order of occurrence from most to least from left to right. The Pareto analysis is intended to help focus the team on the most common type of defect found from the process at any point in time.

The lower left part of the STS is reserved for displaying or noting the result of the team's effort to prioritize potential causes. In this case, the fishbone diagram or Ishikawa strategy is used to help the team dig deeply into why problems are occurring. The combined team member knowledge is critical in the causal analysis aspect of the overall solution attempt. It is expected that different team members will bring different levels of knowledge and different perspectives to bear on the problem. Causal analysis discussions are noted on the fishbone diagrams to help the team members visualize relationships and to help them dig deeper into what or who might be causing the overall problem. The fishbone diagram most commonly considers people, machines, equipment, the environment, materials, and processes as contributors to the overall problem although other prime contributors may be used in the analysis.

The lower right part of the STS is reserved for preventive planning. Using the data, trends, defect analysis (Pareto), and the fishbone results, each team member is expected to take an action item or two to be completed outside of the weekly team meeting. Generally, the weekly team meeting is used to review the STS, the data analyses, and to develop action items that each member can finish during the work week. The team is expected to spend 1 hour in the team meeting and 1 hour outside of the team meeting completing the assigned action item each week. The lower right part of the STS is used to record each action item or assigned task, when the task is to be completed and the initials of the person assigned to complete that particular task. Completion of each task by the agreed upon deadline is critical to the team's overall success. If an individual team member does not complete the action item agreed on, the results of the overall team effort can be jeopardized. Once a team member agrees to complete an action item by a certain deadline, the team member must complete the action item on time.

At the bottom of the STS is a section reserved to add status or other requirement notes. It is critical for the team secretary when filling out the STS to place a date in this section. The STS is part of a critical record keeping system that establishes the organization's approach to valid preventive controls. When kept by date, the STS file for a particular problem may have dozens of records, and these records must be kept by date to establish a clear trail of activities focused on continuous improvement.

The last section to be found on the STS is to record the names of team members who have attended the team meeting each week. Attendance at team meetings is critical to assure that different perspectives are focused on the problem at hand. Overall, the time allocated to food safety process improvement is about 2 hours per week for each team member. Meeting time and the time it takes to complete action items are preventive activities. If no time is spent by employees working on prevention, prevention of food safety issues will not occur.

ESTABLISHING BASELINES

We can understand the STS if we study each section separately. Starting in the upper left corner, the objective is to establish the baseline measurement of the problem we are concerned with and then to track the measurement of that problem over time as we continually experiment with potential causes by removing them or attempting to reduce their impact.

Baselines are important. We can take almost any problem and measure it several times without making any changes to any process. This is usually done with historical data or data that has been collected as part of some ongoing data system.

For example, suppose that lab personnel have been taking samples of raw chicken parts from different production lines. The chicken parts sampled were sent to the lab and tested for enterobacteriaceae such as *Escherichia coli*, salmonella, and campylobacter. Table 5.1 shows the results of such testing from a previous study:

Table 5.1 FSIS Sampling Survey Data [1]

Microorganisms Indicator Organism [1]	Sample Collected at	Number of Samples Tested	Number of Samples Quantifiable [2]	Percent Positive (%)
Aerobic plate count	End of production line	2496	2467	98.84
Enterobacteriaceae	End of production line	2496	2402	96.23
Total coliforms	End of production line	2496	2208	88.46
Generic *Escherichia coli*	End of production line	2496	1554	62.26
Pathogenic organism				
Salmonella [3]	End of production line	2496	657 [3]	26.32
Campylobacter	End of production line	2496	534 [4]	21.39

From the table, at the end of the production line, the testing found 88.45% of 2496 samples had a quantifiable level of total coliforms. *Escherichia coli* showed up 26.32% of the time and campylobacter was quantified on 21.39% of the samples. If the sampling had been going on for some time, we could use those findings to establish a baseline. For instance, we might say that on the average, we expect to find *E. coli* about 62% of the time.

We could draw a line on our STS in the upper left hand box at the 62% level as our starting point. In reality, we would probably measure *E. coli* in the lines over periods of time (maybe every week) and plot the findings in the upper left hand box. The line would go up and down for unknown reasons, but we would expect the average to be about 62% if we made no changes to the process.

MAINTAINING MEASUREMENT VALIDITY

In this example, we have a problem identified (*E. coli* in the raw chicken part production lines) and we know the level of positive findings in our normal process (62%). Although the lab personnel take samples every week, we have an established environmental sampling plan in place. With some discussion with the lab manager and personnel, we would want to get agreement regarding the fact that we would not want sampling or testing procedures to change during our attempts to solve the problem of high levels of contamination in the production line. If the method of sampling or testing changed during our attempts to get control over the problem, we wouldn't know whether changes in our data were because of changes to the test or sampling strategy or due to some changes we made to the production line. Once we begin to establish baseline and trend measurements, we need to assure that our measurement strategy remains reliable and repeatable.

Unfortunately, in some companies, it has been observed that a manager or someone will intentionally change the sampling, measurement, testing, or reporting strategy in an attempt to manipulate the data with the intent of showing "improvement" when there has been no change to the process. Taking samples and analyzing data sometimes provides evidence that processes are not being managed properly and those responsible for such management and control are not capable of or do not know how to control the process properly. Hence, the data is manipulated, generally as a result of pressure felt to "solve the problem" when the individual who is supposed to solve the problem does not know how to solve the problem.

The STS strategy described here is designed to relieve such pressures and make problem solving a team activity. Stabilized and standardized sampling, test, and reporting should continue throughout the entire set of team activities related to the identified problem.

Table 5.2 shows the CFU/mL test results for six manufacturing lines for week 1. There were 30 samples taken overall, one sample taken from each line each workday.

The team's job is now to calculate the daily averages and ranges from the data. If we look only at Monday's data (Table 5.3), we can calculate the overall process average and range for that day.

Table 5.2 Raw Data: 1Sample Set (Week 1)

	Sample Day				
Line	**Mon**	**Tues**	**Wed**	**Thurs**	**Fri**
A	190	320	1200	750	1300
B	0	12	3245	903	140
C	4700	2341	988	750	2309
D	890	933	563	909	1124
E	2409	456	890	3211	11
F	3564	900	2	357	1100

Time →

Table 5.3 Monday Data for Six Manufacturing Lines

Line	**Mon *x***
A	190
B	0
C	4700
D	890
E	2409
F	3564

To calculate the process range, we simply take the highest test result and subtract the lowest test result from that number. The highest test result for Monday was found in line C with a count of 4700. The lowest test result was in line B with a count of zero. 4700–0 = 4700, which is our range for Monday.

Note that an "*x*" is used to represent each score. For example, line A for Monday was 190 CFU/mL. The value of "*x*" for line A on Monday was 190. To determine the average of all Monday scores, we will use the following formula for a sample mean:

$$\text{Sample mean} = \frac{\text{sum of x}}{\text{n}}$$

where x is a score, n is the number of scores, and sum of x is the addition of all the scores together.

If we add up all the Monday scores and divide by the number of scores ($n = 5$), the result is the average raw chicken process contamination score for Monday. If an Excel spreadsheet is being used to help record and control raw data, finding the total for all of Monday's data is easy. The calculations are simplified (Fig. 5.2) by using the summation symbol (arrow).

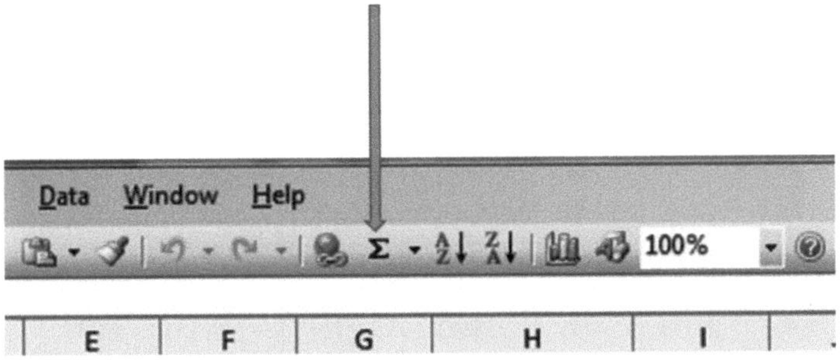

FIGURE 5.2

Excel summation symbol.

Table 5.4 Calculating Daily Averages

Six Lines	Mon	
A	190	
B	0	
C	4700	
D	890	
E	2409	
F	3564	
Day total	11,753	
Day average	1959	=SUM(I12/6)

The daily total (or sum of x) is shown in Table 5.4 as 11,753. When the summed number is divided by the number of samples taken on day 1 (6), the daily average is 1959 CFU/mL.

The rest of the daily averages can be calculated in the same manner and, if interested, line averages can also be calculated as shown in Table 5.5.

For the reader wishing to attempt a couple of challenges, the STS upper left hand corner needs to have daily averages plotted, the overall average calculated and the overall average plotted across the daily averages. Complete the following team or individual exercises:

1. Create a trend plot of the daily averages
2. Calculate and plot the overall average
3. Draw the overall average (baseline) on your plot

You can use the Excel Chart Wizard (Fig. 5.3) line function

Your plot of averages should look similar to Fig. 5.4:

To estimate the overall process average for week 1, you need to add up all daily scores to get the "Day Total" then add the five days total scores together to calculate

Table 5.5 Final Calculations

	Sample Day						
Line Number	**Mon**	**Tues**	**Wed**	**Thurs**	**Fri**		**Line Avg.**
A	190	320	1200	750	1300	3760	752
B	0	12	3245	903	140	4300	360
C	4700	2341	988	750	2309	11,088	2218
D	890	933	563	909	1124	4419	884
E	2409	456	890	3211	11	6977	1395
F	3564	900	2	357	1100	5923	1185
	11,753	4962	6888	6880	5984		
Daily average	1959	827	1148	1147	997		

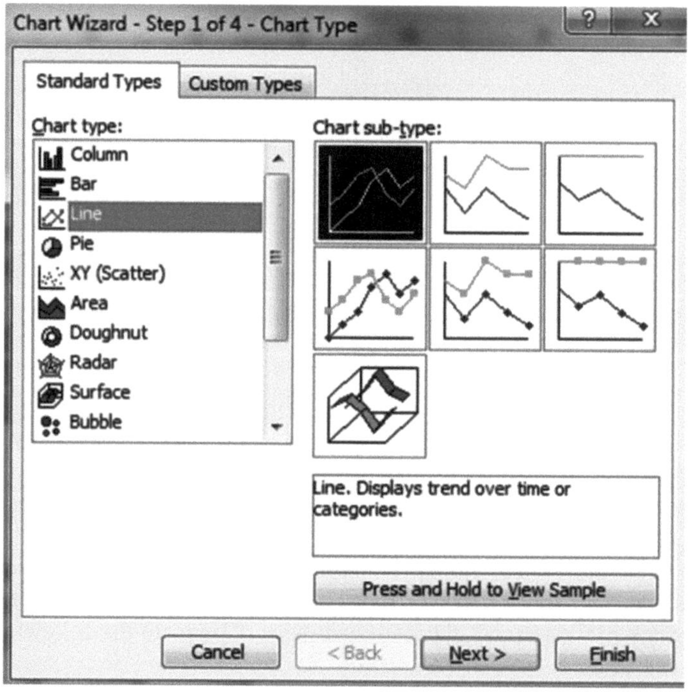

FIGURE 5.3

Excel trend line function.

the week total (36,467) and divide by the total number of scores for the week. There are 5 days and six lines. The total number of scores is five times 6 or 30. Dividing 36,467 by 30 equals 1215.6 (Table 5.6).

Now, plot the overall process average over the daily average trend line as shown in Fig. 5.5.

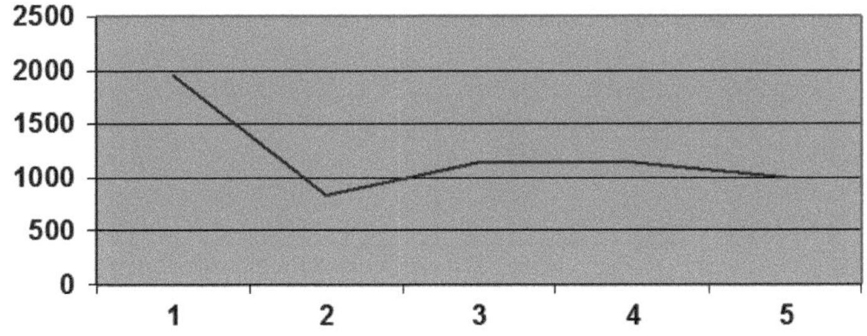

FIGURE 5.4

Basic week 1 trend (Monday through Friday).

Table 5.6 Calculate the Overall Process Average

Line Number	Mon	Tues	Wed	Thurs	Fri	Line Total
A	190	320	1200	750	1300	3760
B	0	12	3245	903	140	4300
C	4700	2341	988	750	2309	11,088
D	890	933	563	909	1124	4419
E	2409	456	890	3211	11	6977
F	3564	900	2	357	1100	5923
Day total	11,753	4962	6888	6880	5984	36,467
Day average	1959	827	1148	1147	997	**1215.6**

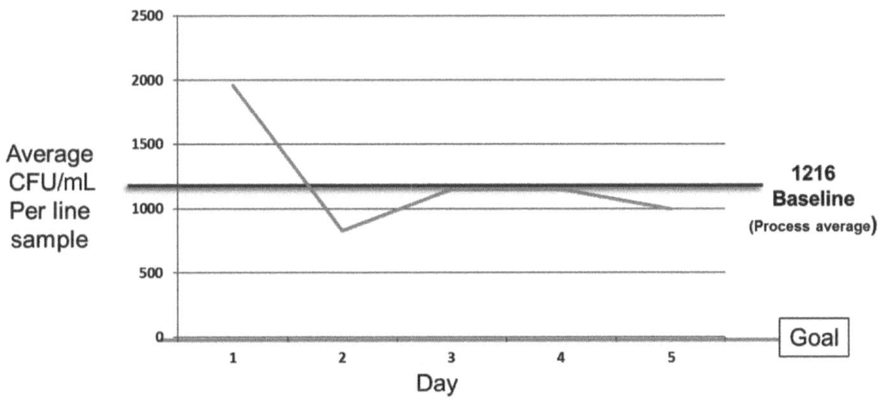

FIGURE 5.5

Estimated process trend and baseline process average.

Table 5.7 Unorganized Bacteria Findings

	% Pos
Campylobacter	27.4
Salmonella	62.3
E. coli	44.9

Table 5.8 Reorganized Bacteria Data

	% Pos
Salmonella	62.3
E. coli	44.9
Campylobacter	27.4

That completes the upper left hand corner of the STS for week 1.

To complete the Pareto analysis (upper right hand corner of the STS), we will use the following data from week 1 (Table 5.7).

From the data, we can see that 62.3% of the samples were tested and found positive for salmonella, 44.9% were positive for *E. coli*, and 27.4 were found positive for campy. We need to create an organized bar chart (Pareto analysis) to help viewers clearly see prioritization of causes (or contributors) to contaminated chicken from manufacturing lines.

Team exercises:

1. Create a bar chart (Pareto analysis) for this data
2. Organize the bars from high to low (left to right)
3. Create a cluster plot of the first week's data for team analysis

When you reorganize the bacteria data, the data should look like Table 5.8.

Using Excel, select the column function in the Excel Chart Wizard (Fig. 5.6) and use the reorganized bacteria data to create a final Pareto analysis.

The final Pareto analysis for week 1 should like Fig. 5.7.

The reason that the Pareto analysis is set up to show the most occurring problem on the left and the least occurring problem on the right is to cause the team members and others to quickly identify the number one issue. In this case, salmonella accounts for a large percent (almost half) of sampling failures. If the team focuses on salmonella and is successful in eliminating salmonella in the process, the overall contamination trend will be greatly reduced thereby yielding great process food safety improvements.

Assuming that salmonella is greatly reduced through team causal analysis and team actions, the next target would be *E. coli*. In reality, a single solution or combination of process changes might go a long way to reducing all three bacterial contaminants. However, generally one problem area needs to be attacked at a time, and the team needs to work with a mind to continuous improvement.

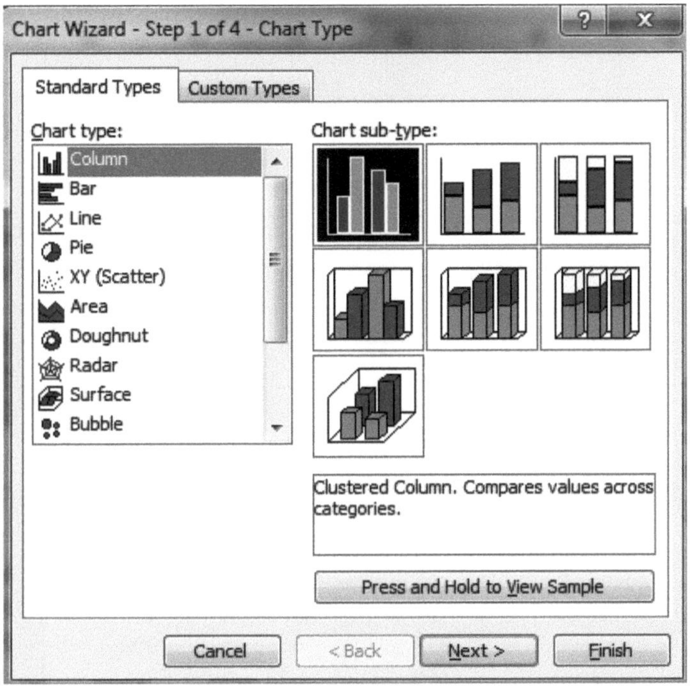

FIGURE 5.6

Excel chart wizard column function.

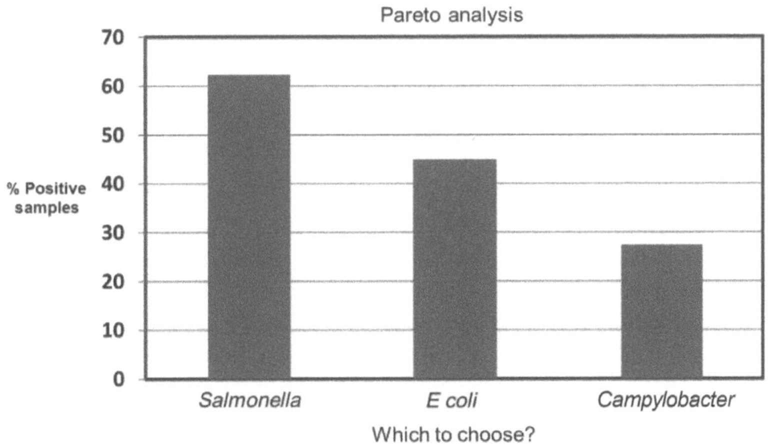

FIGURE 5.7

Week 1 Pareto analysis.

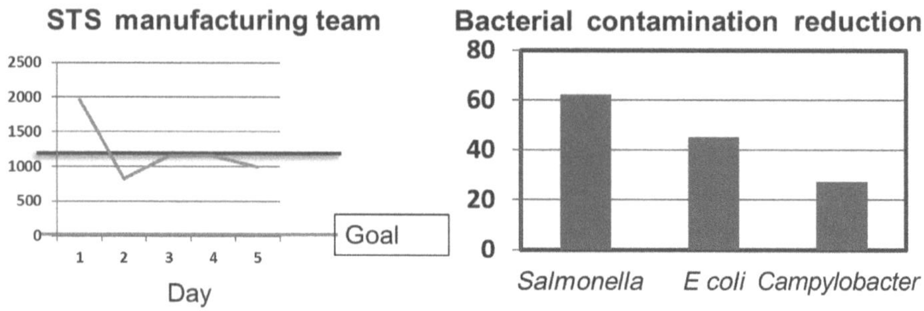

FIGURE 5.8

Week 1 trend and Pareto analyses.

Table 5.9 Raw Sample Data from Week 1

Line Number	Mon	Tues	Wed	Thurs	Fri
A	190	320	1200	750	1300
B	0	12	3245	903	140
C	4700	2341	988	750	2309
D	890	933	563	909	1124
E	2409	456	890	3211	11
F	3564	900	2	357	1100

When the final trend and Pareto analyses are added to the STS, the upper two sections of the STS should look like Fig. 5.8.

With this baseline analysis, the team should hold a team meeting to do the following:

1. Visually inspect the raw data and discuss observations
2. Run a cluster analysis of the raw data and discuss
3. Develop an Ishikawa fishbone diagram to discuss potential causes
4. Develop team action items and record the action plan on the STS.

Review the raw data from week 1 (Table 5.9).

Circle high and low sample values (Table 5.10) in the week 1 data.

Some questions can be discussed among team members in an initial attempt to begin isolating potential causes. For instance, why does Monday have two of the highest contamination scores in lines C and F while line B shows zero contamination? Why do Monday samples indicate that Monday lines are more contaminated than any other day? Also, why does line C show the highest overall line contamination average?

The idea is that different team members who work in these processes might know details about people, maintenance, sanitation, and other issues that managers or

Table 7.10 Identifying High and Low Sample Patterns from Raw Data

	Sample Day						
Line Number	**Mon**	**Tues**	**Wed**	**Thurs**	**Fri**	**Total**	**Line Avg.**
A	190	320	1200	750	1300	3760	752
B	0	12	3245	903	140	4300	860
C	4700	2341	988	750	2309	11088	2218 ← Highest Line
D	890	933	563	909	1124	4419	884
E	2409	456	890	3211	11	6977	1395
F	3564	900	2	357	1100	5923	1185
Total	11753	4962	6888	6880	5984		
Day Average	1959 ↑ Highest Day	827	1148	1147	997		

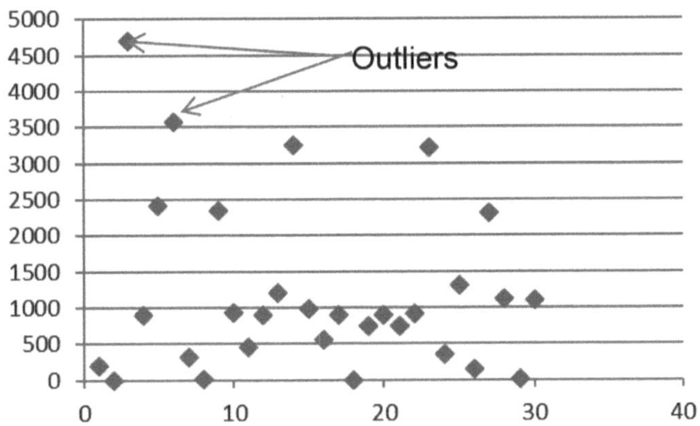

FIGURE 5.9

Week 1 Raw data cluster plot.

supervisors might not know. The team leader can lead the discussion and listen carefully to team member questions and responses.

Are the supervisors or sanitation maintenance practices for different lines different? Were raw chicken parts that were run in line C from a particular farm or source?

If a cluster plot is developed using the Excel function, Fig. 5.9 results. It is easy to identify two high flying outliers.

The cluster plot gives the team a second look at the data. Maybe, there are actually two processes going on as shown in Fig. 5.10. The lower circle seems to indicate that the process has a much average lower contamination level than might have been indicated by the baseline calculation arrived at and plotted on the STS. There are

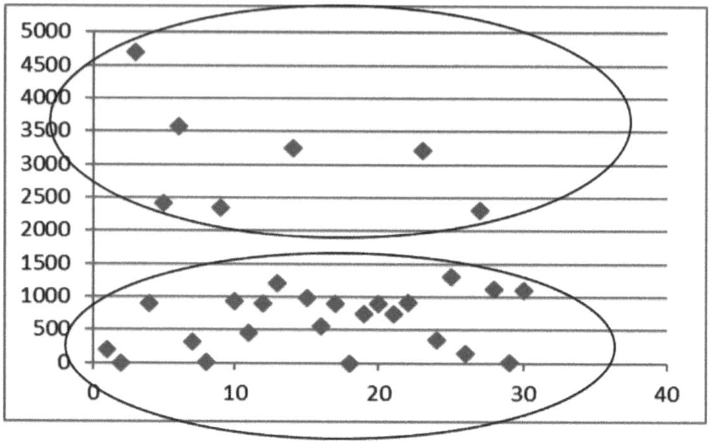

FIGURE 5.10

Identifying process patterns using cluster plots.

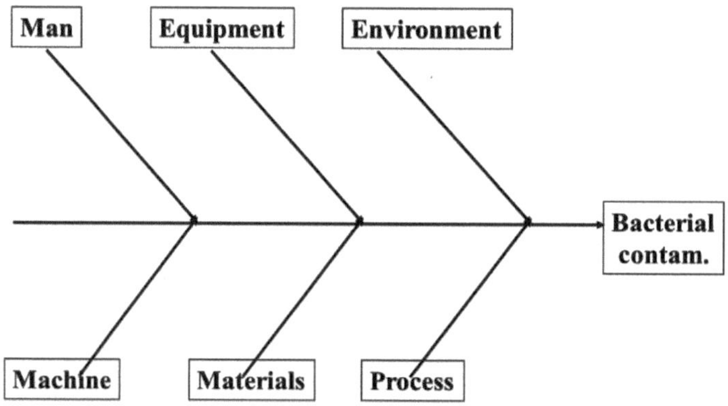

FIGURE 5.11

Fishbone diagram.

several sample findings that seem to be outside of the normal process and are pulling the overall process average up.

Remember from the team discussion that all team members are encouraged to participate and offer suggestions. Suggested causes should be noted in preparation for using the Fishbone (Fig. 5.11) diagram to begin to isolate potential causes. Sometimes, this figure is called the "Five Whys" or the Ishikawa diagram which is named after the initial developer of the idea. Note that at the right side of the fishbone, bacterial contamination is identified as the problem and on each of the fish's ribs are primary potential causes for the contamination. Since manufacturing processes consist of interactions among people, equipment, machines, materials, the environment, and process particulars, the analysis usually begins with those major potential causes. The problem now becomes one of brainstorming by asking the question "Why" over and over until the team believes it may have isolated a cause that they can work to eliminate.

The team uses the fishbone diagram to discuss and isolate likely causes for the process line contamination. In theory, those working on a functional improvement team are all focused on this manufacturing process, and each member comes from a different point of view because each job has a slightly different focus and function.

Suppose that the team was most concerned about equipment and theorized that the contamination was coming from improper sanitation of the equipment. The causal analysis process starts with the question "Why do we have these contaminants?". The team answers that one potential cause is that the equipment is not being sanitized as it should be thereby carrying contaminants from one processing run to the next. The team leader then asks "Why do you think this is true?" and the team members might answer that there is no standard established for the pressure used for cleaning sprays and that different manufacturing lines are being cleaned with varying cleaning spray pressures. The leader now asks "Why is there no standard for the cleaning spray pressure?". The team could answer that engineering did not specify a standard spray pressure or that maintenance personnel did not implement checks to assure that a standard spray pressure was applied across all lines. Another team member notes that neither engineering nor maintenance personnel bothered to train personnel whose job it was to use the sprayers so that they would use the specified spray pressure.

The team leader uses the fishbone diagram (Fig. 5.12) to note the team's concerns and after the first round of questions regarding spray pressure, the team notes after

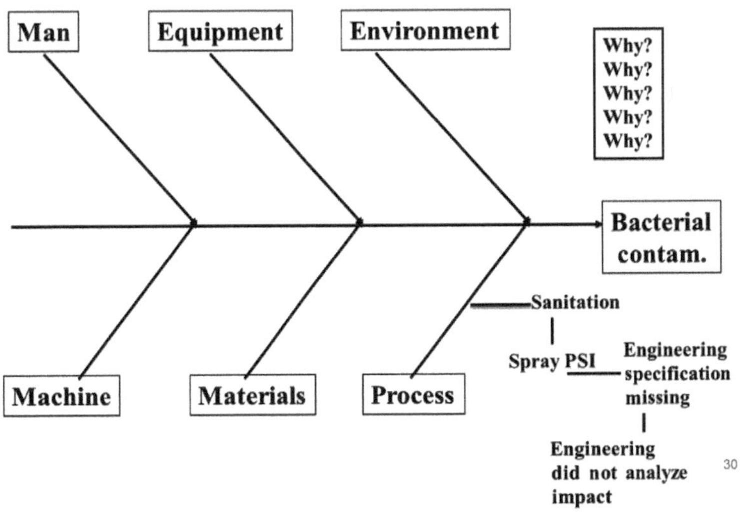

FIGURE 5.12

Causal analysis.

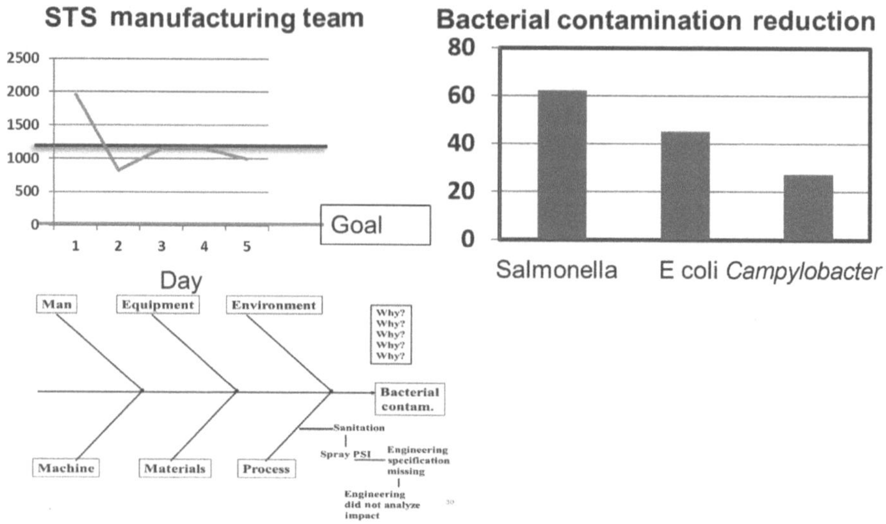

FIGURE 5.13

Manufacturing team STS.

the fifth "Why" that engineering did not take the time to analyze the impact of spray pressures on the removal of bacterial contaminants from the manufacturing line.

This is only round one of the causal analysis, and the team will generally continue for a few rounds listening to other potential causes until several sets of "Why" bones are added to the original diagram.

Once the team has isolated a single potential cause that they tend to agree is the most likely cause and they can take team action to remove that cause, the Ishikawa diagram is copied and added to the STS, thereby completing the third part of the STS (Fig. 5.13).

Notice that the STS is beginning to look like a report card that can be easily explained to other teams or upper management. More importantly, it is an ongoing record of team preventive control efforts that serves as a concise and convenient continuous improvement summary. The STS is an excellent way to show a valid system that employs environmental sampling, statistics, teamwork, and other factors required to validate the operation's preventive control efforts.

At this point, the team is focused on salmonella reduction and believes that there needs to be some attention paid to the spray pressure. There would obviously be additional potential causes identified, but for purposes of this example, the team needs to develop an action plan to attack what they believe to be the cause.

The fourth part of the STS is the preventive action plan located in the middle right hand section. Having chosen to eliminate sanitation spray pressure as a variable, they believe contributes to bacterial contamination in the manufacturing line; the team meeting consists of working on a step-by-step preventive action plan. Brainstorming

Table 5.11 Preventive Action Plan (First Week)

Preventive Action Plan		
Activity	**Deadline**	**Resp.**
Present problem to management	6/1/16	TL
Meet with engineering	6/1/16	JR
Establish PSI Spec	6/6/16	AB
Implement PSI Spec	6/10/16	RS
Run tests	6/10/16	SH
Rerun sampling	6/11/16	ST

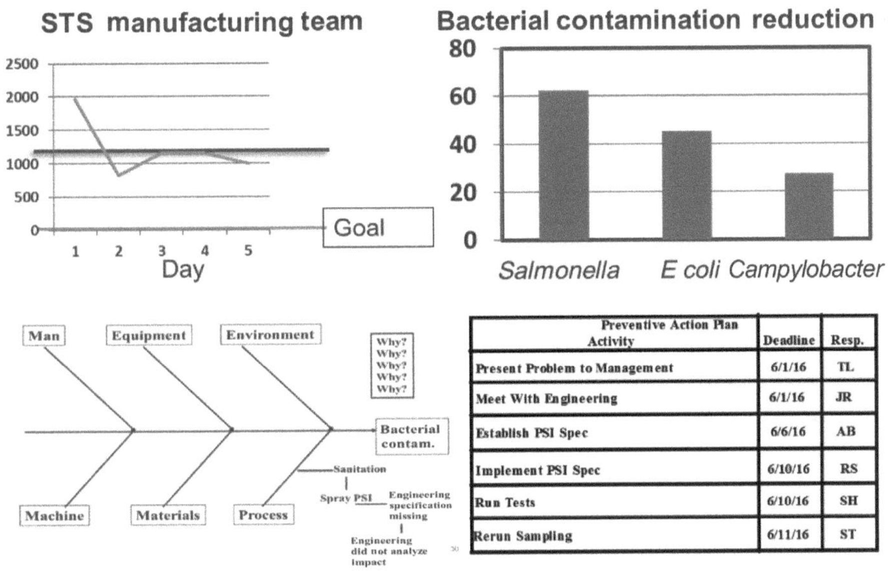

FIGURE 5.14

Adding the preventive action plan to the STS.

the steps required to get a new spray pressure specification established, implemented, and tested, the team knows that new bacteria test sampling needs to be rerun prior to June 11 as shown in Table 5.11.

The preventive action plan is then added to the manufacturing team STS as shown in Fig. 5.14.

To finalize the first week's overall STS, two additional items are added. There is a status section for keeping track of which STS goes first and which ones came later. The status section must include the publication date and which week the plan

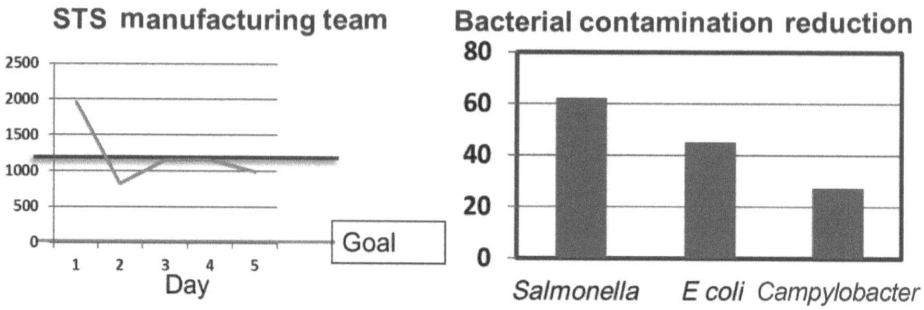

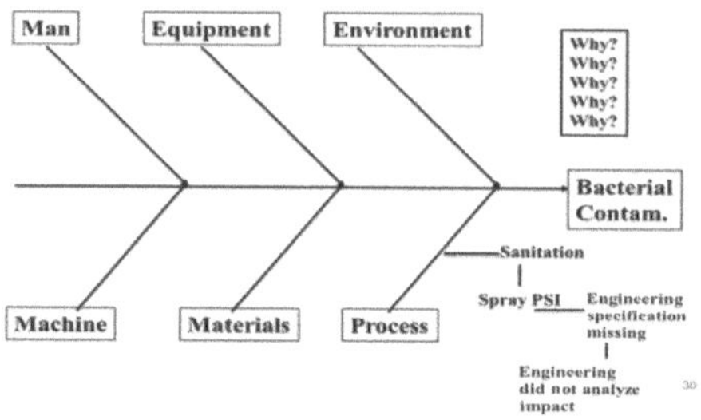

Preventive Action Plan Activity	Deadline	Resp.
Present Problem to Management	6/1/16	TL
Meet With Engineering	6/1/16	JR
Establish PSI Spec	6/6/16	AB
Implement PSI Spec	6/10/16	RS
Run Tests	6/10/16	SH
Rerun Sampling	6/11/16	ST

Status/Other Requirements:	June 1, 2016 - Week 1: Establishing basic causes and plan 1
Team Members:	John Ryan, Richard Stubberfield, Steven Hoch, Alison Day, Michael Carr

FIGURE 5.15

Final week 1 solution tracking sheet.

represents. Also included in this section are notes related to what was accomplished by the team during the week (Fig. 5.15).

The plan is then implemented and new environmental (manufacturing line) sampling for bacterial contamination is completed.

NOTES

1. Lag time: Lag time is a phenomenon that must be considered when looking at data each week. In this example, no lag time is shown. That means that the changes the team made to the spray pressures impacted the lines immediately. Ordinarily, such changes will not show up in sampling data for some time period, perhaps a week or two or more. Teams may be disappointed when reviewing data after making significant process changes and not seeing the impact of the changes evidenced in hard data. Team leaders and members must consider the fact that lag time is the time it takes for the impact of the

process change to actually show up in data. There is a time lag between change implementation and data that might show the impact of the change.

2. Data analysis: When using Excel, sometimes data arranged in one way can cause graphical results such as bar codes or scatter plots to yield incorrect or undecipherable results.
3. Evidence versus proof: Changes to overall trend lines that seem to result from causal analysis and team actions provide evidence to the team that they are on the right track to getting a process under their control. From a scientific perspective, the changes to the process and the corresponding changes that show up in the data provide evidence that the team is on the right track. In statistics, there is no such thing as proof.
4. Continuous improvement: The strategy suggested by the use of the STS is a continuous improvement strategy. When a process that is exhibiting out of control conditions or high levels of hazards, that process cannot usually be brought under control with a quick fix or what has come to be known as "corrective action." Quick fixes do not ordinarily eliminate causes. Continuous improvement practices employ strategies that take time and thought to bring processes under the control of the people responsible for them. Continuous improvement also assumes that out of control processes must be carefully analyzed, are complex and will take considerable time and effort to bring under control. This means that the cycle will be repeated from analysis to planned changes to reanalysis to planned changes over and over again until the team goal is reached or exceeded.
5. Record keeping and reporting: The STS, teamwork, continuous improvement, environmental sampling, hazard analyses, preventive controls, causal analysis, and other issues must be recorded and reported. Under governmental laws, evidence of these activities must show up in for form of historical documentation, record keeping, and reports. The STS becomes a critical and comprehensive document that fulfills many governmental requirements for record keeping and reporting and should be made part of the overall document control procedures and processes.

The results of the sampling are shown in Table 5.12.

Table 5.12 Week 2 Data Sampling Results

Line Number	Mon	Tues	Wed	Thurs	Fri
A	320	190	750	1300	1200
B	45	1165	933	900	2132
C	3267	890	563	827	1124
D	412	1190	1428	900	0
E	457	764	864	988	469
F	784	764	800	563	911

Table 5.13 Second-Week ParetoAnalysis

Bacteria	% Pos
Salmonella	33.2
E. coli	40.6
Campylobacter	25

Table 5.14 Week 2 Test Results

	Line Number	Mon	Tues	Wed	Thurs	Fri	Line Total	Line Avg.
	A	320	190	750	1300	1200	3760	752
	B	45	1165	933	900	2132	5175	1035
After Change One	C	3267	890	563	827	1124	6671	1334
	D	412	1190	1428	900	0	3930	786
	E	457	764	864	988	469	3542	708
	F	784	764	800	563	911	3822	764
	Day Total	5285	4963	5338	5478	5836		
→	Day Average	881	827	890	913	973		

The data were also analyzed for which bacteria tested positive in each manufacturing line. Table 5.13 shows the second-week Pareto analysis (after the first process change from the preventive action plan).

EXERCISE

Week 2 and all subsequent evolutions of the changes follow the same calculation and plotting procedures reviewed above. Using the week 2 (post changes) data shown above,

1. Calculate the daily averages and plot them on the baseline chart (weeks 1 and 2)
2. Recalculate and plot the overall 2-week process baseline (total plot for weeks 1 and 2)
3. Run a Pareto analysis and reorganize it from high to low
4. Run a cluster plot for all raw data
5. Rerun the fishbone exercise discussing new or additional potential causes

Table 5.14 shows the raw data for six manufacturing lines for week 2. The daily averages and the line averages are also calculated. The day averages show less variation than they did in week 1. The range of the daily averages is from 827 on Tuesday to a high of 973 on Friday ($R = 973 - 827 = 146$). Before any line changes were

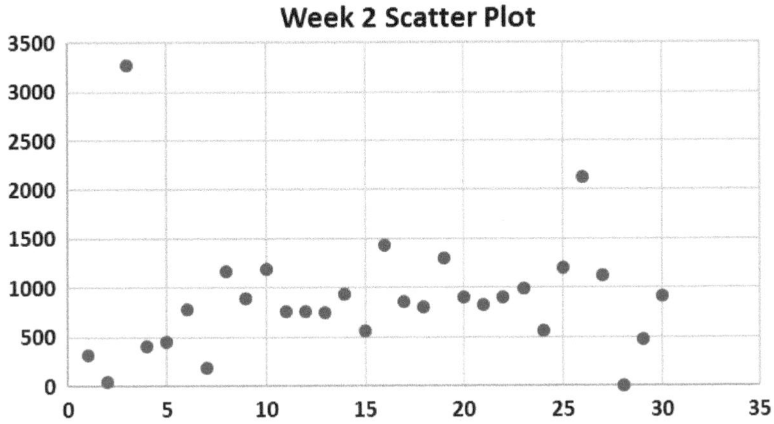

FIGURE 5.16

Week 2 scatter plot.

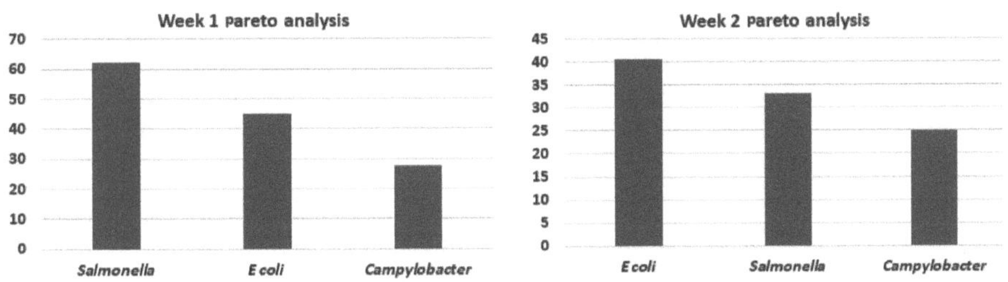

FIGURE 5.17

Weeks 1 and 2 Pareto analyses.

made in week 1, the day range was from 827 to 1959 or $R = 1132$. So, there is some evidence that our change to the process by standardizing the pressures used to sanitize the line may be resulting in less variation. Also, the highest score in week 2 was 3267. A couple of low scores show up on Monday in line B and Friday in line D.

If we run a week 2 scatter plot (Fig. 5.16), we see that there is quite a bit less variation. Something happened on Monday in line C that should be discussed to stimulate the fishbone discussion. Someone on the team may know what caused line C to have such a high count on Monday. The team could also discuss the low scores (line B on Monday and line D on Friday) to determine if any special treatment happened on those lines during the week.

Fig. 5.17 shows the results of the Pareto analysis for weeks 1 and 2 when the data is rearranged to show the highest bar on the left and the shortest bar on the right. If we put the weeks 1 and 2 Pareto analyses side by side, we can see that salmonella has

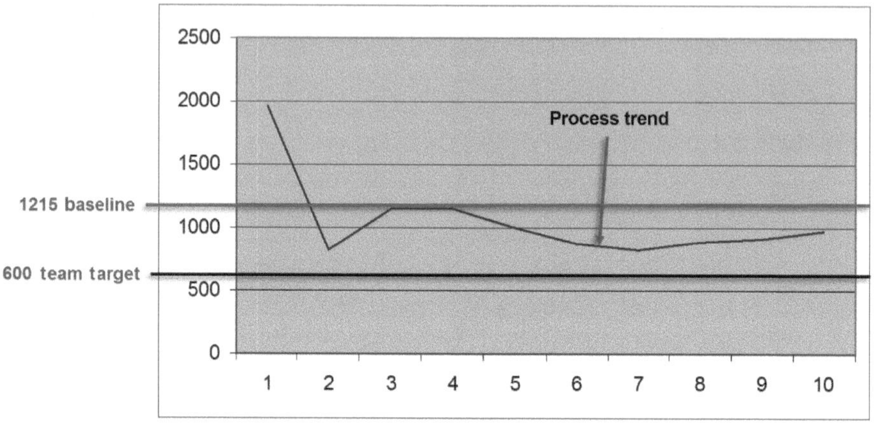

FIGURE 5.18

Weeks 1 and 2 trended on the chart.

been reduced enough to eliminate it from consideration as the top priority. Perhaps, the standardization of spray pressures has had an impact on salmonella contamination. On the basis of the data, salmonella has dropped from a level of 62.1 in week 1 to 33.2 in week 2. That's almost a 50% drop. There is some evidence that spray pressure standardization has helped reduce salmonella levels.

The week 2 daily averages shown in Fig. 5.17 are now plotted on the trend chart. The trend chart now shows both weeks 1 and 2 data points. Fig. 5.18 shows the 2-week trend line, the process baseline measurement (1215 CFU/mL) and a team improvement target (600 CFU/mL).

Notice that the data line has dropped below the process baseline indicating that there might be some reduction in the overall bacterial hazards. If the team feels confident that it can identify other causes and implement needed changes, it might be time to establish an overall goal for an acceptable bacterial contaminant. Recall that the salmonella level dropped by almost 50% from the first process change. It would not be unreasonable for the team to establish an overall 50% reduction target from the baseline. At 1215 CFU/mL for all contaminants, setting a first stage team target at a process average of 600 CFU/mL might be a good starting point. Setting targets keeps the team focused on making incremental and continuous changes in an effort to get improved control over the process and as the team achieves more and more success, the target can be reset to tighten the process further.

Fig. 5.19 shows the beginning of the week 2 STS with a new trend line, team target and Pareto analysis.

The team will continue completing the STS by going through the fishbone and team planning exercises. The STS will be completed during each week's team meeting.

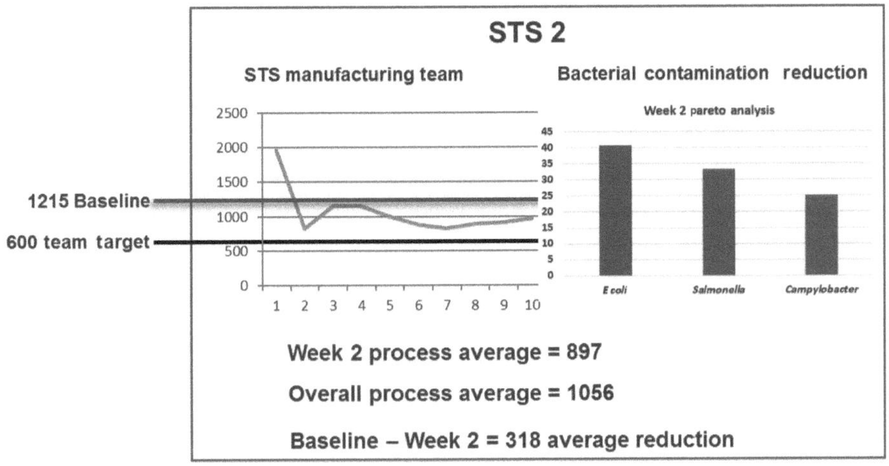

FIGURE 5.19

Week 2 STS.

BASIC STATISTICAL PROCESS CONTROL (SPC) CONCEPTS

Does anyone in the food industry remember or know of W. Edward Deming's 14 points?

Here is a list of Deming's 14 points first published in "Out of the Crisis" (4). Take a minute to read them and think how they apply to the food supply and our control over how food systems may or may not be managed from the farm to the consumer.

The following are the 14 points of Deming:

1. "Create constancy of purpose toward improvement of product and service, with the aim to become competitive, to stay in business, and to provide jobs.
2. Adopt the new philosophy. We are in a new economic age. Western management must awaken to the challenge, must learn their responsibilities, and take on leadership for change.
3. Cease dependence on inspection to achieve quality. Eliminate the need for inspection on a mass basis by building quality into the product in the first place.
4. End the practice of awarding business on the basis of price tag. Instead, minimize total cost. Move toward a single supplier for any one item, on a long-term relationship of loyalty and trust.
5. Improve constantly and forever the system of production and service, to improve quality and productivity, and thus constantly decrease costs.
6. Institute training on the job.
7. Institute leadership. The aim of supervision should be to help people and machines and gadgets to do a better job. Supervision of management is in need of overhaul, as well as supervision of production workers.
8. Drive out fear, so that everyone may work effectively for the company.

9. Break down barriers between departments. People in research, design, sales, and production must work as a team, to foresee problems of production and in use that may be encountered with the product or service.
10. Eliminate slogans, exhortations, and targets for the work force asking for zero defects and new levels of productivity. Such exhortations only create adversarial relationships, as the bulk of the causes of low quality and low productivity belong to the system and thus lie beyond the power of the work force.
    a. Eliminate work standards (quotas) on the factory floor. Substitute leadership.
    b. Eliminate management by objective. Eliminate management by numbers, numerical goals. Substitute leadership.
11. Remove barriers that rob the hourly worker of his right to pride of workmanship. The responsibility of supervisors must be changed from sheer numbers to quality.
12. Remove barriers that rob people in management and in engineering of their right to pride of workmanship. This means, inter alia, abolishment of the annual or merit rating and of management by objective.
13. Institute a vigorous program of education and self-improvement.
14. Put everybody in the company to work to accomplish the transformation. The transformation is everybody's job" [2].

There is a good deal of discussion nowadays about food quality versus safety. Deming is well known for helping to improve quality, but can the quality concepts he espoused do the same for food safety? If you re-read his 14 points, you might come to realize that our food supply chain is in need of exactly the types of changes recommended by Deming 30 years ago. Food safety and food quality go hand in hand. Both rely on and can be seriously impacted by the food industry and its ability to improve services.

You should have noticed that all of Deming's 14 points are focused on management attitudes and actions. Some specific management contributors to poor food quality systems were discussed in Chapter 1, Background: Understanding Common and Assignable Causes, Laws and Costs to give the reader a perspective focused on what needs to be done industry-wide.

From Deming's perspective, 85% of quality problems are caused by management actions or inactions and are represented by common or system causes, whereas 15% or so come from what he calls "assignable causes." Certain programs that will soon impact preventive controls as they are applied to food safety are based on the ideas that both management and assignable causes must be addressed if food safety programs in production, processing, packing holding, distribution, transportation, retail, and restaurants are to resolved.

BASIC CONCEPTS FOR ASSIGNABLE CAUSES

SPC is focused on assignable causes. SPC allows for an objective measurement, tracking and analysis of process trends.

In this section, SPC and Six-sigma are covered to provide a basic statistical foundation in support of valid preventive controls. SPC and Six-sigma are just a couple of the tools from the quality side that can be easily applied to food safety issues. Both quality and food safety issues result from a lack of control. The objective of the team approach, the STS, SPC, and Six-sigma are all the same: To objectively quantify, analyze, and eliminate causes for problems so that people may attempt to get control over them. The assumption that people, with management responsibilities or not, can get control over processes to prevent problems from recurring is basic to quantitative approaches. The statistical or quantitative approach merely takes the emotion out of the issues.

Fig. 5.20 represents what is known as a theoretical normal process distribution of sample means attained from sampling in the raw chicken line. When we looked at the STS, we calculated the means for each set of samples for the six manufacturing lines each day. We ended up with five daily averages (means) each week and we plotted those sample means on the STS trend chart.

In Fig. 5.20, the average (or mean) of all samples is 1959 CFU/mL. The curved line represents the assumption that if all samples were analyzed (maybe thousands), and the sample means were piled up without the bell shaped (normal) curve, most of the scores would be near the 1959 average, whereas fewer and fewer scores were a good deal lower or higher than the average. A statistician would say that the probability of finding a sample mean as high as 5000 would most likely be found because of some specific or assignable cause (5000 is far above the 1959 average). There would be far less than one chance in 100 that a sample mean that high would be found if the process was under control or without either a managerial cause or assignable cause for the high score.

Indeed, Fig. 5.21 is a breakdown of the likely distribution of sample means. With the average or norm in the middle, the figure shows that one would expect 99.74% of all sample means to gall between the two points shown on the curve. Those two points are normally represented as ±3 standard deviations. 95.44% of the sample means would fall between ±2 standard deviations and 68.26% of the sample means would fall between ±1 standard deviation. Only a very small percent (100 − 99.74 = 0.26) of the sample means would fall beyond ±2 standard deviations. The point being that process samples can be statistically analyzed this way, and if we know how to plot or trend sample means like we did with the STS, we can begin to determine whether or

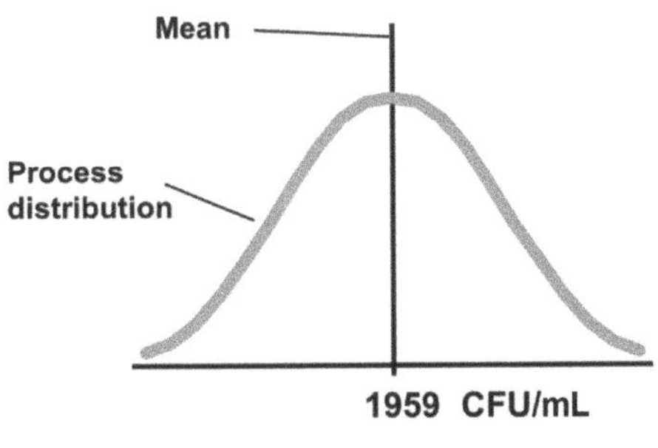

FIGURE 5.20

Normal distribution of sample means.

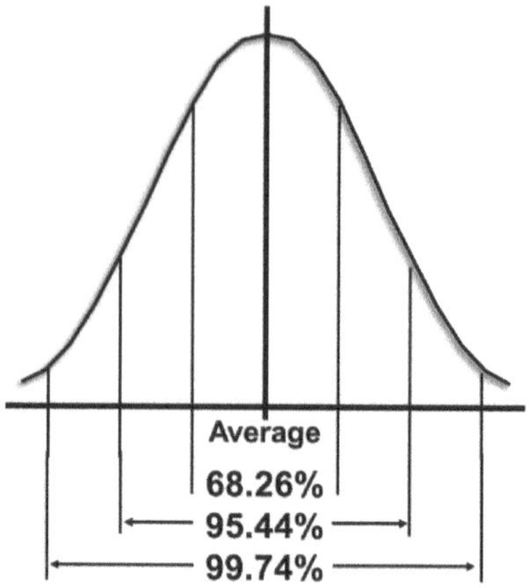

FIGURE 5.21

Likelihood of sample means distribution.

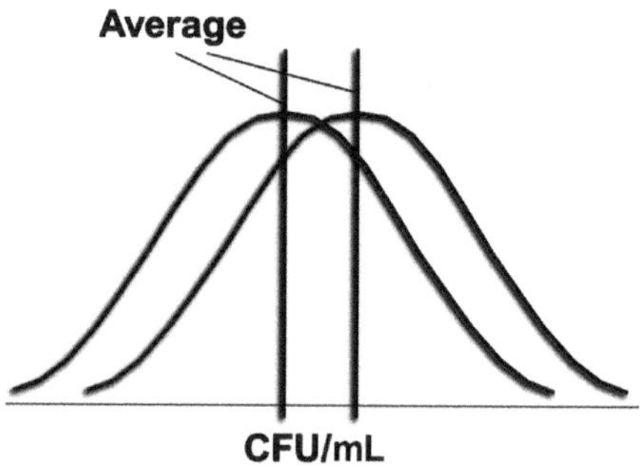

FIGURE 5.22

Shift in the average.

not we have achieved some type of process control through the changes we make to procedures, ingredients, spraying, sanitization, or whatever else we might be doing to control any particular process.

If the process we were sampling shifted to a higher average for some reason (we made some intentional change), the average of the distribution might shift to a higher level as shown in Fig. 5.22.

Another effect of a change we might make to a process could be to squash the distribution somewhat as shown in Fig. 5.23. In this case, fewer sample means would be found in the center, and the standard deviation would be larger meaning that our process is likely to be less under control.

Of course, many other changes might occur due either to a team's intentional changes or due to factors beyond the team's control. A third example is shown

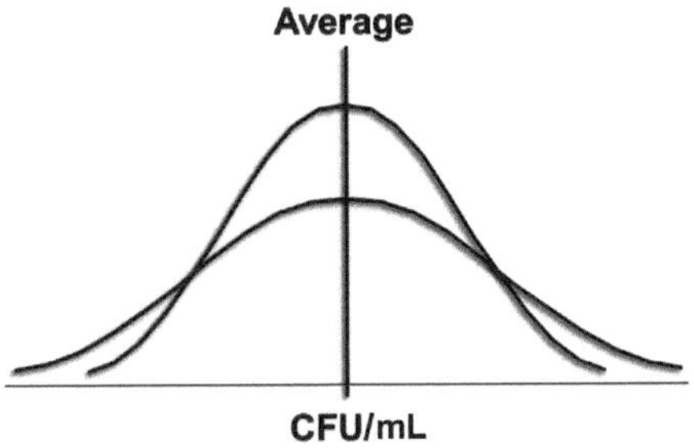

FIGURE 5.23

Greater spread in the process measurements.

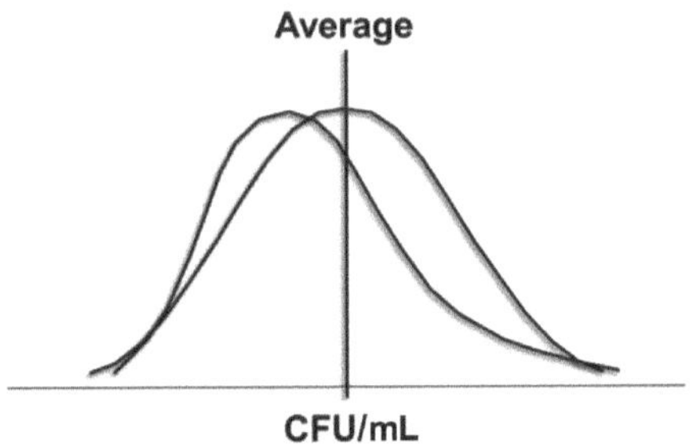

FIGURE 5.24

Distribution is no longer normally shaped.

in Fig. 5.24 where the shape of the distribution has changed and is now skewed (a higher proportion of sample means are found on the left or lower scores, but the mean or average of the distribution remains the same).

In statistics, we generally assume that sampling distributions are normally shaped.

If we can visualize the turning of the frequency distribution on its side as shown in Fig. 5.25 and we plot the sample means around an average line, a new picture emerges. From our data, we can also calculate the upper and lower control limits (LCL) as shown in the figure. Usually, we would draw an "Average" line on a piece of paper, then we would draw (from our calculations) an upper control limit (UCL) line and a lower control limit LCL line.

From the figure, it can be seen that the Monday, Tuesday, and Wednesday plotted points are not all between the UCL and the LCL. Monday's average sample mean falls between the Average and the UCL, Tuesday's average sample mean falls between the average and LCL lines, and Wednesday's sample mean falls below the LCL.

The control limits are like the standard deviations discussed above and as such, we would expect all measured means to ball between the UCL and the LCL if the process were in 99.74% control. When a point falls either above the UCL or below

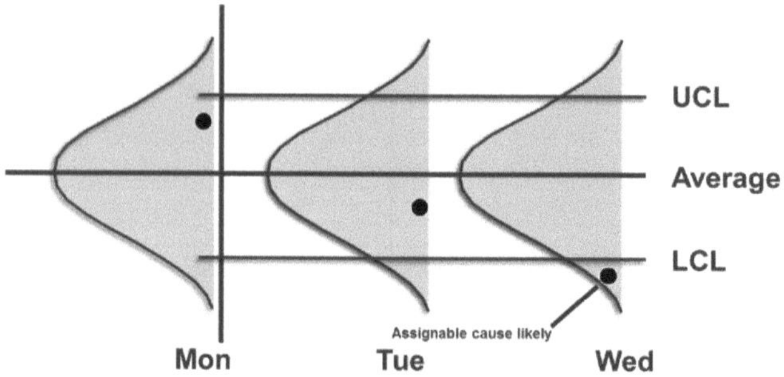

FIGURE 5.25

Plotting the daily sample means.

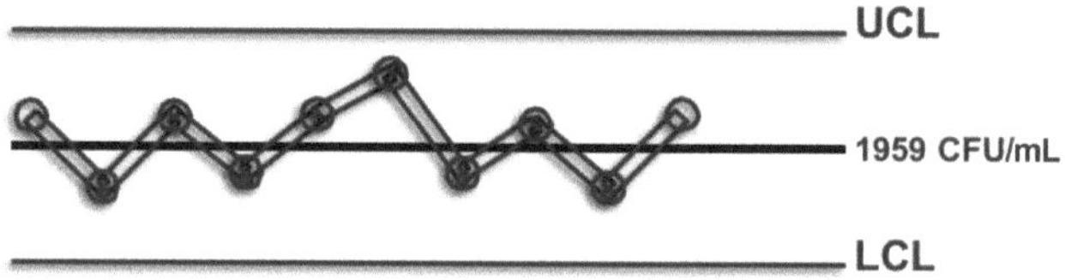

FIGURE 5.26

Process trend in control.

the LCL, things have gone out of control, and we need to begin looking for what is called an assignable cause.

If we expand the concept to an ongoing set of measurements, we will begin to see a trend line that allows everyone to quickly know whether or not the process is in a state of control. Fig. 5.26 illustrates a series of 10 plotted points. Each of the small circles represents the average score found on a day when calculated as shown during the STS exercise. The 10 points are joined together by a double line (although a single line is fine) to show the trend. The figure shows that all points are spread rather uniformly above and below the process average line with no point exceeding the limits set by the UCL or LCL. This process appears to be in a state of statistical control.

If we assume that the team has made some change to the process in an attempt to bring the CFU/mL averages under control, we might see a trend chart that looks like Fig. 5.27. In this case, most of the plotted points are between the process average (1959 CFU/mL) and the LCL. All points are between the UCL and the LCL, but because of the fact that we have multiple points in a row that are below the average line, we must conclude that the process has shifted because of some assignable cause (out intentional process change). Of course, if the team made no change to the process and the trend line shifted to below the average line, we would still conclude that the process has changed and was out of control. This trend represents a shift similar to that shown using the normal distribution explanations above. The process curve

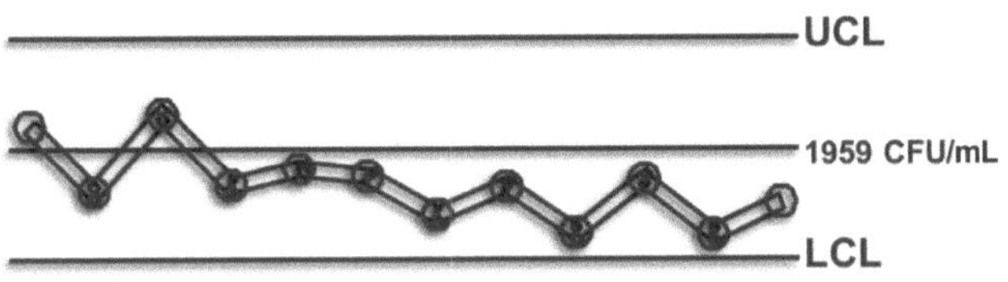

FIGURE 5.27

Process shift.

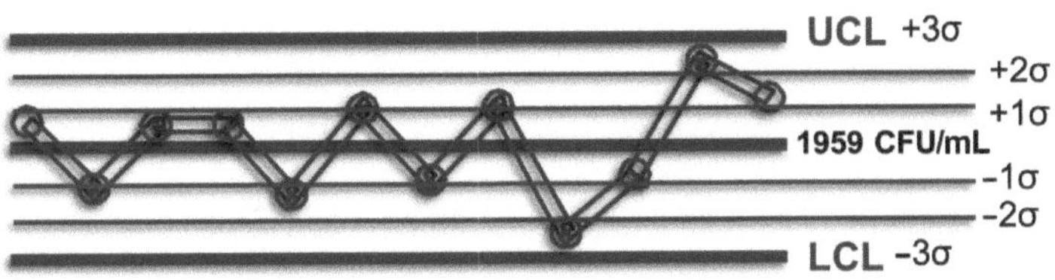

FIGURE 5.28

Envisioning 1–3 standard deviations above and below the process average.

has shifted and a new process average has emerged indicating the process is out of control.

There are some basic rules that are commonly used to interpret SPC chart trend lines.

SPC rule 1: Nine consecutive points fall on the same side of the centerline means the process is out of control.

Fig. 5.27 shows nine consecutive points falling on the same side of the mean (centerline).

There are many possible trends that might occur to stimulate the team's thinking. Fig. 5.28 shows another pattern. The first eight plotted means are randomly distributed above and below the 1959 CFU/mL average, but points 9–12 show more variation in daily averages.

Taking our discussions about the application of standard deviation concepts to the control chart and recalling that we have converted the normal sampling distributions from a vertical perspective to a horizontal one, the trend chart can be divided above and below the 1959 CFU/mL line into three standard deviations above the centerline and three standard deviations below the centerline. Recall that there is less and less likelihood that a point would be calculated and plotted the further one gets from the centerline.

Fig. 5.29 shows a process that exhibits even more variation. Notice the last five consecutive points (sample averages) above the average 1959 CFU/mL line. Four out of five of those consecutive sample means mean the process is out of control on the basis of rules 2 and 3.

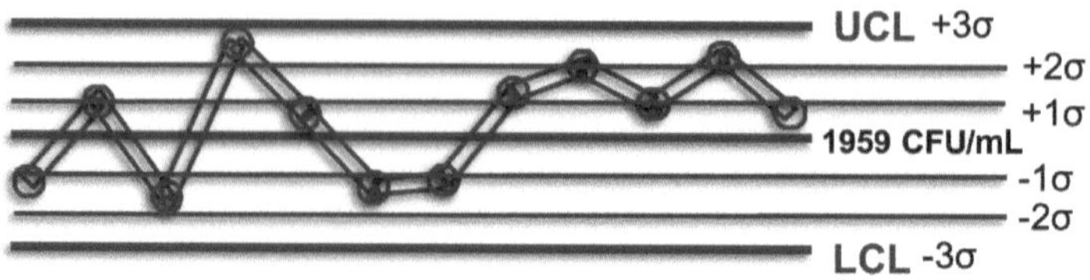

FIGURE 5.29

Out of control process.

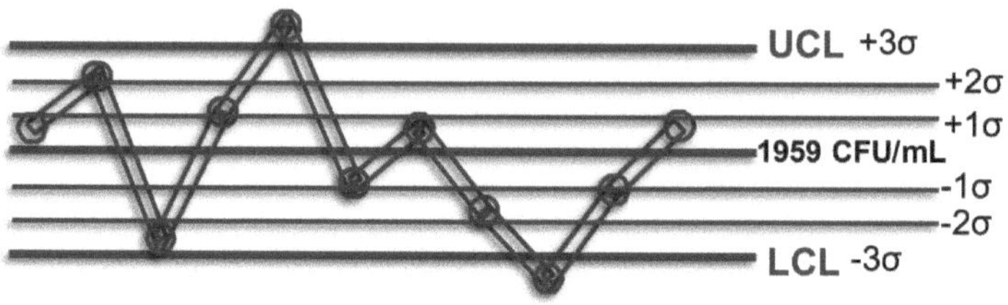

FIGURE 5.30

Outside of control limits.

SPC rule 2: Four out of five consecutive points fall beyond the 1σ limit on the same side of the centerline.

SPC rule 3: Two out of three consecutive points fall beyond the 2σ limit on the same side of the centerline

Fig. 5.30 exhibits even more process variation with two points outside of each of the UCL and LCL. This brings up SPC rule 4.

SPC rule 4: Any single data point falls beyond either the upper or LCL.

For those desiring a more complete SPC review, download and save the Western Electric Statistical Quality Control (SQC) Handbook at this link (341 pages, free): http://www.contesolutions.com/Western_Electric_SQC_Handbook.pdf [3].

SIX-SIGMA BASICS

For the past 20 years or so a new program has been brought into the statistical arena that is now beginning to be seen on the food safety scene. The program and statistical approach is known as Six-sigma. The idea can be understood on the basis of the reader's understanding of the three standard deviations shown in the SPC charts above.

A normally distributed process such as that shown in Fig. 5.31 exists with a LCL of 800, average of 1959 and UCL at 2700.

If a new process distribution emerged because of changes in the process such as that depicted in Fig. 5.32, everything found below the LCL or above the UCL would

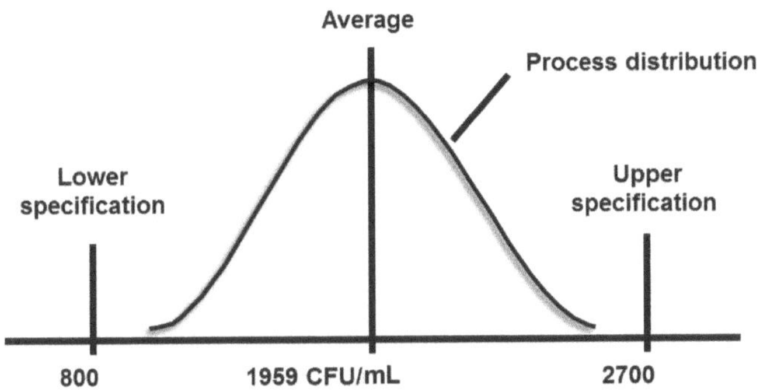

FIGURE 5.31

The Three-sigma process.

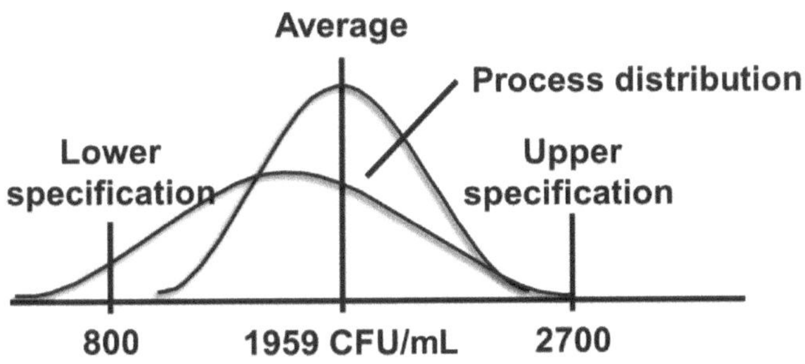

FIGURE 5.32

Shifted and flattened process.

mean an out of control condition existed. In this case, exceeding the LCL would be a good situation because the team is targeting a reduction in bacterial CFU/mL.

The idea behind Six-sigma is that if a company or team focuses its attention on continual improvement, the distribution can be continually narrowed until the probability that negative sample averages are outside of the control limits would be zero, and the company would be saving large sums of money by bringing the process under control.

In Fig. 5.33, Two, Four, and Six-sigma distributions are shown. The tighter a company is able to control a process through improvement cycles, the lower the probability that any of the product or measured variable will exceed the UCL or LCL.

Tied to this idea is the fact that the more a problem persists or the more defective product is produced, the greater the loss in dollars. The principal is illustrated through the Taguchi loss function as illustrated in Fig. 5.34. A process capable of producing product in the middle of the specification or close to the mean with no product outside of the control limits is less likely to cost a company money than a product or process that has not been a subject of continuous improvement.

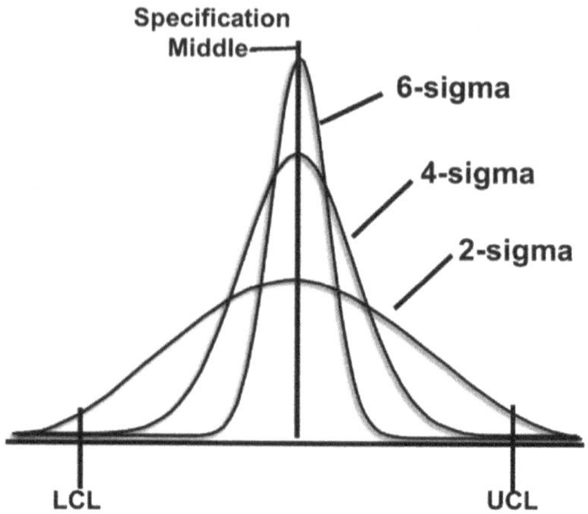

FIGURE 5.33

Two, Four, and Six-sigma distributions.

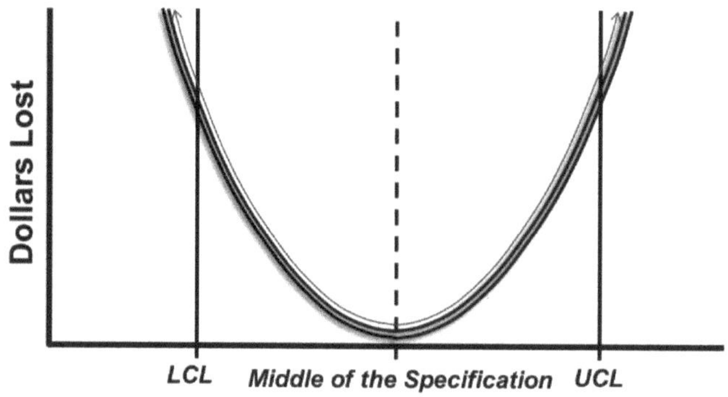

FIGURE 5.34

Taguchi loss function.

MEAN AND RANGE CHART CALCULATIONS FOR CONTINUOUS DATA

In many cases, measurements or sample results will be taken when the type of data can be continuously measured.

Table 5.15 shows a continuous data set from 5 days. Four samples are taken from each area each day. The task is to calculate the range (R) and the average for each set of samples.

To calculate the range of data for each day, one must inspect the four samples from day 1 to determine the highest and lowest sample finding. The R is calculated

Table 5.15 Dataset

Sample Number	Sample				R	$\bar{x}$
	1	2	3	4		
1	0.5014	0.5022	0.5009	0.5027		
2	0.5021	0.5041	0.5024	0.5020		
3	0.5018	0.5026	0.5035	0.5023		
4	0.5008	0.5034	0.5024	0.5015		
5	0.5041	0.5056	0.5034	0.5039		

Table 5.16 Calculating the range of samples for each day

Sample Number	Sample				R	$\bar{x}$
	1	2	3	4		
1	0.5014	0.5022	0.5009	0.5027		
2	0.5021	0.5041	0.5024	0.5020		
3	0.5018	0.5026	0.5035	0.5023		
4	0.5008	0.5034	0.5024	0.5015		
5	0.5041	0.5056	0.5034	0.5039		
			0.5027–0.5009			=0.0018

by subtracting the lowest daily sample result from the highest daily sampling result as shown in Table 5.16.

The resulting R is then placed in the data set as shown in Table 5.17.

Calculating the mean for each daily set of samples is shown in Table 5.18. All daily results are added together and divided by the number of daily samples (4). The resulting average (mean) is placed in the data set as shown.

All sample range and average calculations are completed and placed in the data set as shown in Table 5.19. In addition, the average range for the 5 days is found by adding all daily range results together and dividing by the number of days (5). The overall average is found in a similar manner.

The resulting range, average range, sample, and dataset average results are used to plot control charts and in the calculations of upper (UCL) and lower (LCL) limits. Taking the average range (0.0021), the UCL and LCL for ranges can now be calculated using the formulae shown below. The value for D_4 comes from a table found in the back of any SPC book. The table is reproduced here

$$\bar{R} = 0.0021$$

$$\mathrm{UCL}_R = D_4\bar{R}$$

$$\mathrm{LCL}_R = D_3\bar{R}$$

Table 5.17 Adding the Range result to the Data Set

Sample Number	Sample 1	2	3	4	R	$\bar{x}$
1	0.5014	0.5022	0.5009	0.5027	0.0018	
2	0.5021	0.5041	0.5024	0.5020		
3	0.5018	0.5026	0.5035	0.5023		
4	0.5008	0.5034	0.5024	0.5015		
5	0.5041	0.5056	0.5034	0.5039		
		0.5027–0.5009				=0.0018

Table 5.18 Calculating Sample Daily Averages

Sample Number	Sample 1	2	3	4	R	$\bar{x}$
1	0.5014	0.5022	0.5009	0.5027	0.0018	0.5018
2	0.5021	0.5041	0.5024	0.5020		
3	0.5018	0.5026	0.5035	0.5023		
4	0.5008	0.5034	0.5024	0.5015		
5	0.5041	0.5056	0.5034	0.5039		

0.5027 – 0.5009 = 0.0018
(0.5014 +0.5022 + 0.5009 + 0.5027)/4 = 0.5018

Table 5.19 Calculating Data Set Average Ranges and Means

Sample Number	Sample 1	2	3	4	R	$\bar{x}$
1	0.5014	0.5022	0.5009	0.5027	0.0018	0.5018
2	0.5021	0.5041	0.5024	0.5020	0.0021	0.5027
3	0.5018	0.5026	0.5035	0.5023	0.0017	0.5026
4	0.5008	0.5034	0.5024	0.5015	0.0026	0.5020
5	0.5041	0.5056	0.5034	0.5047	0.0022	0.5045
					$\bar{R} = 0.0021$	
						$\bar{\bar{x}} = 0.5027$

Table 5.20 Control Chart Factors

Size of Sample (n)	Factor for UCL and LCL for x-Charts (A_2)	Factor for LCL for R-Charts (D_3)	Factor UCL for R-Charts (D_4)
2	1.880	0	3.267
3	1.023	0	2.575
4	0.729	0	2.282
5	0.577	0	2.115
6	0.483	0	2.004
7	0.419	0.076	1.924

***R*-Charts** $\bar{R} = 0.0021$ $D_4 = 2.282$ $D_3 = 0$

$$\text{UCL}_R = D_4\bar{R}$$
$$\text{LCL}_R = D_3\bar{R}$$

$$\text{UCL}_R = 2.282\ (0.0021) = 0.00479$$
$$\text{LCL}_R = 0\ (0.0021) = 0$$

FIGURE 5.35

Calculating the UCL and LCL values.

The values for D_3 and D_4 come from a table found in the back of any SPC book. The table is reproduced here as Table 5.20. For a sample size of four, the value for D_3 is equal to 0, and the tabled value for D_4 is 2.282 as shown by the circles in the table.

The table values are plugged into the formulas, and results can be calculated as shown in Fig. 5.35. The resulting value for the UCL is 0.00479. The resulting value for the LCL is 0.

The resulting R-chart with UCL, LCL, and average R for the five samples is shown in Fig. 5.36.

To calculate the UCL and LCL for the mean chart, the same control chart factors table is used to determine the results. The formulae for the mean chart UCL and LCL are shown in Fig. 5.37.

Using the control chart table, the sample size of four indicates that the A_2 value is 0.729 as shown in Table 5.21. By plugging the values for the overall data set mean (0.5027), A_2 (0.729) and the data set average range (0.0021) into the formulas, the UCL and LCL are calculated.

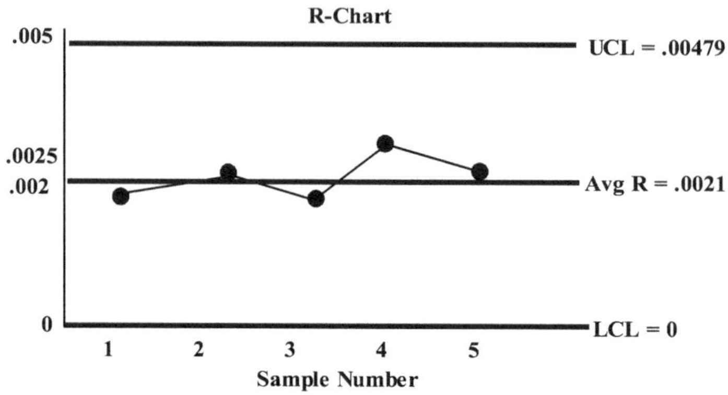

FIGURE 5.36

Final *R*-chart.

$\bar{X}$-Charts $\bar{R} = 0.0021$, $\bar{\bar{x}} = 0.5027$

$$UCL_{\bar{x}} = \bar{\bar{x}} + A_2\bar{R}$$
$$LCL_{\bar{x}} = \bar{\bar{x}} - A_2\bar{R}$$

FIGURE 5.37

Mean chart UCL and LCL calculations.

Table 5.21 Control Chart Table

Size of Sample (*n*)	Factor for UCL and LCL for *x*-Charts (A_2)	Factor for LCL for *R*-Charts (D_3)	Factor LCL for *R*-Charts (D_4)
2	1.880	0	3.267
3	1.023	0	2.575
4	0.729	0	2.282
5	0.577	0	2.115
6	0.483	0	2.004
7	0.419	0.076	1.924

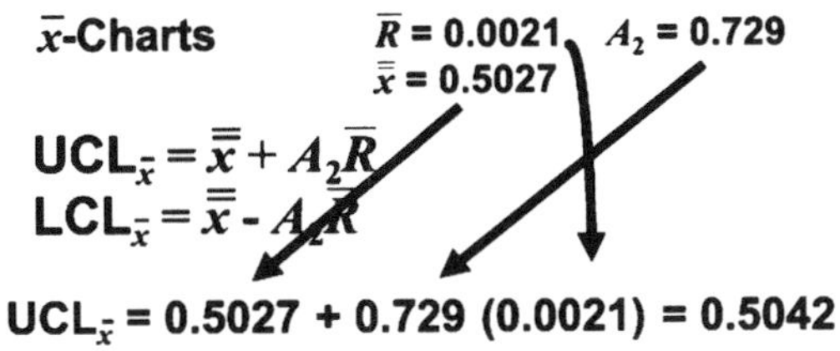

FIGURE 5.38

Calculating the UCL for the mean chart.

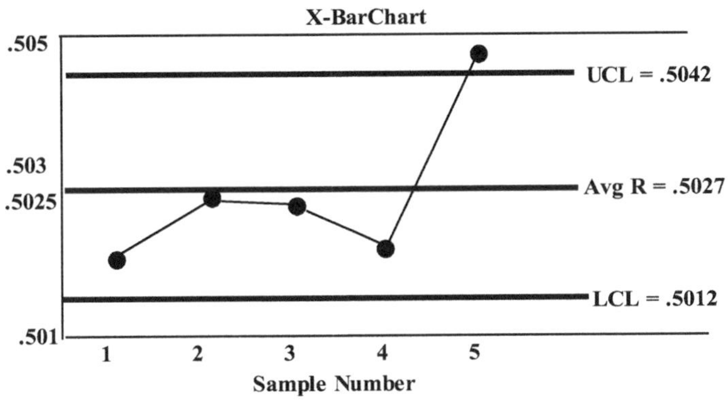

FIGURE 5.39

Plotted *X*-bar chart with UCL and LCL.

Fig. 5.38 shows the values as they are plugged into the formula for calculating the mean chart UCL.

The final results for the calculation of the UCL and LCL are shown below.

$$UCL_x = 0.5027 + 0.729(0.0021) = 0.5042$$

$$LCL_x = 0.5027 - 0.729(0.0021) = 0.5012$$

Fig. 5.39 shows the *X*-bar chart with upper (UCL) and lower (LCL) control limits, the average *R*, and plotted points.

CHARTS FOR ATTRIBUTES

Control charts for attributes are used to analyzed percentages of defective product (*p*-charts) in samples taken usually from inspection or test processes.

Although there are many different types of SPC charts available for study and analysis, there is another chart called a "*p*" chart that allows for the analysis of percentages of defective products such as might be of interest in food sampling schemes.

Table 5.22 includes 15 samples taken from 3382 single tomatoes. The number of improperly accepted tomatoes for each sample number shows up as an error count. For instance, sample 1 had one rejected tomato in the sample. Over the 15 samples that were taken, 28 defective tomatoes were found from the overall batch.

The type of data shown in Table 5.22 lends itself to analysis using *p*-charts, in this case a *p*-chart for varying sample sizes. There were 15 samples taken. Sample sizes ranged from 193 to 250. The table shows that a total of 3382 units were analyzed and 28 on an average, 0.83% of those were found defective.

The average number of defectives found in a large sample set is calculated in the following manner:

$$\overline{p} = \frac{\text{Total defectives}}{\text{Total observations}}$$

When the proportion defective was plotted and upper and LCL were calculated, the resulting *p*-chart looked like Fig. 5.40

The *p*-chart UCL and the LCL were calculated using the following formulae:

$$\text{UCL}_p = \overline{p} + z\sigma_p$$

$$\text{LCL}_p = \overline{p} - z\sigma_p$$

$$\sigma_p = \sqrt{\overline{p}(1-\overline{p})/n}$$

Table 5.22 *p*-Chart Data Analysis

Sample Number	Sample Size	Defects Found	Proportion Defective
1	208	1	0.0048
2	225	3	0.0133
3	201	3	0.0149
4	236	1	0.0042
5	220	3	0.0136
6	244	1	0.0041
7	247	1	0.0040
8	245	1	0.0041
9	250	1	0.0040
10	227	0	0.0000
11	234	2	0.0085
12	227	6	0.0264
13	213	2	0.0094
14	212	1	0.0047
15	193	2	0.0104
Total	**3382**	**28**	**0.0083**

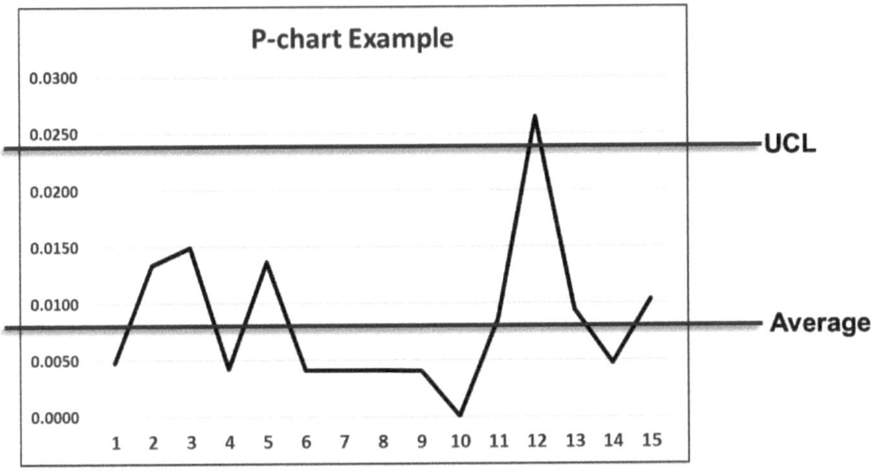

FIGURE 5.40

p-Chart example.

There are many other types of control charts, each one used for different purposes.

Most modern text books focused on statistical analysis for operational improvements include software packages that can be used to help set up spreadsheets or include useable software as part of the purchase price.

CYCLE TIME ANALYSIS

The food industry is perhaps the single industry that is on top of trying to assure that food is delivered well within shelf life or expiration limits. Generally speaking, inventory turns are very high and the time from the farm to the store is minimal.

Regardless, the Food and Agriculture Organization of the United Nations (11 May 2011) estimates the following:

- "Roughly, one-third of the food produced in the world for human consumption every year—approximately 1.3 billion tonnes—gets lost or wasted, according to an FAO-commissioned study.
- The industrialized and developing countries dissipate roughly the same quantities of food—respectively 670 and 630 million tonnes.
- Every year, consumers in rich countries waste almost as much food (222 million tonnes) as the entire net food production of sub-Saharan Africa (230 million tonnes).
- Fruits and vegetables, plus roots and tubers have the highest wastage rates of any food.

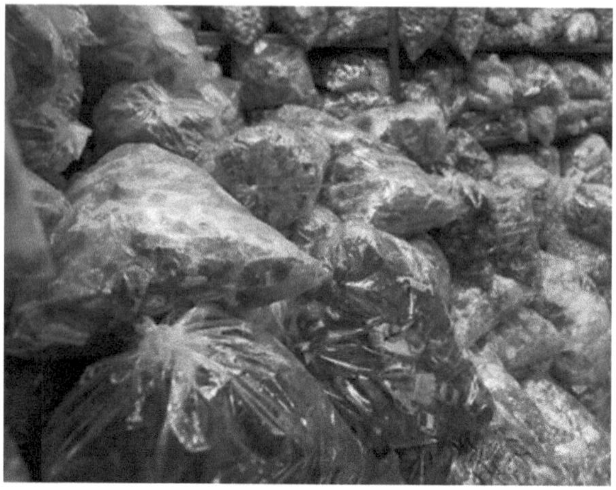

FIGURE 5.41

Unsold product.

- The amount of food lost or wasted every year is equivalent to more than half of the world's annual cereals crop (2.3 billion tonnes in 2009/2010)." [5]

GLOBAL FOOD LOSSES AND FOOD WASTE

Fig. 5.41 illustrates piles of excess or obsolete inventory that go unsold as a result of such waste.

A LOOK AT SOME ASSOCIATED COSTS

Of equal importance are the wasted resources that go along with wasted food. Assuming we use 30% to estimate wasted food. The water pesticides, herbicides, fertilizers, transportation, distribution, processing, handling, and other associated costs went into the landfill along with the food. Companies worrying about slim profit margins need to take a very close look at handling and inventory wastes to figure out why such margins are so low.

If we apply some basic cost analyses to each operational supply chain step, we can begin to see the potential for some serious cost savings.

The questions quickly become "where is the inventory" and "what can we do"?

Starting at a farm, Fig. 5.42A–D illustrate potential losses. Beginning on the left, if a farm has a 30% or 30-lb loss for a 100-lb harvest and the sale of fresh tomatoes is set at about $1/lb, the ship out loss is 30 lb and the ship out weight is now 70 lb or

$70 with a loss of $30. Add to that the cost of inspection ($8 per hour), overhead at $0.05/lb and transportation costs at $0.15/lb, the supply chain losses add up quickly.

The total yield and sales losses on the initial 100 lb is $46.

Following the same logic through distribution (Fig. 5.42B at $25.10), processing (Fig. 5.42C $40.59) and retail (Fig. 5.42D at $39.22), the losses roll up through the supply chain.

Table 5.23 adds up the costs across all four supply chain phases. The overall loss as a percentage of the initial 100-lb harvest ends up showing a total loss of $895 or a whopping 16.86%.

Inventory is a critical issue and as far as controlling such costs is concerned, it can become the difference between companies able to control such costs and those unable to control such costs.

The analysis is a bit simplistic, but consider the factors noted in Table 5.24 that can accrue on the basis of FDA rejected shipments.

When relabeling, re conditioning, detention, seizures, destruction, examination, inspection, testing, lack of proper documentation, and other such expenses are

(A)

1

							Co sts				Total Loss
Incoming Farm Operation # 1	Yield Loss %	Yield Loss #	New Shipout Weight	Reason	Per lb Sales Price	Shipout Value	Yield Losses Shipout $ Loss	Inspection At $8 per hour	Overhead at .05 per Lb	Transport at $.15 per Lb	
100	30	30	70	Packout	$1	$70	$30.00	$2.00	$3.50	$10.50	$46.00

(B)

2

							Co sts				Total Loss
Incoming Distribution Operation # 2	Yield Loss %	Yield Loss #	New Shipout Weight	Reason	Per Lb Sales Price	Shipout Value	Yield Loss Shipout $ Loss	Inspection At $8 per hour	Overhead at .05 per Lb	Transport at $.15 per Lb	
70	10	7	63	Culling	$1.50	$95	$10.50	$2.00	$3.15	$9.45	$25.10

(C)

3

							Co sts				Total Loss
Incoming Process Operation # 2	Yield Loss %	Yield Loss #	New Shipout Weight	Reason	Per lb Sales Price	Shipout Value	Yield Losses Shipout $ Loss	Inspection At $8 per hour	Overhead at .05 per Lb	Transport at $.15 per Lb	
63	15	9.45	53.55	Rejected	2.95	$157.97	$27.88	$2.00	$2.68	$8.03	$40.59

(D)

4

							Co sts				Total Loss
Incoming Retail Operation # 2	Yield Loss %	Yield Loss #	New Shipout Weight	Reason	Per Lb Sales Price	Shipout Value	Yield Loss Shipout $ Loss	Inspection At $8 per hour	Overhead at .05 per Lb	Transport at $.15 per Lb	
53.55	15	8.03	45.52	Albert	3.5	$159.31	$28.11	$2.00	$2.28	$6.83	$39.22

FIGURE 5.42

(A) Farm level loss calculations. (B) Distribution loss calculations. (C) Processing loss calculations. (D) Retail loss calculations.

Table 5.23 Rolled Up Supply Chain Costs

	Loss	Summary
	Yield/Wt	$96.49
	Inspection	$8.00
	Ohead	$11.60
	Transport	$34.81
Loss summary		$150.90
Sales potential at 100 lbs		$895.00
Loss as percentage of 100 lb sales		16.86

potentially added moving the right inventory in the right condition becomes a critical market issue.

From a business perspective, regardless of food safety or food security, inventory is money.

Any person in any company can take a walk around the company and look at different piles of inventory. When you look at raw materials, work in process (WIP) and outgoing inventory pretend you are standing in a bank vault looking at heaps and piles of money. Money that could be used to pay better benefits or salaries, invest in new products, better control systems, or other investments that would help to improve the company's operations or longevity.

For both vegetable commodities and products and animal commodities and products, the report outlines the following areas noting that causes and preventive practices must be applied throughout the entire supply chain from origin to consumer:

1. Agricultural production
2. Post-harvest handling and storage
3. Processing
4. Distribution
5. Consumption

The report notes that the overall supply chain (production to retailing) is significantly more wasteful worldwide than consumers, industrialized nations lead in wasting foods, agriculture, and food processing lead in food losses.

The report also notes several contributing causes:

"In industrialized countries foods gets lost when production exceeds demand"

"High 'appearance quality standards' from supermarkets"

"Poor storage facilities and lack of infrastructure cause post-harvest losses in the developing countries"

"Unsafe food is not fit for human consumption and therefore is wasted"

Table 5.24 FDA Rejected Shipment Information

Added	Costs From	FDA International Rejected Shipments					
	Relabeled Documentation Traceability	Recondition	Refusal Registration	Detained w/FDA	Seized	Destruction Holding	Examination GMP/GAP inspections

"Disposing is cheaper than using or re-using' attitude in the industrialized countries"

"Lack of processing facilities causes high food losses in the developing countries"

"Large quantities on display and a wide range of products/brands in supply lead to food waste in the industrialized countries"

"Inadequate market systems cause high food losses in the developing countries"

"Food wasted at consumer level is minimal in the developing countries"

"Abundance and consumer attitudes lead to high food waste in the industrialized countries"

The report offers a number of preventive suggestions including communication, cooperation and organization among farmers, consumer surveys (to forecast needs and wants), increased investment in infrastructure and transportation, educating food chain operators in food handling, establishing and educating food chain operators in safe food handling practices, establishing markets for substandard (but safe) foods, improving market systems, and increasing public awareness of the problem.

Though the problem of wasted food is not new, some assumptions are clear:

1. All food ages
2. All food has an expiration date (regardless of label information)
3. All food sits in inventory at different times and in different places
4. As food ages, the likelihood that it will be subject to spoilage or contamination increases
5. Preventing aging, spoilage, or contamination (under the right controls) means that food must move from production or processing to the customer in the shortest time possible
6. Controlling food cycle times is a critical preventive strategy for both food safety and food security

In this section, the power of cycle time analysis is explored as a quantitative tool for reducing the time it takes food to go from a farm to the consumer or reducing the time it takes the food to go through any single food process.

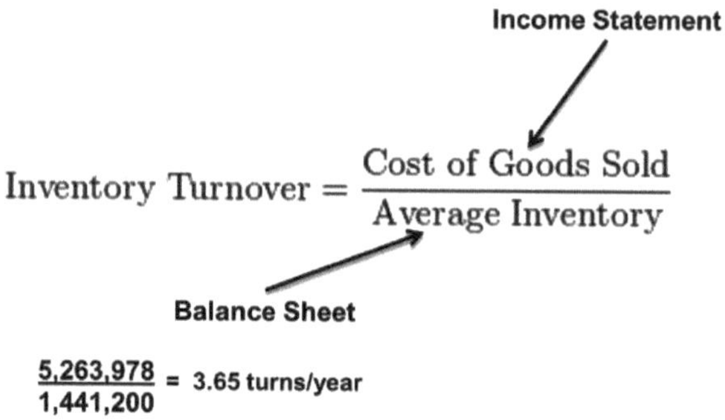

FIGURE 5.43

Inventory turns analysis.

In the case of the food supply stream, cycle time analysis can be said to have at least two goals:

1. Reduce the time it takes to preserve food quality and establish improved food security
2. Prevent food safety problems from excessive and obsolete food items
3. Establish an ideal cycle time for the process
4. Reduce wait times to zero

Inventory turns is a common strategy for financial analysts to determine company health. Fig. 5.43 summarizes how to calculate inventory turns.

The calculations are simple. The cost of goods sold is found on the company income statement and is divided by the average inventory figure that can be found on the company balance sheet. In Fig. 5.44, the company exhibits 3.65 turns per year which can be interpreted to mean that from the time the product is ordered to the time the product has gone through all company processes and been paid for, the company receives payment on their expenses about every 3.3 months.

Fig. 5.44 illustrates a basic cycle time analysis. In a process that takes 11 hours, the analysis shows that about 4 hours (36.4%) waiting while the actual time it takes to handle and process the product is 7 hours (64%). The processing time stand is shown as a dotted line while the average wait time is depicted as a solid line.

The process begins with a simple process flowchart showing each process step from input to process output as shown in Fig. 5.44.

The illustration shows that the product goes through five processes as shown in Fig. 5.45. For example, the time taken by process 1 is 1.0 hours but the product waits for the next process approximately 30 minutes. Inspection of the analysis shows that the wait time between process step 3 and process step 3 is 2 hours. That wait time has a square drawn around it to highlight it as the longest wait time established in the process.

Note that the analysis can be set up for any time period (hours, days, or months) allowing cycle time analysis to be used for any just about type of process.

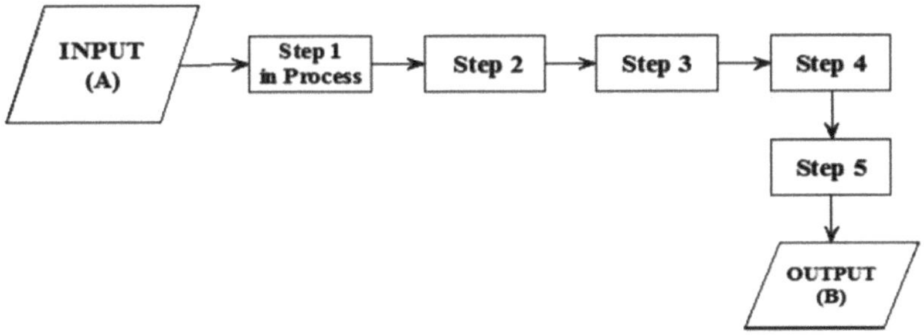

FIGURE 5.44

Simple input to output process (steps 1 through 5).

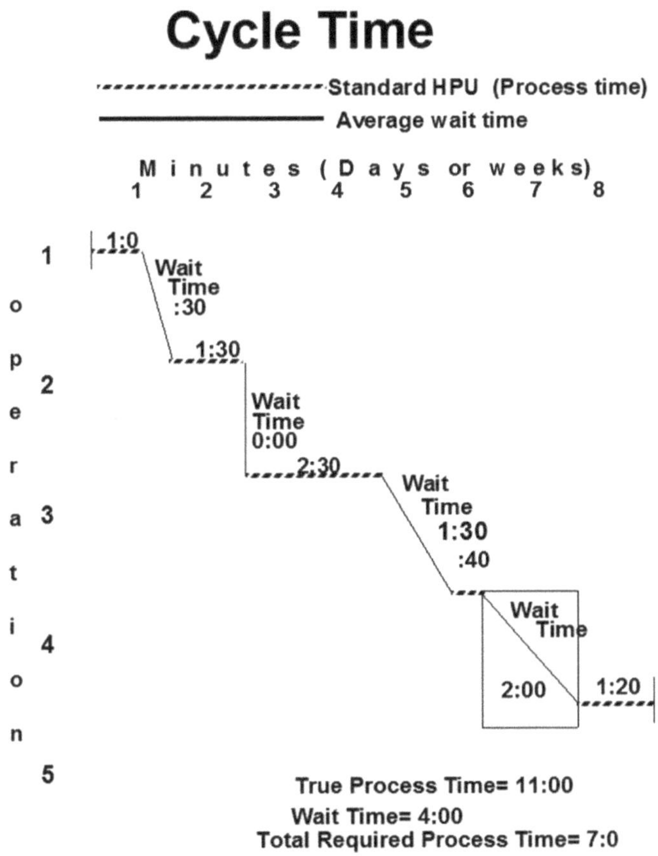

FIGURE 5.45

Illustrated cycle time analysis.

DATA COLLECTION

For cycle time analysis, the time for each process step and each wait time must be measured. This is done with a stopwatch by measuring the process and wait times over between 20 and 30 batches of product going through the process. A batch could be a bin, or pallet or a larger quantity of product. A Process Tracking (Fig. 5.46) sheet is attached to each batch that allows the person receiving the batch to record the time received and the time finished at each process step. Once 20 or 30 batches have gone through the process, the process step entry and exit times is used to determine the average or mean time taken in the process step or while waiting.

The Process Tracking Sheets has a box to include notes taken for each tracking sheet. The individual managing the process tracking sheet is expected to include any observations of the process that might be important for team members to know.

Process Tracking Sheet

Team Name__________ **Measurement Number** __________

Date __________ **Process Name** __________

Name of Person Doing the Measurement __________

Process Step 1
Process Time ______
Wait Time ______

Process Step 2
Process Time ______
Wait Time ______

Process Step 3
Process Time ______
Wait Time ______

Process Step 4
Process Time ______
Wait Time ______

Process Step 5
Process Time ______
Wait Time ______

Observation Notes

All Process Steps (Total)
Total Process Times ______
Total Wait Times ______

All Process Steps (Total)
Average Process Times ______
Average Wait Times ______

FIGURE 5.46

Process cycle time process tracking data collection sheet.

Assume that 30 process timing sheets are collected from 30 batches. An excel spreadsheet is used to record times from all 30 sheets (Fig. 5.47).

Using each data sheet, enter the time in and time out for each process step. Subtract the time in from the time out to determine the process time. As the batch arrives at Step 2 through n, calculate the wait time by determining the difference between the ending time out from the previous step and the time in from the current step.

There are a number of potential issues to be investigated. These include:

- Bottlenecks (in processes)
- Administrative redo's (paperwork)
- Inventory Pileups
- "Not enough time"
- Takes too long!
- Late deliveries
- "I need more people!"
- Working long days?

We can take the data from the illustrated analysis and create a Pareto analysis similar to what we do on the STS. Fig. 5.48 illustrates the cycle time analysis for this illustration. The figure shows, as usual, that the wait and process times are arranged from left to right in terms of the time each process stem and wait time take based on process time measurements. The Pareto analysis is transferred to the STS.

The next step becomes one of measuring cycle times and plotting inventory trends over time as shown in Fig. 5.49. Fig. 5.49 illustrates a breakdown of total inventory (top line) raw materials (line with steep upwards slope below the total line), work in process and finished goods (FGI). These trends show a company with increasing total inventory over a 4-year period.

The trends show that inventory is increasing, primarily due to raw materials. This may be contributed to over ordering with a lack of regard to the company's ability to process WIP.

Data Sheet Number	Step 1				Step n			
	In Time	Out Time	Process Time	Wait Time	In Time	Out Time	Process Time	Wait Time
1								
2								
3								
4								
5								
.								
.								
.								
.								
n								

FIGURE 5.47

Recording data on the excel spreadsheet.

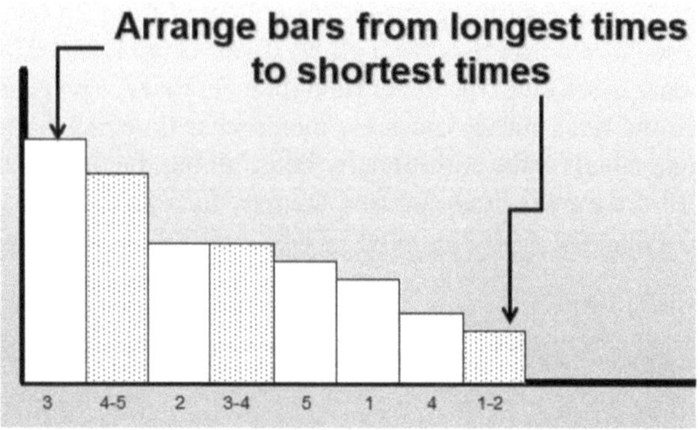

FIGURE 5.48

Cycle time Pareto analysis.

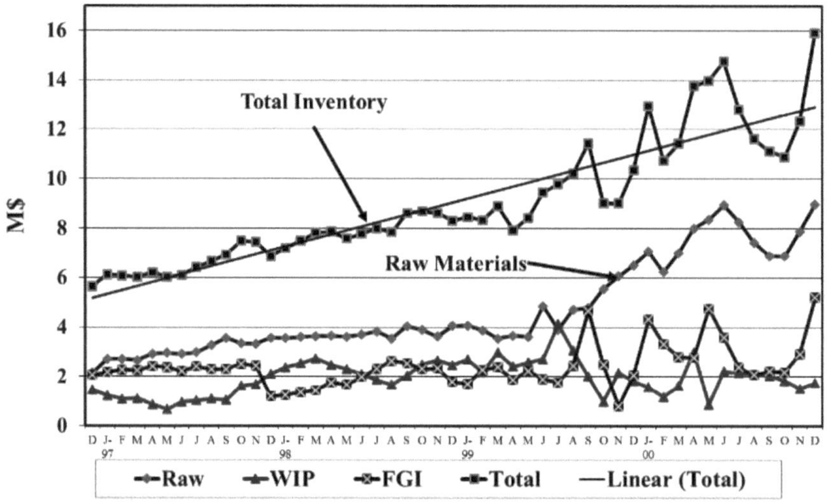

FIGURE 5.49

Analyzing inventory with a simple trend analysis.

CYCLE TIME ANALYSIS IS A TEAM ACTIVITY

The team approach can be used to establish trends, target improvements, the Pareto analysis, causal analyses and team action items in an effort to get control over the inventory trends. Usually, a CC team is established among functional managers who work together to reverse inventory trends using the STS as shown in Fig. 5.50.

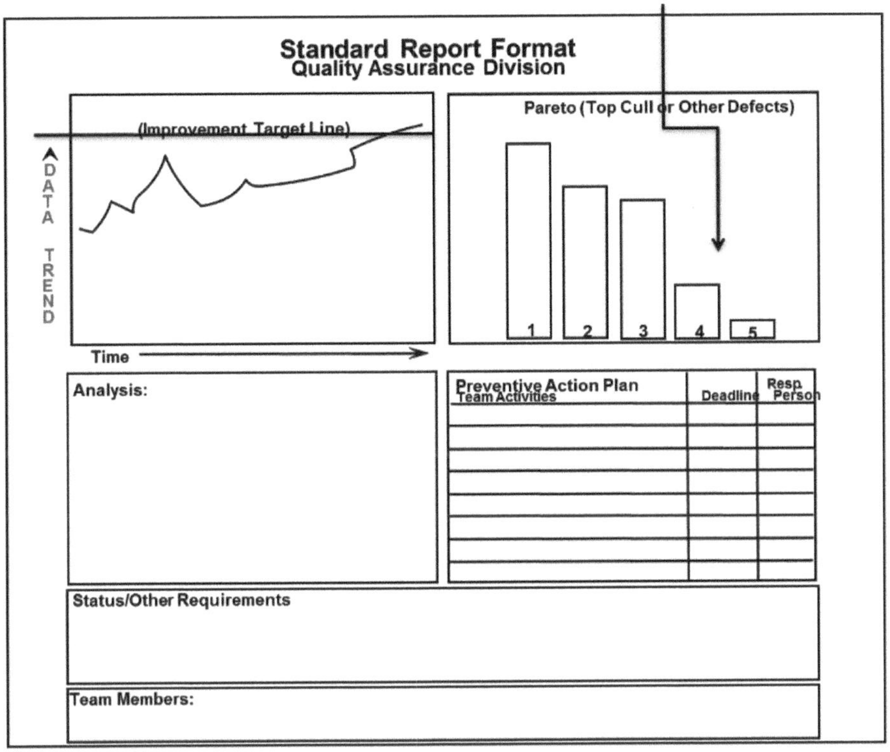

FIGURE 5.50

Solution tracking sheet (STS).

The CC team can consider the following list of potential causes:

- Line bottlenecks
- Reduce steps in the process
- Reduce movement and handling
- Synchronization (line balance)
- Simplify process operations
- Combine steps or operations
- Eliminate steps or operations
- Identify and eliminate wasted movements
- Reduce overproduction
- Eliminate unnecessary production steps such as inspection and test
- Reduce transportation and handling
- Reduce excessive inventory
- Reduce excessive motion

Causes can be team analyzed using the fishbone diagram found on the STS as shown in Fig. 5.51.

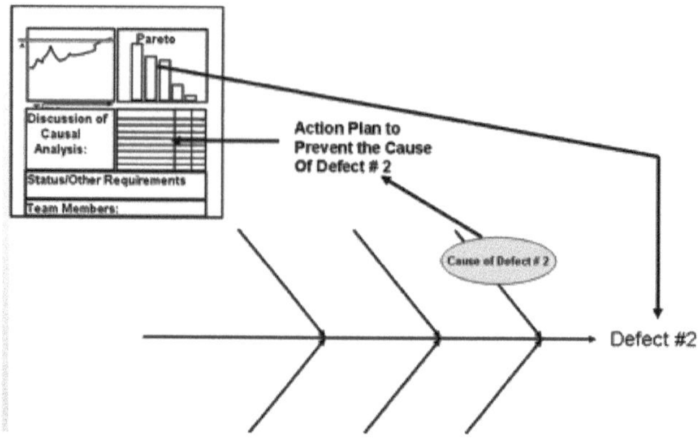

FIGURE 5.51

Process improvement trend.

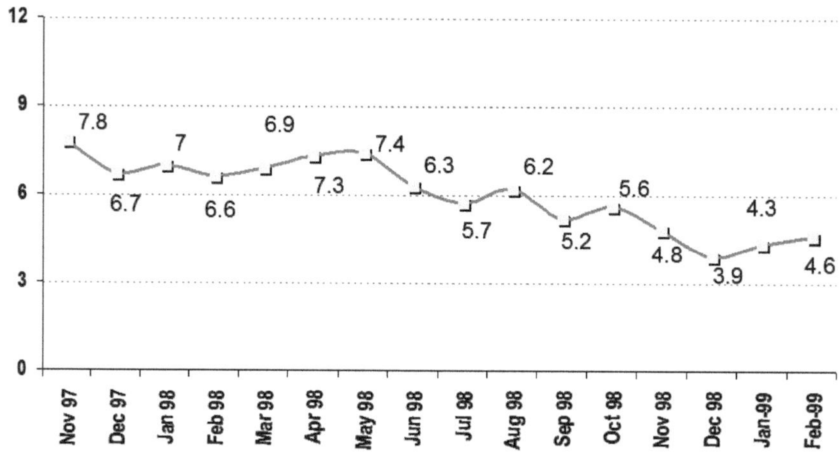

FIGURE 5.52

Sample CC team inventory control continuous improvement trend.

Fig. 5.52 is an illustration of one team's success over time to continually improve the overall inventory trend that is transferred to the STS.

THE IDEAL CYCLE TIME

The ideal cycle time is the time it takes to process one unit with no wait times between process steps. In other words, a continuous flow similar to what might be observed in automated processing.

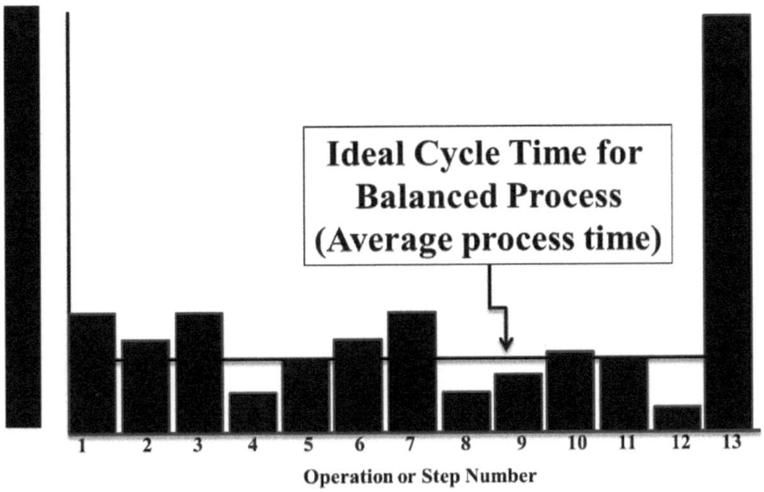

FIGURE 5.53

Establishing an ideal process time for each process step.

Fig. 5.53 shows one team's cycle time analysis with an ideal cycle time established as an average process time for each operation step.

The cycle time analysis steps can be summarized as follows:

1. Calculate inventory turns
2. Establish a cycle time team (CAT) for the process
3. Make sure management supports the teams
4. Flowchart the process
5. Identify process and wait areas in the process
6. Measure the process times and the wait times
7. Perform calculations using an Excel spreadsheet
8. Plot the process and wait times on the STS
9. Set up the Pareto analysis on the STS
10. If possible, determine causes for the longest wait time
11. Have the team work on eliminating the cause using the STS
12. When the longest wait time in the process has been eliminated, work on the next longest wait time
13. Re-measure the process times and the wait times in the new process
14. Re-do steps 6–11 until wait time is equal to the target hours per unit (wait time = 0)

REFERENCES

[1] <http://www.fsis.usda.gov/wps/wcm/connect/a9837fc8-0109-4041-bd0c-729924a79201/Baseline_Data_Raw_Chicken_Parts.pdf?MOD=AJPERES>, June 6, 2016.

[2] <https://www.deming.org/theman/theories/fourteenpoints>, June 9, 2016.
[3] Statistical Quality Control Handbook, Western Electric Company, 1958 First Edition, Printed in the United States of America by The Mack Printing Company, Easton Pennsylvania.
[4] J.R. Evans, D.L. Olson, Statistics, Data Analysis and Decision Modeling, second ed., Prentice Hall, Upper Saddle River, NJ, 2003, p. 257.
[5] <http://www.fao.org/docrep/014/mb060e/mb060e00.pdf>, June 27, 2016.

CHAPTER

Preventing cross-contamination through the supply chain

6

While the food and drug administration (FDA) food safety modernization Act (FSMA) preventive control rules distinguish between food contact (allergen cross-contact) and cross-contamination (unintentional transfer of a foodborne pathogen from a food to another food), in this chapter, no such distinction is made.

The Minnesota Department of Health defines cross-contamination as "Cross-contamination is the physical movement or transfer of harmful bacteria from one person, object or place to another. Preventing cross-contamination is a key factor in preventing foodborne Illness."

The Minnesota website describes what to do when shopping, refrigerating, preparing, and serving food and focuses on bacterial cross-contamination in kitchens and food processing (Fig. 6.1). The picture illustrates what most people have been informed about when it comes to cross-contamination. The plastic cutting board is used to cut up chicken (salmonella potential) with a knife that is later used on the same cutting board to prepare tomatoes and lettuce for a salad. Theoretically, the salmonella from the chicken is carried by the knife onto the lettuce and tomato. Unfortunately, the chicken will be cooked and the cooking provides a kill step due to the high temperature. Also unfortunately, the lettuce, and tomato will not be cooked and will invisibly carry the salmonella that was transferred by the knife into the salad and into the eater.

Such perspectives limit our view of the overall impact of food contamination through the food supply chain.

Fig. 6.2 shows a river with observable contamination flowing downstream. If the picture of the river was a picture of the food supply chain, far up that river, one might imagine a farm around the bend and that farm might be the source of the foam flowing down the river. Notice how the foam spreads through the river and, in the foreground, the foam seems to disappear.

The picture illustrates what happens when hazardous food enters the food supply chain. Once hazardous food enters the supply chain, all downstream operations become holders, packers, processors, and transporters of the contaminated food. Of equal importance is the fact that everything the food touches also becomes contaminated, and the contaminant can readily be transferred from the original contaminating product to other food products going through the same process.

Validating Preventive Food Safety and Quality Controls. DOI: http://dx.doi.org/10.1016/B978-0-12-810994-6.00006-7

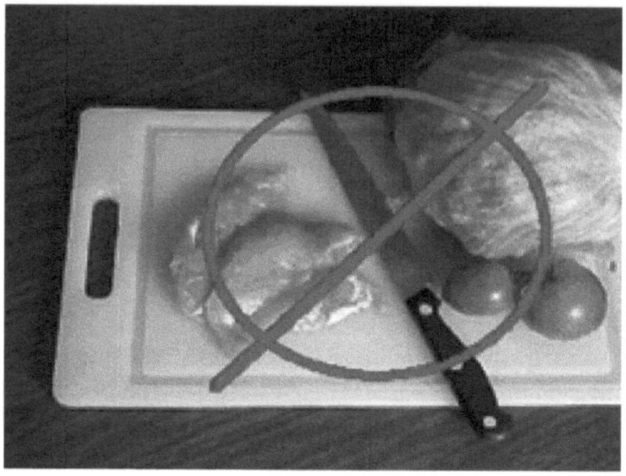

FIGURE 6.1

The most common conception of cross-contamination [1].

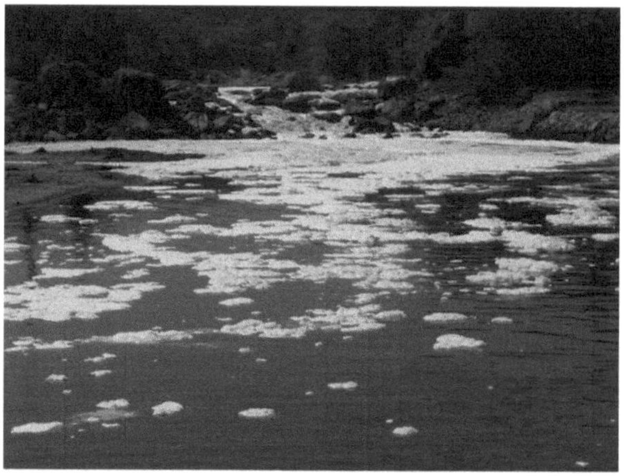

FIGURE 6.2

The river of no return.

Although the river is the main transporter of the hazard, all downstream food operations are impacted whether they know it or not. For most of those food operations, the contaminant remains unseen but has the potential of contaminating everything it comes in contact with—Packing and processing lines, restaurant areas, processing lines, trucks that carried the food, home kitchens, retail shelves, distribution centers, pallets, trays, bins, tools, people, conveyors, and load and unload equipment.

The river illustrates how easy it is for cross-contamination to occur. As the impacted food travels downstream from the farm, it carries the contaminant through all food operation processes.

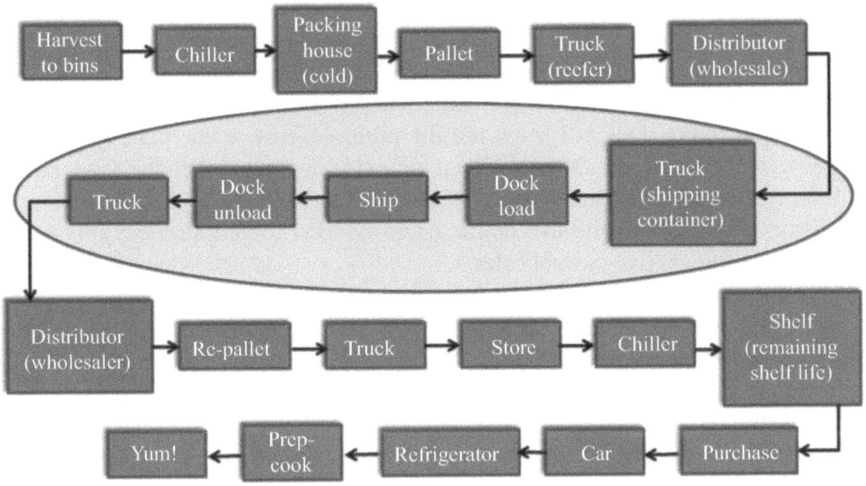

FIGURE 6.3

Supply chain product flow.

Preventive controls for cross-contamination are a critical aspect the food industry and must be able to detect, intercept and control, track back to the source, and eliminate through determination of causes and the implementation of valid preventive approaches.

Many industries have suffered from this free flowing cross-contamination phenomenon. Many industries have found that they must put systems in place to detect and control the potential impact of such contaminating flows. The food supply chain is no different. Cross-contamination through supply chains is not new nor is the need to identify and prevent such contaminants.

Consider the Chipotle example described in this book. Contaminants from farms have flowed through the entire supply chain into restaurants to end up causing human illness. Unlike the foamy river, the contaminants that flowed through the Chipotle supply chain were invisible.

Fig. 6.3 illustrates a normal food product flow through the supply chain. Starting at the farm harvest in the upper left, food normally goes through a chiller to remove field heat after which it ordinarily moves into a packing house where it may be placed in cases or further packaged. Once palletized, the food is forklifted or conveyed into a reefer truck that transports it to a distributor. Once at the distributor, the pallets are usually moved into coolers to await order fulfillment. When an order comes in, the food is reloaded into shipping container that is loaded onto a truck and, in this case that illustrates trans-oceanic shipment, goes onto a dock where it waits on the dock for loading. Once loaded, the container moves across the ocean where it is unloaded and placed into another truck for movement to a distributor. When an order is received from a store or restaurant, the product is reloaded onto another pallet along with many dissimilar products, trucked to the store and placed in a cooler if it is temperature sensitive. Finally, the product is placed onto a market shelf for purchase, transportation home, and storage until cooked.

What that figure does not show are the multiple bins, trays, pallets, and other devices used to carry food. Often such equipment is in contact with the food making, the food carried surface contact tools. Whenever food and surfaces come in contact, entirely new and more aggressive sanitation of the food contact surfaces are required that fall under preventive control rules.

The 17 steps in the figure include multiple handling operations by many people while also requiring a variety of tools and equipment that are all capable of cross-contamination.

Common cause (CC) teams are assigned the responsibility of defining a general system designed to identify, prevent, and eliminate cross-contamination sources from suppliers and throughout company processes. Functional improvement teams (FIT) are assigned the responsibility of preventing and eliminating specific sources of cross-contamination within each part of the process within their sphere of control.

CROSS-CONTAMINATION ON FARMS

If we consider what types of contaminants may enter the food supply chain at the farm, here are a few observations:

- Genetically modified organisms (GMO) crops cross-contaminate nearby crops (genetic pollution)
  - Pollen drift
  - Insect pollination
  - Horizontal gene-transfer (weeds)
  - High potential impact to organic and other nearby farms
- Bacteria
- Herbicides
- Fertilizers
- Pesticides

The GMO industry would like to assume that things like pollen drift, cross-contamination from birds, inspect pollination, and the spread of weeds do not cross-contaminate crops. Perimeters are often established around GMO farms to prevent such occurrences, but it is not likely that inspects, weed seeds, birds, and pollen can be kept only within the perimeters of GMO fields.

GMO farm or not, the same potential cross-contamination situations occur on all farms that supply the contaminants to downstream food processes. Add the normal bacteria, herbicides, fertilizers, and pesticides from the farms to the equation and the potential for cross-contamination through all supply chain steps begins.

By walking through packing houses or distribution centers that contain packing houses and by following the food flow through the operation, one will often come across a wash step where produce, as an example, is theoretically washed to remove dirt and chemical residues. To analyze a company's process for prevention in wash operations, samples of the water pre and post-wash should occasionally be tested for chemicals and bacteria. Preventive practices would require such testing and adjustment of the process until low levels of contamination are found in the wash water.

It should be obvious that any hazardous material that comes in from the field will end up in the wash system, and if the system does not filter out or otherwise remove the contaminant, the wash system becomes increasingly polluted. Dirty wash water in packing houses is a problem similar to a person taking a bath after several other people have taken a bath in the same wash water. The last person to take a bath in dirty wash water is not likely to get very clean.

Fig. 6.4 illustrates a more common origin of potentially deadly contaminants at the farm level.

In the picture, birds are seen nesting on citrus harvest bins that have been left in fields between harvest seasons. There is no doubt that the bins are loaded with bird feces, rats, rat nests, rat urine and feces, and other contaminants can be easily transferred to the product to be placed in them.

The harvest process itself can introduce hazardous adulterants into the food supply chain that later impact all supply chain processes through cross-contamination. Fig. 6.5 depicts how the harvest process itself can introduce hazardous adulterants into the food supply chain that later impact all supply chain processes through cross-contamination. Fig. 6.5 shows a common harvest process that hand picks while loading product into cases sitting on the ground.

Unknown to the workers, both the cases (that will later go onto pallets and into trucks) are a potential source of hazardous contaminants that can be distributed undetected world-wide.

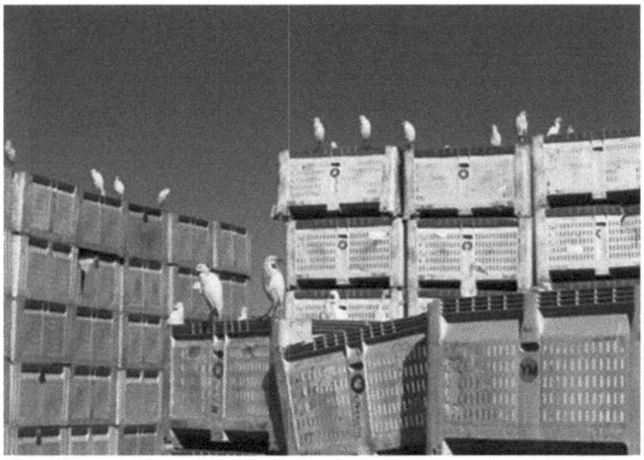

FIGURE 6.4

Source contamination at the farm level.

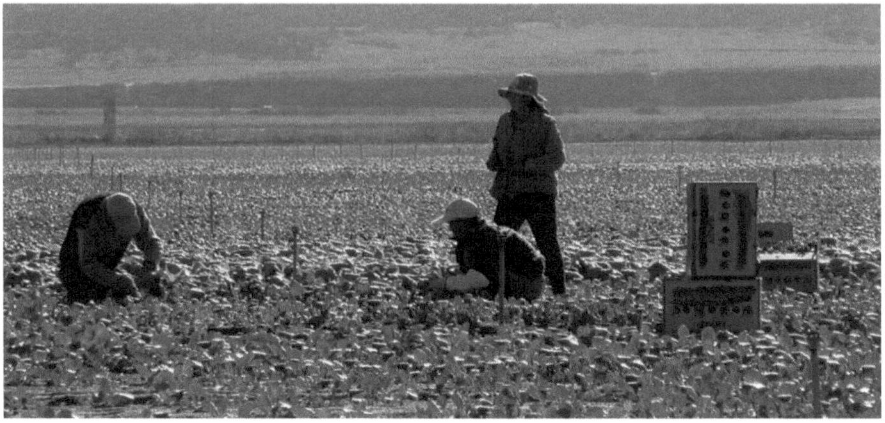

FIGURE 6.5

Harvest.

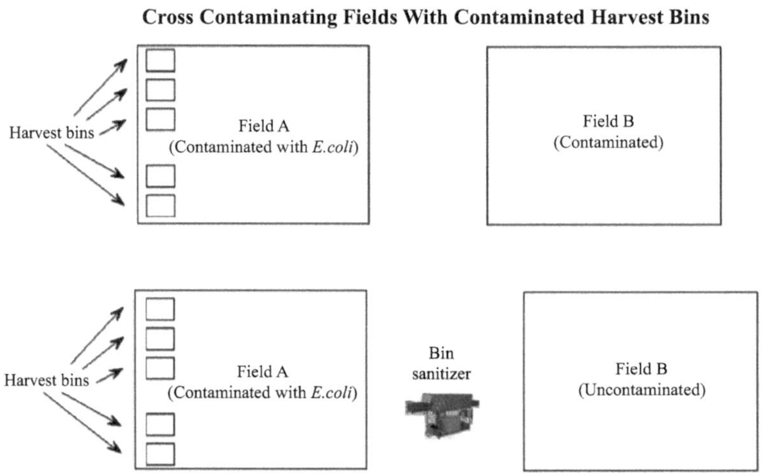

FIGURE 6.6

Cross-contamination in crop fields.

A simple illustration of field cross-contamination is shown in Fig. 6.6. As dirty harvest bins that have been field contaminated are moved from contaminated fields (field A) into uncontaminated fields, the contaminants are dragged into the uncontaminated field on the bins contaminating field B. The lower part of the illustrations shows a field bin sanitizer placed between fields A and B. The sanitizer helps to prevent contaminants in field A from contaminating field B.

Fig. 6.7 shows a close up of the bin sanitizer. In this case, the dirty bins are input at one end, sanitized and come out the other end. The figure shows also shows how bin

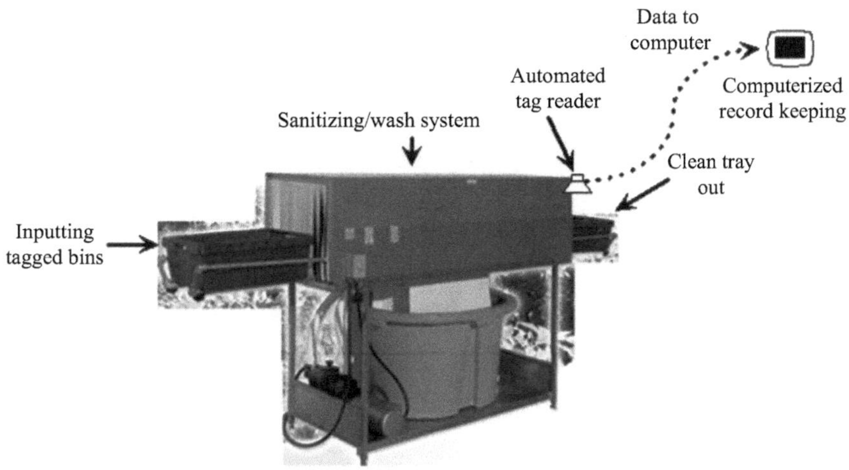

FIGURE 6.7

Details of a bin sanitizing system.

cleaning sanitation records may be maintained using small RFID tags embedded in each individual bin. As the bins exit the sanitizer, an RFID reader reads the bin ID number and locates the place of the sanitizer using Bluetooth-enabled global positioning system (GPS) technology. The time and date of the wash are also recorded in a record that shows when and where the bin was washed. The bin ID number, wash location, and wash time/date are all wirelessly sent to a computer for record keeping and analysis.

For farms or others that also test the bins for sanitation as part of an overall preventive process control system, the data can be used to continually improve the bin cleaning process.

Fig. 6.8 shows other citrus harvest bins, in this case wooden, loaded with harvest citrus prior to processing. There should be no doubt that the contaminants on the citrus, either from the birds, rats or other field contaminants are easily transferred to the product.

PACKING HOUSES

Although most packing houses contain no or very few cross-contamination preventive controls, many of them employ different zones for product input, wash, packing, and cooling. Fig. 6.9 shows produce coming in from a harvest on the left. The produce goes through an opening serving as a pass through from the dirty fields into a wash operation and through packing lines. A conveyor then carries food through a second pass through and into a cool, clean zone where clean product is stored until being picked up by a delivery truck. Shown are three zones: Two dirty zones (incoming from the field and outgoing to the truck), a clean zone number 2 where wash and packing occur, and a cool clean zone number 3 where final product awaits pickup.

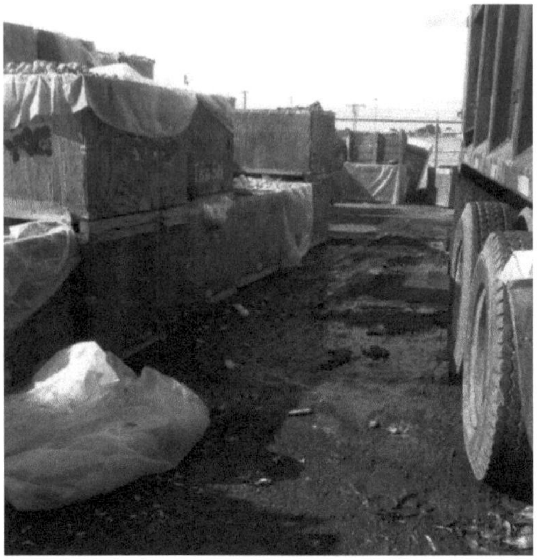

Packing houses

FIGURE 6.8

Post-harvest handling contamination.

At the bottom of the figure, both people and trays and pallets enter zone 2 under controlled conditions. Humans may be required to wear hair nets, face masks, gloves, and clothing covers in an attempt to keep clothing contamination from the produce. Trays, pallets, and bins are washed or even de-sanitized prior to being passed into the packing area. Both are attempts to keep field dirt and hazardous adulterants from entering the packing house and serving as sources of cross-contamination.

Although the packing house example above is rather simplistic, large producers commonly employ much more extensive controls through wash, pack, and ship operations than that shown above, whereas other packers either ignore or simply do not care about much more than getting the product to market.

As food is moved from the packing house and into distribution, it should be obvious that the trucks carrying from the farm to the packing house or distribution center may become contaminated and are, therefore, potential sources of farm level or packing house contaminants. Fig. 6.10 shows a portable trailer cleaning system that is towed behind a pickup truck to various farm locations. Based on established cleaning procedures, the truck trailer may be inspected and cleaned with specified disinfectants at specified intervals using such portable cleaners.

In some cases, it is advisable to determine whether or not the wash operation can be validated as a preventive control. This can be done by sampling the trailer bed and walls using a system that can detect food residues (as a basic test). The test procedure should become part of a farm's (or any other perishable food transportation process) environmental sampling plan and procedures.

The testing of the trailer bed is shown in Fig. 6.11.

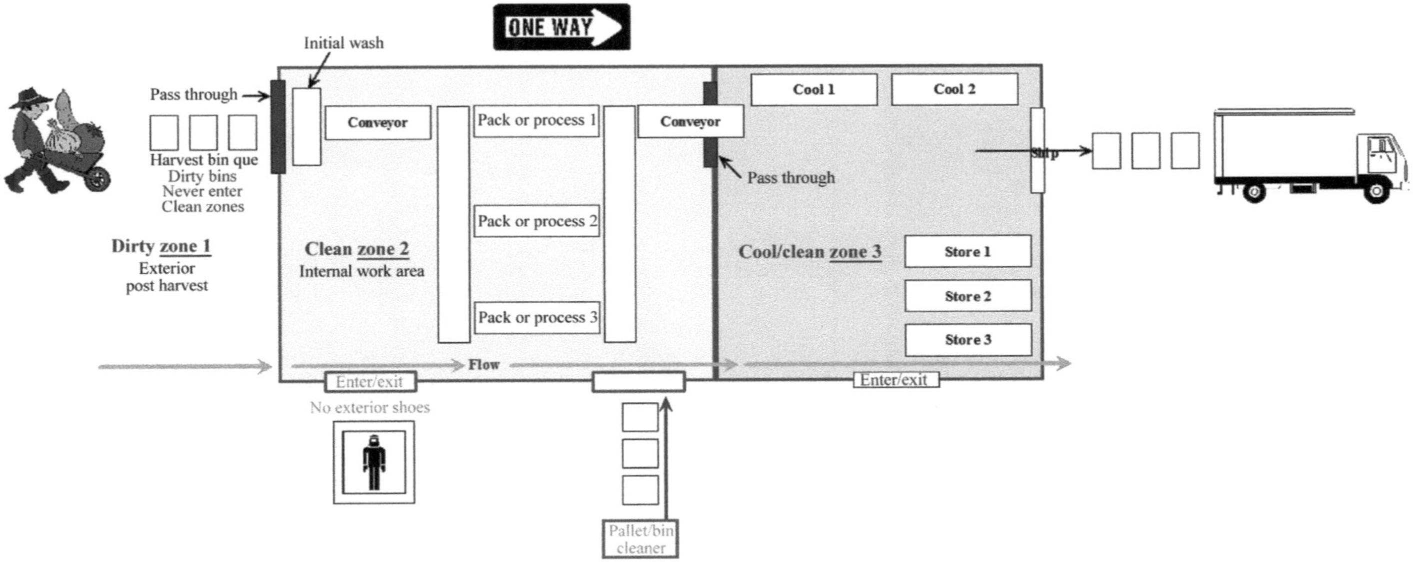

FIGURE 6.9

Contamination control through the packing house.

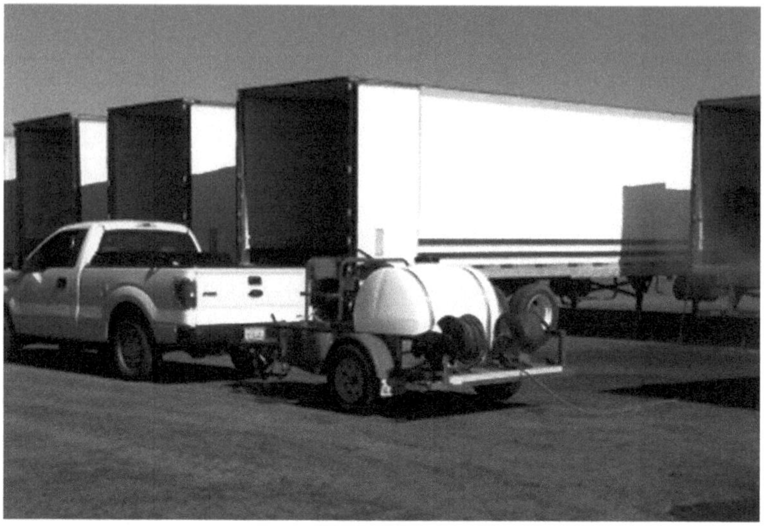

FIGURE 6.10

Farm trailer washing.

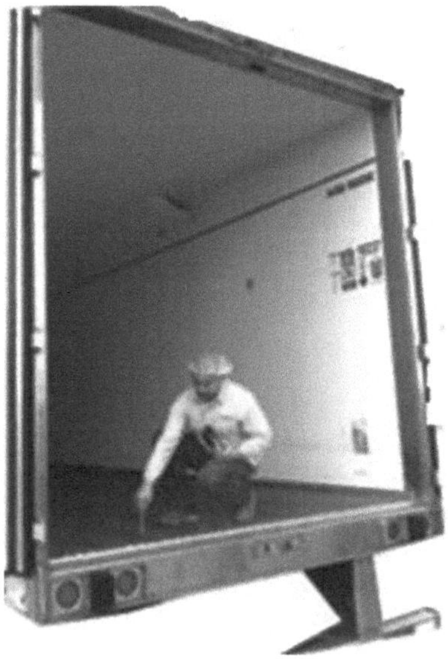

FIGURE 6.11

Environmental sampling in perishable carrying truck trailers.

One of the most common and lowest cost initial testing procedures is known as ATP or adenosine triphosphate. ATP is a surface cleanliness tester (see chapter: Environmental Monitoring and Sampling). The idea is not to test every trailer after every wash, but to use the system to determine whether or not the wash process (frequency, water pressure, etc.) is keeping potential cross-contaminating bio-hazards under some level of control.

Regardless of whether or not testing is part of the preventive process controls designed to prevent cross-contamination, record keeping is required. Date, time, location, test results, and other data must be collected and maintained. It is preferential to select and implement a testing system tied to computer, database, and analytic capabilities. By doing so, a process control team or quality personnel can analyze the data to determine whether or not the process is under control, establish preventive procedures, and validate the process's ability to reduce, eliminate, and control bacterial hazards.

FOOD PROCESSING OPERATIONS

During food processing and other operations, controls may be established and maintained using colors to designate the specific personnel, took, handling, and processing sanitation and temperature requirements for various facility areas. Fig. 6.12 illustrates a sample sketch of a processing operation that is being managed according to different preventive sanitation and temperature controls based on the location and need to protect food products from contamination.

In this case, the dirty areas requiring ambient sanitation controls are shown in yellow. As food enters the operation from the field and as food is in the shipping process,

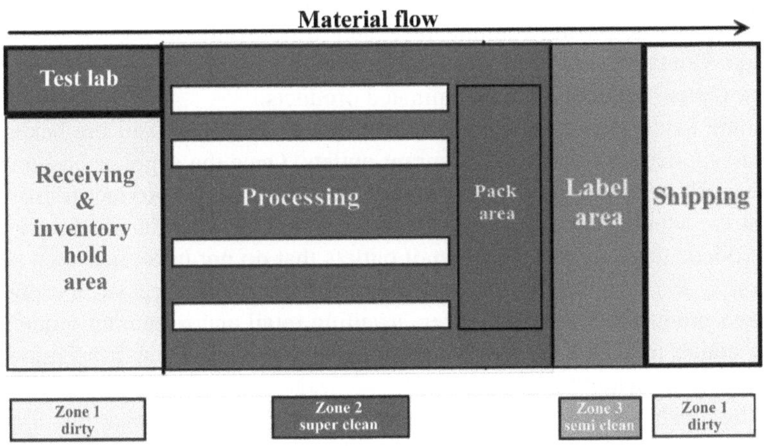

FIGURE 6.12

Color coding the processing operation.

sanitation conditions may be minimal until the product is washed and enters zone 2. The test lab, processing, and packing area are designated as zone 2 and are colored red. All personnel and equipment in the red zone 2 have the highest level sanitation controls based on the company's food safety plan and procedures. Ordinarily, the tools and equipment used in the lab, processing, and packing operations should be maintained in a sanitary condition and controlled to prevent their use in yellow or gray zones. An intermediate zone 3 is established for package protection and is shown as a gray area. Clean shipping pre-shipping controls are established in zone 3. Pre-shipping operations may contain storage of shipping packaging in sanitary conditions. Once the product is protected with clean packaging (completely enclosed by a container), it is moved into the shipping area.

Note that, assurances need to be established so that no tools or equipment are allowed to be moved from any zone to another zone. This would include forklifts, floor jacks, and other mobile equipment, though zone product movement can be accomplished using conveyors.

DISTRIBUTION CENTERS

Distribution centers can become a prime source of cross-contaminants. Many distribution centers do not wash fresh product after harvest. That means that they send unwashed product directly into restaurants and retail outlets unwashed. As such, contaminants are brought in from the field, moved into the distribution centers, and are stored in coolers to await order processing when the pallets of cases are broken down to fulfill store orders. Individual cases are taken from several different pallets and placed on a store-delivery pallet after which the new pallet is placed in a reefer and sent by truck to the store.

In the cases where unwashed produce is in the delivery process, the distribution center as well as tools and equipment related to transportation operations are also unwashed. Contaminants from any single incoming batch can easily be transferred onto new pallets with other uncontaminated products.

In some cases, the distribution center may deliver frozen and pre-baked product from suppliers to retail and restaurant outlets. Once the supplier has developed products such as baked goods, sandwiches and the like, the product is frozen and stored at the supplier awaiting delivery to large regional distribution centers. Most of the produce that can be seen in retail outlets that do not have their own bakeries is processed and delivered this way. Once at the distribution center, the pre-baked and frozen product is stored in freezers awaiting retail and restaurant orders. When an order comes in, pick lines are set up on the central floor of the distribution center similar to that shown in Fig. 6.13.

The figure shows that pallets are set up on both sides of the pick line. Each pallet contains a different product from a different supplier. A conveyor line runs down the middle of the two pallet lines and order fulfillment personnel read each order as delivery trays come down the line. Each order fulfillment person reads the order and

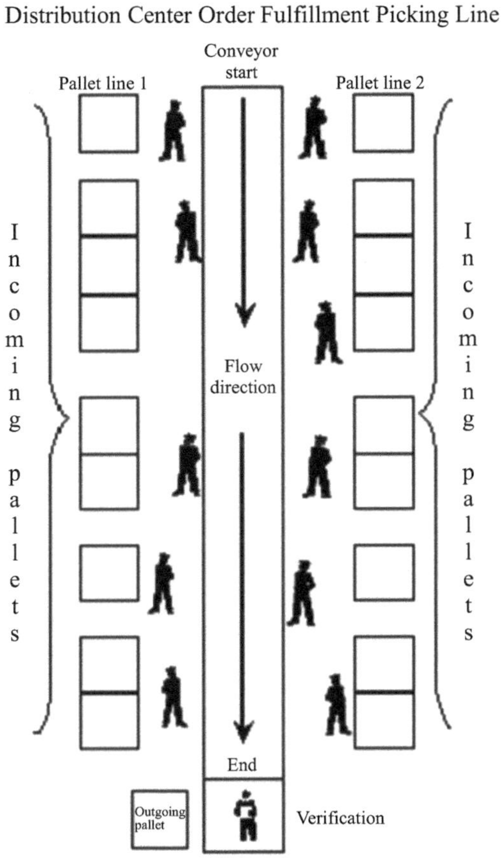

FIGURE 6.13

In process tray.

picks the appropriate amount of each product and places that quantity on the tray that is moving down the conveyor. At the end of the line, a quality department employee checks the written order against the product on the tray. Once the tray has passed inspection, the retail delivery tray (Fig. 6.14) is placed on a loading rack to await pickup and loading into delivery trucks.

It should be noted that in many cases, once the food has left the freezer prior to being placed in the pickline, the food is left on the pallets for some period of time in ambient temperatures to allow the food to defrost. In some cases, temperatures in the pickline can reach over 100° during hot weather.

More importantly, the trays going down the line to have the picked order placed on them rarely go through any type of sanitation process. Furthermore, the delivery trays are not stored in any type of sanitary condition and are often left open to the

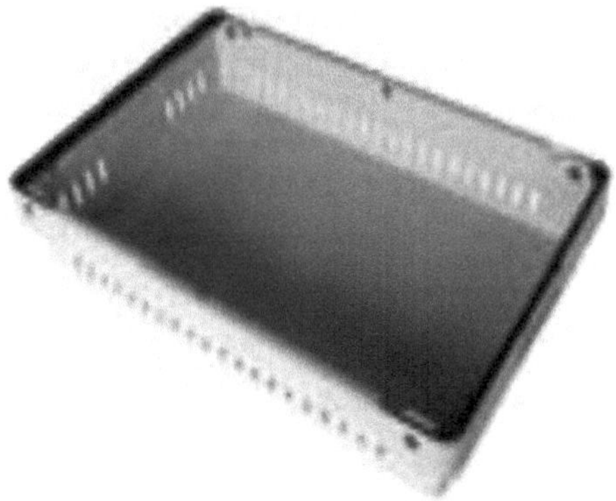

FIGURE 6.14

Store delivery tray.

environment. In other words, clean food is placed on dirty trays. As the trays are dirty, the bottom of food and food packages becomes contaminated from the trays. This contaminant is then loaded onto delivery racks and moved into delivery trucks. The trucks deliver the trays to retail outlets and restaurants where the trays are carried into food storage and sales areas. The contaminants from the trays moves onto display case shelves where it continues to reside until the product is purchased, and the contaminants are carried into homes to rest in refrigerators, on sinks and on dining tables.

The lack of a wash process for delivery trays can, in similar instances, become a prime source of contaminant flow. A preventive process would establish sanitation conditions for the delivery trays and, even perhaps, the racks in the delivery trucks. This would mean that in the distribution center, a tray wash process would be set up. In addition, some basic way of testing for bacterial and chemical hazardous materials would also be established. Validation of the tray cleaning process would mean washing the trays and occasionally taking a single or more trays, doing surface tests for contaminants (environmental sampling), and adjusting wash process variables (temperatures, spray pressures, type of sanitizer) until the process is stable and has contaminants under control.

Consider also that regardless of what process is followed for keeping the distribution center clean, unless the upstream bakery delivers food in a clean delivery process, the contaminated stream will begin with them. Even if delivery trays are sanitized, they must be stored under conditions that prevent them from becoming contaminated while awaiting use.

Moving back upstream to the bakery or product supplier, if the food is delivered dirty trays or on dirty pallets that move into the distribution center, contaminants are moved from the supplier into the distribution center floors. Similarly, using unclean packaging allows for food in direct contact with the packaging to become contaminated at the source.

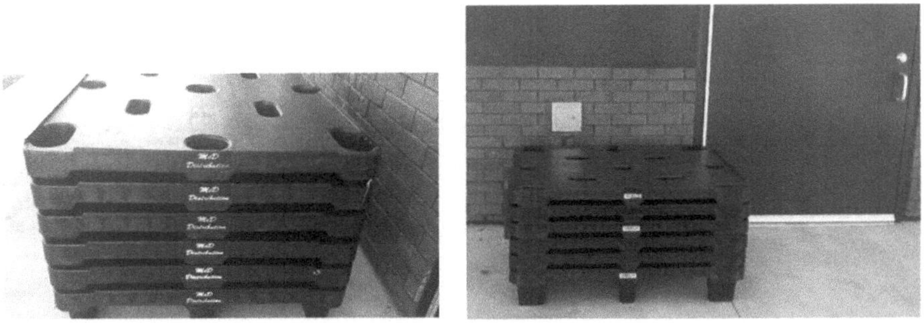

FIGURE 6.15

McDonald's tray delivery.

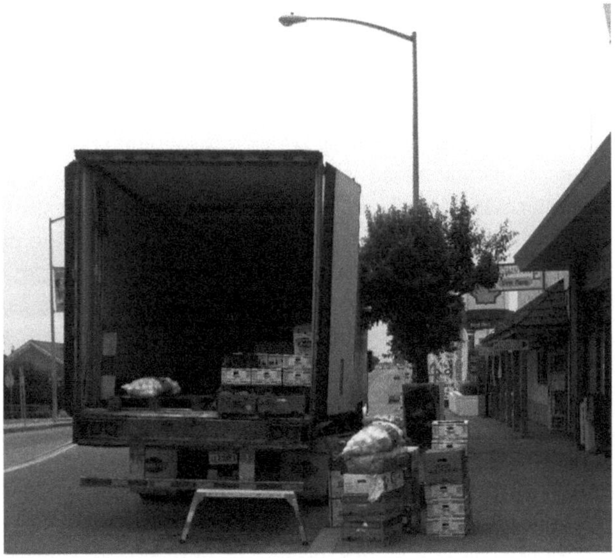

FIGURE 6.16

Illegal food delivery.

McDonald's has taken the issue seriously and implemented a plastic tray system that allows for delivery of foods into retail outlets to be delivered on clean trays (Fig. 6.15). Each tray contains a bar code for tracking and for the collection and storage of data related to when and where the tray was last washed. The trays are also designed with short legs on them to keep the food some inches off the ground.

The McDonald's delivery system can be compared with that shown in Fig. 6.16. In this case, food is placed in stacks on the sidewalk that is often used for dog delivery systems, oral discharges, and such.

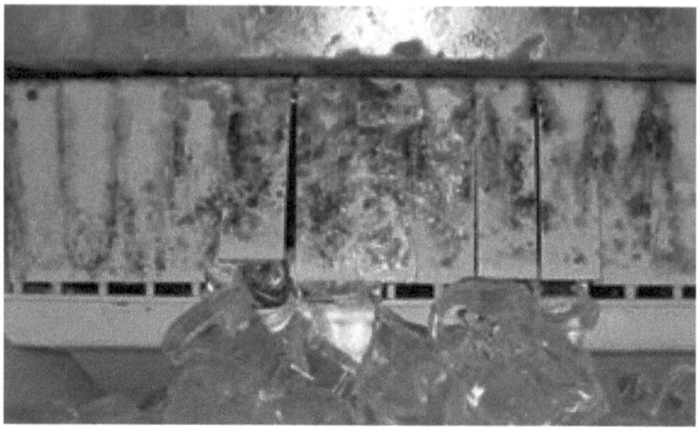

FIGURE 6.17

Dirty ice maker.

ICE COOLING SYSTEMS

Many packing or holding operations may not have sufficient cooling capacity during harvest times. In such instances, ice is used as a coolant. The ice is often uploaded to a drip system under which fresh produce may be palletized or sitting in piles. As the ice above melts, the cold dripping water is expected to cool the produce below. Whether or not the ice is tested for contaminants is anyone's question, but preventive practices would require testing the ice and controlling the process. Fig. 6.17 shows how even a simple ice maker can contaminate ice.

At the end of the supply chain, one could easily assume that the ice in Fig. 6.17 was used to keep fish cold on supermarket shelves.

In the case of restaurant cross-contamination (Chipotle), initial track back and recall operations will focus on who ate what, when, and where. The restaurant enters the Center for Disease Control's cross-hairs and becomes the primary target for an investigation. The news hits the press, the value of the company's stock falls and consumers, fearing for their own health, frequent competitor restaurants. Most of the time, we never hear about chemical cross-contamination. Chemical cross-contamination from pesticides, herbicides, and fertilizers seems to be a taboo subject despite great speculation about the impact such chemicals might have and working diligently on prevention, detention, and protection from chemical contaminants seems to be placed on the back-burner as far as food safety is concerned.

The recession that hit the world in 2008 onward inadvertently created problems for the food supply chain. Many governments, seeking to reduce costs and cut back on the size of governmental staff, reduced or eliminated produce sampling, and testing in distribution centers. Government health personnel in some places were previously taking samples of produce as it arrived at the distribution center before it could escape into the supply chain. Some of these government workers took the samples back to government labs for testing and required that the produce be kept out of distribution until test results were completed, and the product could be cleared for distribution or returned to the farm due to contaminants. As the government agencies were required to test the product for chemicals, many of them had established their own very expensive testing labs. Due to the economic pressures, to reduce the size of government and save money, health agencies, while looking at their budgets and due to pressure from farms and distributors, simply eliminated the labs thereby making testing for chemicals at a distributor's incoming operations a thing of the past.

From a food safety perspective, the changes resulted in a severely backwards move.

As discussed above, cross-contamination is commonly mistakenly only associated with the transfer

1. of bacteria
2. in kitchens and food processing.

The fact is, cross-contamination may include many types of hazardous adulterants and it begins with

- the wind or water on the farm,
- moves into harvest bins,
- continues through product wash and packing,
- moves into truck trailers and shipping containers,
- flows into distribution centers and coolers,
- resides on store or super market shelves, and
- long before it is a problem in restaurant, retail outlet or home kitchens.

There are many ways for containers and foods to become contaminated, but little attention is paid to control one source of contamination from getting into or onto the next product to inhabit containers used to move food through the supply chain. These include the following:

- Dirty or contaminated product
- Water
- Trays
- Packaging
- Bins
- Utensils and tools
- Food handlers

For instance, Food Safety News published a report entitled "Studies Find Reusable Produce Containers Often Contaminated." In two studies, 43% of the containers used by farmers that were being sanitized exhibited excessive levels of fecal contamination and failed United Kingdom (UK) food safety standards for food surfaces. Harvest bins and other small containers used to transport foods from one operation to another, all have food in contact with the interior surfaces of the container. Prevention would not require not only sanitizing the container, but also testing the interior surfaces of the container to bring sanitation processes under valid preventive controls [2].

(A) (B)

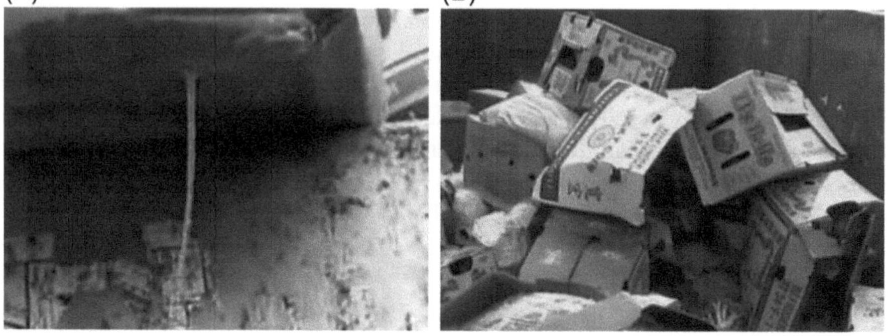

FIGURE 6.18

(A) Defrosting chicken. (B) Contaminated produce.

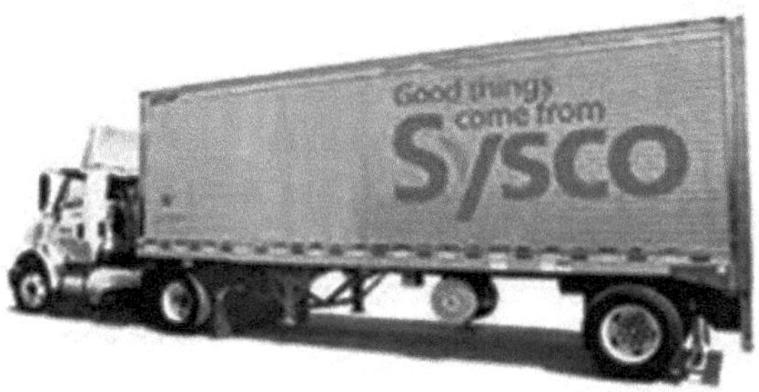

FIGURE 6.19

Do good things come from Sysco? [4].

National broadcasting company (NBC) News's special reporters Jeff Rossen and Leonor Ayala published an article in 2012 that highlighted the fact that Indiana state police were stopping trucks with reefers on the trailers and measuring the inside temperatures.

From Rossen, "On our first stop we found trouble; police said the truck's refrigerator wasn't working properly. By law, the food should have been at a cool 41°; some of it was pushing 60! There were yogurts in there too, for kids, all destined for a dozen grocery stores.

The driver told us he was actually relieved the cops stopped him: 'I'm glad that it didn't make it.' His company told us it monitors food temperatures carefully, and that, the unit was working when the truck left the warehouse, claiming the driver would have disposed of bad food before delivering it."

Fig. 6.18(A) and (B) illustrates one type of problem. Frozen chicken is defrosting in Fig. 6.18(A), and the juice from the frozen chicken was dripping onto the produce stacked below it. Chicken often contains salmonella that is killed when the chicken is cooked. Unfortunately, the lettuce, broccoli, and other produce stored under the chicken do not always get cooked. The result is salmonella laden produce that goes onto kitchen preparation surfaces (thus contaminating the surfaces and tools) and is then tossed into the salad. This is a simple process that can be defined and easily prevented.

The state police found chicken stored above fresh product open to the environment. The chicken had defrosted, and the chicken juice was draining down onto the produce. There is a reasonable probability that any bacteria that was now proliferating because of the heat was being actively transferred from the chicken through the dripping blood and juice down onto the produce.

In our kitchen example above, the problem of cross-contamination in the kitchen was highlighted when knives were used to cut raw chicken then used again to cut lettuce and tomatoes. The cross-contamination potential in that kitchen example and the cross-contamination that could occur in the heated truck trailer are identical.

Such cases are what the new FSMA rules classify as economically motivated adulteration or economically motivated adulteration (EMA) [3].

A highly publicized case involving Sysco is another example of EMA. Sysco reportedly delivers food to over 400,000 food operations across the United States and Canada (Fig. 6.19). In a news report concerning some questionable Sysco deliveries in the San Francisco Bay area, the Midwest and Canada, NBC investigative unit reporters found that the company was unloading reefer trailers into the type of storage sheds you and I would use for storing excess furniture. Found in the sheds were milk, chicken, raw meats, produce, and other perishables on their way to be delivered to restaurants and retail outlets. The reporters measured shed temperatures as high as 81° and observed Sysco sales people picking up loads of food, placing the food into the trunks of their cars and moving the food to their customers. The California Department of Public Health fined Sysco $19 million dollars and Sysco claimed to reorganize to prevent a recurrence. The potential for cross-contamination and the threat to overall food safety were significant.

As late as 2016, one of the America's major US trucking companies provided the author with information regarding the new ability of Arizona state police to monitor truck load temperatures with newly acquired technology. Though preventing food safety problems is their primary objective, by stopping food safety problems, prevention of cross-contamination also occurs.

Some religions, most notably the Jewish and Islam religions, maintain strict food safety standards to prevent contamination and cross-contamination through their food distribution processes. Jewish food is known as Kosher, and food transport tanks about to transport Kosher foods cannot carry any nonKosher foods for the previous three trips. Kosher foods also tank cleaning after each trip using high temperature steam clean all in the name of the prevention of cross-contamination.

Muslim foods (Halal) have established guidelines for strict cleanliness in all food processing and transportation, manufacturing, and environmental controls and require good manufacturing practices to be classified as Halal. Halal guidelines is also called as Codex General Guidelines on labeling claims [5].

THE KICKERS: RAW LIQUID EGG CROSS-CONTAMINATION AND OTHER OUTBREAKS

The potential for cross-contamination during transportation operations abounds. In 1994 a salmonellosis outbreak occurred in which ice cream mix became contaminated during transport in tanker trucks that had previously hauled raw liquid eggs. That outbreak affected an estimated 224,000 persons nationwide and clearly established a need for legal control over the transportation of hazardous foods in interstate commerce.

Some of the other outbreaks that led the law are noted by the FDA below:

> *"In 1974, an incident involving contamination of a component of food for animals in a rail car occurred. This case, which FDA investigated after receiving reports of several sickened dogs, involved corn gluten used in dog food. The corn gluten was determined to have been transported in a rail car that had been previously used to transport lead monoxide. Samples taken of the dog food in which the corn gluten was used revealed that it was contaminated with lead monoxide at levels ranging up to 28,000 parts per million. A Class I recall was issued for the dog food and other food for animals manufactured at the same plant within the same time period. Additionally, FDA successfully prosecuted the carrier involved in this incident."*

"In July 1999, an outbreak of *Salmonella* Muenchen occurred in 15 States and 2 Canadian provinces with more than 300 cases reported (66 FR 6138 at 6172, January 19, 2001). The product was fresh orange juice, a portion of which was imported. Several serotypes of *Salmonella* were isolated from tanker truckloads of juice tested at the United States/Mexican border. In such circumstances, there is a potential that *Salmonella* from one contaminated shipment could contaminate future shipments [6].

In 2007, the Motor Carrier Division of the Michigan State Police reported 22 cases of illegal and unsafe food transport on Michigan highways during 2006 [7]. The report listed findings such as:

- Raw poultry hanging from the roof inside the cargo area of a truck, with juices dripping onto open boxes of produce below, and with juices from the raw poultry dripping out onto the pavement from under the rear cargo box doors. The food was being transported in an unrefrigerated truck with an internal temperature greater than 70°F;
- Truck(s) with no refrigeration unit;
- Truck(s) with the refrigeration unit turned off or not working; and
- Truck(s) with a working refrigeration unit that was not set at the correct temperature."

These outbreaks and others resulted in the FDA issuing the "Implementation of Sanitary Food Transportation Act of 2005." In that document, the FDA noted the following [8].

CROSS-CONTAMINATION THROUGH THE SPREAD OF PORCINE EPIDEMIC DIARRHEA VIRUS

Harvest facilities serve as a source of contact between many swine farms with different health statuses. This study suggests that collection points, such as harvest facilities and livestock auction markets, can be an efficient source of contamination of transport vehicles that return to pig farms and likely played a role in rapidly disseminating porcine epidemic diarrhea virus (PEDV) across vast geographic regions shortly after PEDV was first identified in the United States. These data also suggest that the contamination of loading ramps and transport vehicles leaving the harvest facilities increased as the prevalence of PEDV—Positive transport vehicles and virus load coming into the facility increased. In other words, the sick pigs loaded by ramps and conveyors and the truck trailers became loaded with impacted pit feces. When the next group of piglets was loaded using the dirty ramps and conveyors or hauled and carried in dirty trucks, the virus was transferred from the transportation equipment to the piglets that were not sick thereby increasing the spread of infection through cross-contamination. The newly impacted piglets were then delivered to other farms not previously exposed to the virus resulting in contamination of the clean farm and the illness and death of a new set of animals.

The results of this study suggest that proactive disease control measures should include improved sanitation, hygiene, and segregation practices at collection points to limit the spread of the agent early in the outbreak.

This study of PEDV transmission by fomites should serve as an example of the risks that a modern, highly technical animal protein industry may encounter during a novel disease introduction [9].

ALLERGENS

Under preventive control rules in the United States, the food and drug administration (FDA) food safety modernization act (FSMA) rules, allergens become a focus primarily because allergens impact a significant percentage of the population, and when unidentified allergens escape into the population, the media is quick to jump on the escape and the associated consequences. Thus, allergens are specifically identified within cross-contact rules where allergen cross-contact is defined as "the unintentional incorporation of a food allergen into a food." It should be noted that intentional adulteration is included in other FDA rules [10].

A quick review of FDA recall lists clearly illustrates the fact that allergen labeling is a primary cause for issuing recall notices.

Any substance that can trigger a hypersensitive or allergic reaction in sensitive humans can be called an allergen.

Eight foods account for 90% of all food-allergic reactions in the United States. There are no cures for food allergies. These include the following:

Peanut
Tree nuts
Milk

Egg
Wheat
Soy
Fish
Shellfish

While eating allergens is not dangerous to most of the human population, the impact that allergens may have on humans may depend on, the individual's age, health, how much of the allergen is consumed, whether or not the eaten product is raw, cooked, or processed, other foods eaten with the allergen and the condition of the eater.

Peanut allergens are well known but cannot always be avoided because they tend to be included or become part of other unsuspected sources. For instance, peanut allergens can often be found in the following:

Thai, African, Asian, and Mexican dishes
Sauces such as chili sauce, hot sauce, pesto, gravy, mole sauce, and salad dressing
Sweets such as pudding, cookies, baked goods, pies, and hot chocolate
Egg rolls
Pancakes
Specialty pizzas
Some vegetarian food products, especially those advertised as meat substitutes
Foods that contain extruded, cold-pressed or expelled peanut oil, which may contain peanut protein
Glazes and marinades
In addition, in some kitchens or restaurants, many foods are cooked in peanut oil that goes undetected by the consumer.

ALLERGEN CONTROL RESOURCES

Allergen problems associated with food-contact surfaces are of critical importance when it comes to preventive sanitation practices. Under Current Good Manufacturing Practices allergens, cross-contact is specifically called out under requirements for storage and handling of cleaned portable equipment and tools (tables, slicers, trays, bins, mixing kettles, etc.) [7].

Within any food manufacturing environment, there are some issues to consider including the identification of the adulterant and failure to disinfect after allergen process use. Manufacturing processes including internal transport, storage, packing, labeling, and training clearly fall under preventive controls. General process control planning, verification, and validation are required for such processes. This means that the best approach is to flow chart the process, specify each input, process step, and output on separate food safety and food quality flowcharts, control points, test requirements, denote standard operating procedures (SOPS) and work instructions (WI), recall and establish an excel spreadsheet to define all critical process steps and the requirements for all process steps as outlined in Chapter 4, Developing a Preventive Controls Plan: Food Safety and Quality. It is important to remember that under cross-contamination requirements all tools and equipment used in the process should also be addressed in the plan.

A good source of information related to allergen problems is the foodsafety.gov recall website. As an example in January, 2016 the list included the following allergen related recalls:

Allergen recalls (misbranding)

"Fresh Express Announces Precautionary Recall of a Limited Quantity of 12 oz. Baby Spinach Due to Possible Allergen Exposure

Fresh Express Incorporated is voluntarily issuing a precautionary recall of 350 cases of 12 oz. Fresh Express Baby Spinach with a Product Code of G010A17A and Use-By Date of January 24 due to a possible exposure to a tree nut allergen (almond). Fresh Express representatives are already coordinating with stores to remove the recalled product from retail stores where distributed, primarily in Eastern and Southeastern states."

Other allergen related recalls on January 19, 2016 included the following:

Blendtech Issues Allergy Alert on Undeclared Milk Allergen in Uncle Buck's Fish Batter Mix—Original

Kermit, Inc. Issues Allergy Alert on Undeclared Soy and Anchovies in Various Barbecue Sauces

Giant Eagle Youngstown Voluntarily Recalls New Year's Pretzels from Select Stores Due to an Undeclared Walnut Allergen [11].

In the European Union, FoodDrink Europe has established guidance to help food manufactures to manage allergens. FoodDrink Europe provides a free 85-page download for users that can be useful when reviewing and planning allergen control systems. Table 6.1 includes the guidance document table of contents to review for usefulness.

The intent of the FoodDrink guidance is "To provide sound, evidence-based and consistent information on good practice in risk management of allergenic foods and certain food intolerances (hereafter referred to as 'allergen management') for food producers of foodstuffs intended for sale to the general population" [12].

A couple of other allergen resources are to be found at the University of Nebraska at Lincoln. And their website (http://www.allergenonline.com) provides information on 744 taxonomic-protein groups with proven allergen involvement. The university's Institute of Agriculture and Natural resources provides allergenic foods and their allergens [13].

Readers may also check the World Health Organization and International Union of Immunological Societies [14].

In 2005, the FDA published good information regarding allergen labeling in the form of an online advice document entitled "Food Allergen Labeling and Consumer Protection Act of 2004 Questions and Answers". The document provides answers to

Table 6.1 FoodDrink Table of Contents

2. Risk management processes
2.1. Overview
2.2. People
2.3. Supplier management
2.4. Raw materials handling
2.5. Equipment and factory design
2.6. Production process and manufacturing controls
2.7. Consumer information
2.8. Product development and change
2.9. Documentation and record-keeping
3. Cleaning and cleaning validation
3.1. General
3.2. Cleaning methods
4. Analytical methods and their application
5. Key Principles of allergen risk management

29 consumer questions and multiple links to other information sources. The Federal Food, Drug and Cosmetic Act requires that that the label of a food that contains an ingredient that is or contains protein from a "major food allergen declare the presence of the allergen in the manner described by the law." In this document, the FDA establishes legal requirements to assure the listing of all ingredients and the word "contain" if any ingredient in the food product contains an allergen [15].

FOOD SUPPLY CHAIN CROSS-CONTAMINATION AND DISTRIBUTION OF CONTAMINANTS DURING FOOD TRANSPORTATION OPERATIONS

Transportation operations may be viewed as the bloodstream through which food flows from origin to destination. Any potential contamination source anywhere in the supply chain now becomes a potential contributor. Farm to fork, this bloodstream has a potential that has not taken seriously. In the same manner that a human's blood stream will move viruses and bacteria from a single source throughout the whole body, transportation processes distribute contaminants throughout the food supply chain.

Hazardous chemicals, bacteria, and physical objects do not ordinarily originate in food shipping containers, on transportation equipment, in rail cars, or in food carrying truck trailers. They migrate through the food supply blood stream through transportation processes.

Considering how contaminants can flow through food distribution processes, it is clear that any time food is in the process of moving from one spot or place to another,

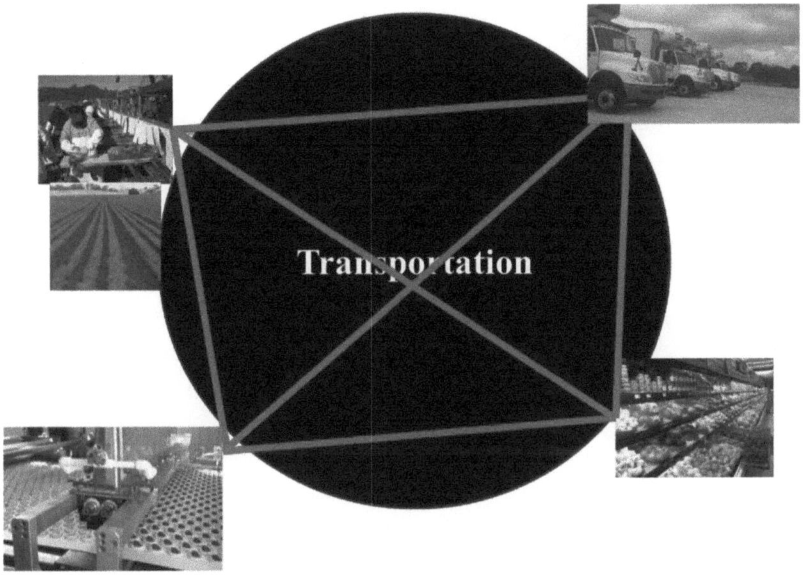

FIGURE 6.20

The black hole.

the contaminants get a free ride. Any and all containers used to move food from one place to another becomes potential carriers of the contaminants as well and if not properly maintained, those carriers become cross-contaminated and transfer the contaminant from one product in one food movement process to the next product in the next food movement process.

The US FDA defines transportation as movement of food in commerce by motor vehicle or rail vehicle and focuses on what they call food not completely enclosed by a container, in other words, perishables. But, what do we know about what goes on when food is actually in the transportation process. For the most part, it is a bit of a black hole (Fig. 6.20).

For the most part, the identity, location, and condition of what are basically perishable foods when the condition of such food is on the road is unknown, ignored, mismanaged, or, in the case of some companies, properly managed.

Consider what may be commonly observed during a walk through a food supermarket. On one side, one would usually see produce a bakery and perhaps a deli, all containing foods not completely enclosed by a container or subject to temperature control requirements. At the rear of the market are seen fish, meat, packaged deli items, and milk and dairy products. These are also foods either not completely enclosed by a container (Fig. 6.21) or requiring temperature controls. Continuing our walk around the supermarket perimeter to the other side, we can see many other temperature-controlled products such as eggs, cheeses, etc. Somewhere near the

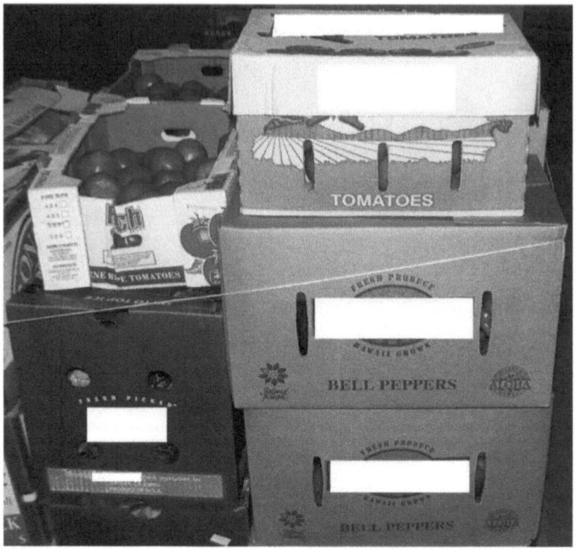

FIGURE 6.21

Food not completely enclosed by a container.

dairy section, it is not uncommon to find frozen food products such as pizzas, ice cream, and frozen foods and dinners. Basically, most of the perimeter of the supermarket contains foods that come under FDA FSMA food transportation regulations.

In the middle of the market are packaged products that are usually completely enclosed by a container and require no temperature controls. These foods are exempt from FDA FSMA food transportation regulations.

Containers that move the food from one place to another may be defined as any device used to transport food or food products. Containers may include bins, pallets, trucks, tankers, truck trailers, shipping containers, rail cars, planes, and other similar devices.

As food load and unload processes include things like conveyors, ramps, forklifts, and people, anything that potentially touches the food can also become contaminated and has the potential to pass the contaminant from the previous batch to the next.

A maintenance station can be defined as any operation involved in the sanitation of carriers, carrier equipment, or containers. Maintenance stations can become critically important in a preventive control system because they provide an opportunity to intercept and stop potential contaminants to the container as a cross-contaminating vehicle.

The FDA FSMA rules on the sanitary transportation of human and animal foods provide separate requirements for shippers, carriers, and receivers. Under these rules, a carrier is defined by the FDA as a "person who owns, leases, or is otherwise ultimately responsible for the use of a motor vehicle or rail vehicle to transport food" (private truck fleets, private fleet truck drivers, contracted drivers, distributors, leased vehicles).

The goal of the act, as stated by the FDA is to "require that all transportation operations be conducted under such conditions and controls as are necessary to prevent the food that they are transporting from becoming filthy, putrid, decomposed, or otherwise unfit for food, or being rendered injurious to health from any source during transportation operations."

Using the FDA's FSMA definition for a carrier, it becomes clear that the carrier and carrier operations can become a primary source for cross-contamination during the distribution of food contaminants.

Although many carriers have instituted excellent sanitation controls for containers (especially truck trailers), others have ignored the potential problem. Under the FDA FSMA rules on the sanitary transportation of human and animal foods, many new legal requirements have been levied on carriers in an effort to prevent contaminants from moving from one place to the next. The final law applies to carriers, shippers, receivers, and loaders engaged in transportation operations whether or not the food is being offered for or enters interstate commerce.

Among these spectrum of issues implied by the rules are requirements covering:

- Food not completely enclosed by a container
- Shippers, carriers, and receivers
- Frozen and temperature controlled foods
- Food shipped by rail or road
- Knowledge of bacteria, chemical, and physical hazards
- Vehicle and equipment design for clean ability
- Preventive control of hazards that can impact food during food load, unload, and transportation operations
- Preventive and corrective action
- Misuse of disinfectants and sanitizers
- The impact of not cleaning bins, trays, pallets, and other tools and equipment used in carrier operations
- Cross-contamination during transportation operations
- Employee personnel hygiene and wash stations
- Impact of temperature variation on bacterial hazards
- Vehicle, container, and trailer traceability and reporting systems
- Reefer failures and reefer failure record keeping
- Container maintenance (seals, doors, etc.)
- Lack of container maintenance, improper or missing container security systems, accidents, and recalls
- Establishing critical parameters and measurement; standards for management
- Validation of preventive controls
- Sanitation
- Temperature controls and monitoring (vehicles, trailers, and shipping containers),

- Procedures
- Record keeping and retention
- Audit and certification
- Training
- Sanitation and wash systems and procedures
- ATP and bacteria testing, inspection and re-inspection requirements
- Equipment calibration
- Maintenance of MSDS sheets
- Statistical analysis and records retention
- Contracts of carriage and agreements between shippers and carriers
- Transportation system assessment strategies
- Deadlines for full compliance
- Waiver application

In addition, the final rules on the Sanitary Transportation of Human and Animal Foods establish mandatory training requirements for all carrier personnel engaged in food transportation operations. Training certificates are required for all carrier personnel engaged in transportation operations upon hiring and as needed thereafter and such training will cover the following areas:

- Responsibilities of the carrier under the final rules
- Awareness of potential food safety problems that may occur during food transportation
- Basic sanitary transportation practices to address those potential problems

The FDA's rules apply to shippers, carriers, and receivers for food transported in the United States by road or rail. Air and ship are excluded from the rules simply because once a plane or ship lands, the food must be transported by road or rail to its next destination.

The rules define a shipper as "A person who initiates a shipment of food by motor vehicle or rail vehicle."

Keep in mind that any food handling operation other than restaurants or retailers are basically classified as shippers who eventually move food out of their operation and ship it to someplace else.

Conversely, someone must receive the food and according to the FDA, that operation is defined as a "receiver" or "Any person who receives food after transportation, whether or not that person represents the final point of receipt for the food."

Between the times that food is in a truck trailer or in a container, the food is being handled, moved, and might go through other processes. This brings up the FSMA definition for transportation equipment which means "equipment used in transportation operations other than vehicles." Under the rules, transportation equipment used in transportation operations can include things like "bulk and nonbulk containers, bins, totes, pallets, pumps, fittings, hoses, gaskets, loading systems, and unloading systems (Fig. 6.22). Transportation equipment also includes a railcar not attached to a locomotive or a trailer not attached to a tractor."

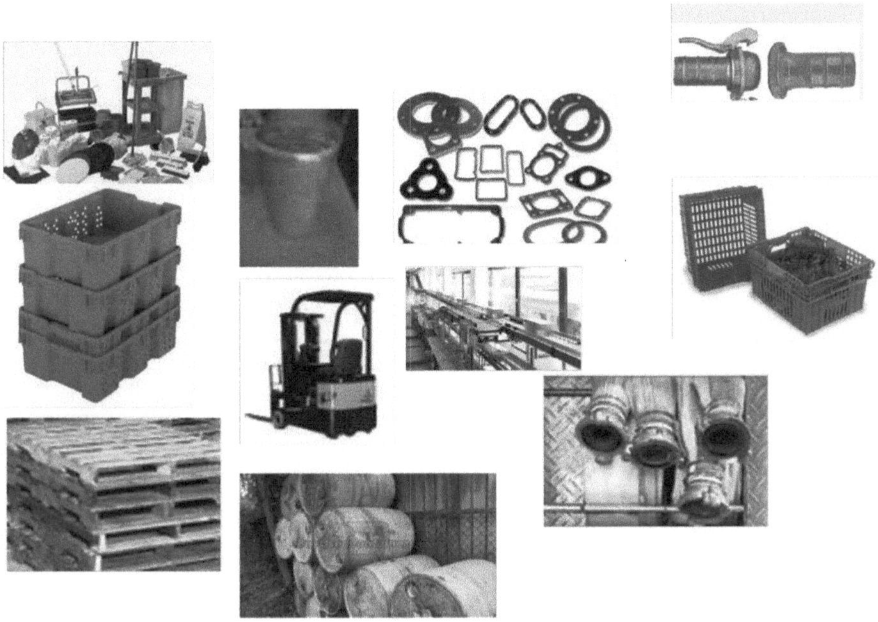

FIGURE 6.22

Transportation equipment.

(A) (B)

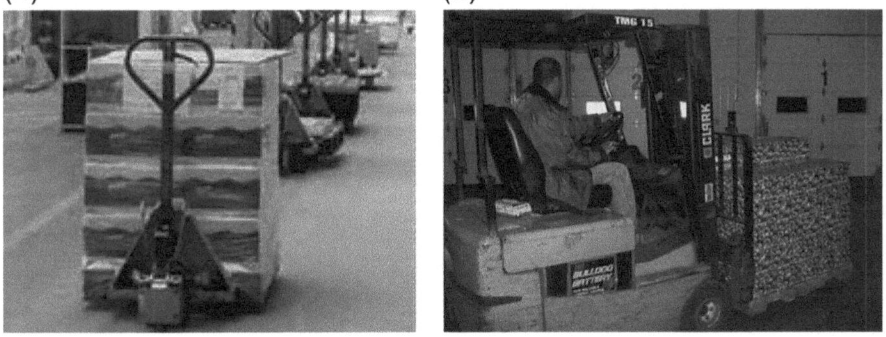

FIGURE 6.23

(A) Floor Jack. (B) Fork Lift.

Also included are floor jacks and fork lifts (Fig. 5.23(A) and (B)).

They further define transportation operations to mean "means all activities associated with food transportation that may affect the sanitary condition of food including cleaning, inspection, maintenance, loading and unloading, and operation of vehicles and transportation equipment.

Transportation operations do not include any activities associated with the transportation solely of shelf stable food that is completely enclosed by a container, compressed food gases or live food animals. In addition, transportation operations do not include any transportation activities for raw agricultural commodities that are performed by a farm."

SANITATION PROCESSES

Regardless of the place in the food supply delivery process, sanitation is critical. To develop procedures for assuring that such kill steps are established as part of a company's preventive controls, there are many factors to be considered in anticipation of sanitation process development. The following list includes some of important considerations:

- Type of food soils, biofilms, and other contaminants
- Solubility of contaminants
- Fat
- Protein
- Carbohydrate
- Mineral salt
- Microbiological films
- Lubricating greases and oils
- Surface composition
- Surface finish
- Surface condition
- Environmental conditions (waste)
- Chemistry of detergents
- Physically active ingredients
- Ionic surfactants
- Nonionic surfactants

Furthermore, conditions listed above would cause one to be faced with a number of sanitizing process choices including:

- Thermal requirements
    - Cold
    - Steam
    - Hot water
- Chemical to be used
- Regulations to be followed
- Customer specifications to meet
- Nonionic surfactants

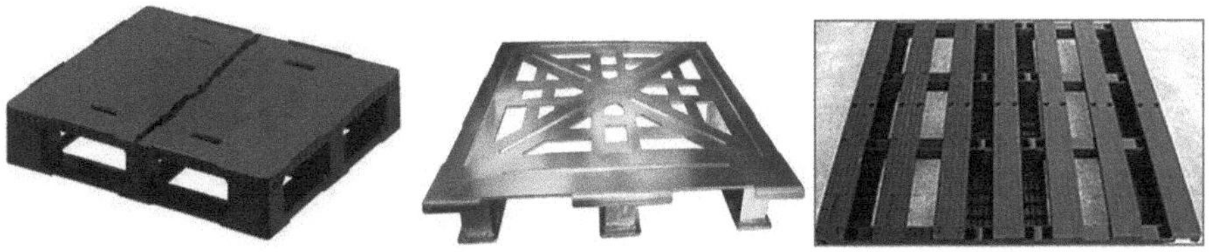

FIGURE 6.24

Cleanable plastic and aluminum pallets.

Such complex conditions would seem to require company personnel to ask suppliers for guidance when developing sanitation processes capable of providing an appropriate sanitation procedure that assures a kill step when required.

There are many ways for containers and foods to become contaminated, but little attention is paid to controlling one source of contamination from getting into or onto the next product to inhabit containers used to move food through the supply chain.

Dirty or contaminated product, packaging, water, trays, pallets, packaging, bins, utensils and tools, and food handlers all provide sources of cross-contamination in the supply chain. Solutions are quickly becoming available in anticipation of changing food safety requirements. As an example, plastic and aluminum pallets, that meet different specifications, are lightweight and washable are currently available (Fig. 6.24).

Some of these pallet designs also allow for the insertion of temperature recording devices that record temperatures, humidity conditions, and track the location of the pallet thus establishing control conditions through food supply chain processes. Fig. 6.25 shows a radio frequency identification or RFID-enabled tag embedded in the base of a plastic pallet. The tag is read by readers established at entry and exit doors on shipping docks, coolers and even in food carrying vehicles.

Of equal importance are newer wash systems designed to lower costs and provide sanitation flexibility for farm and on road vehicles, shipping containers, and trailers. Fig. 6.26 shows two types of automated trailer and container interior wash systems. Priced around $7000, the systems allow for adjustments of the spray pressure, water temperature, and also provide the user the opportunity to automatically dispense chemicals during disinfecting and sanitizing cycles. The systems are computer controlled. Operationally, they move unassisted into and out of the container being cleaned altering between wash, rinse, disinfectant, and other prescribed cycles.

Perhaps, the most common type of interior wash is simply to find a truck wash station along a highway. The problem is that far and few truck wash operations are set up to do interior wash. Those capable of interior wash generally offer only cold water rinses at a single spray pressure using manually operated hoses.

Container pre and post-washout inspection procedures are generally required to determine what type of washout is required based, again, on potential hazardous cross-contaminants. A partial sample pre and post-inspection procedure is shown below.

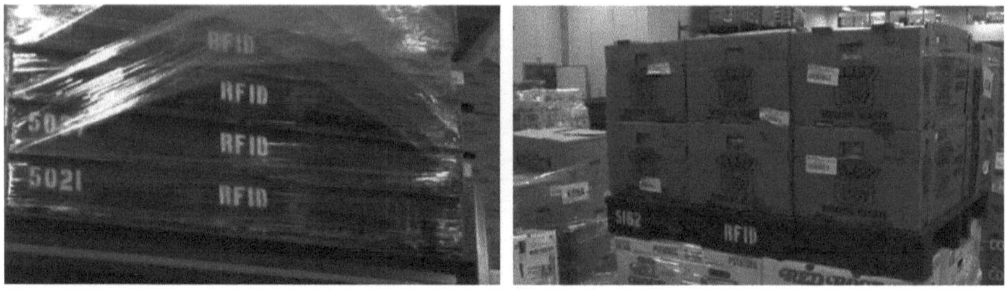

FIGURE 6.25

RFID-enabled pallet temperature recording device.

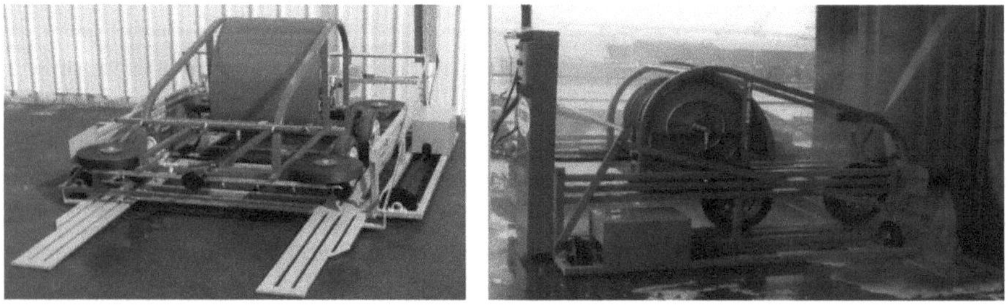

FIGURE 6.26

Robotic container, vehicle, and trailer wash systems.

STANDARD OPERATION PROCEDURE

Sanitized Container Washout Operation
Procedure for Initial Inspections and Contaminate Washout

Version XXX

OVERVIEW

Shipping container contamination can become a source of produce and/or carton cross-contamination. Containers are inspected upon arrival to determine if materials that pose a significant concern for cross-contamination are present. If so, then the container receives an additional wash and sanitation procedure prior to the normal washout and cleaning procedure. This procedure is followed regardless of the comments made by the truck driver.

Materials of concern can include, but are not limited to:

1. Blood
2. Animal pieces

3. Insect infestations
4. Chemicals
5. Rotten produce

PROCESS

1. The rear doors are partially opened and an odor check is done. This is done by an individual who basically sniffs the air. Any off odor is recorded and will lead to the double cleaning of the container.
2. The individual who enters the containers inspects the floors and Side walls for any signs of unusual contamination. The inspection results are recorded.

   If a source of a contaminate is found:

1. The concrete area just outside the rear doors is treated with dry quaternary amine (QUAT) powder.
2. The area with the contaminate is washed down with hot water and sprayed with QUAT 600–800 ppm.
3. The container is then washed using the "Standard Process."
4. The concrete area outside the rear doors is thoroughly washed and sprayed with QUAT 600–800 ppm.
5. If no source of contamination is found the *"Standard* Container Washout" is used.
6. All information is recorded onto the "Pre-inspection and post-inspection Container Form."

Notice that the procedure establishes record keeping requirements.

Fig. 6.27 shows a simple flowcharted truck trailer washout procedure. Specific spray pressure, temperature, and chemical cleaning requirements can be added to the flowchart based on product and customer hazard prevention requirements. The flowchart shows the trailer initial inspection (record keeping is required), a decision made based on the type of cleaning process the trailer requires (standard versus exception) and the basic city water washout at 180°F followed by any required chemical treatment, re-inspection, and the issuance of a compliance document to the driver. Not shown are any requirements for ATP or other food residue or bacterial testing that may be required to confirm that the wash operation (as defined) provides preventive control results that are valid in terms of the type of food being hauled.

Taking the flowchart above and detailing it into a written procedure is another option for defining washout operational requirements. A partial procedure is shown below.

STANDARD CONTAINER WASHOUT PROCEDURE

Version—XXX

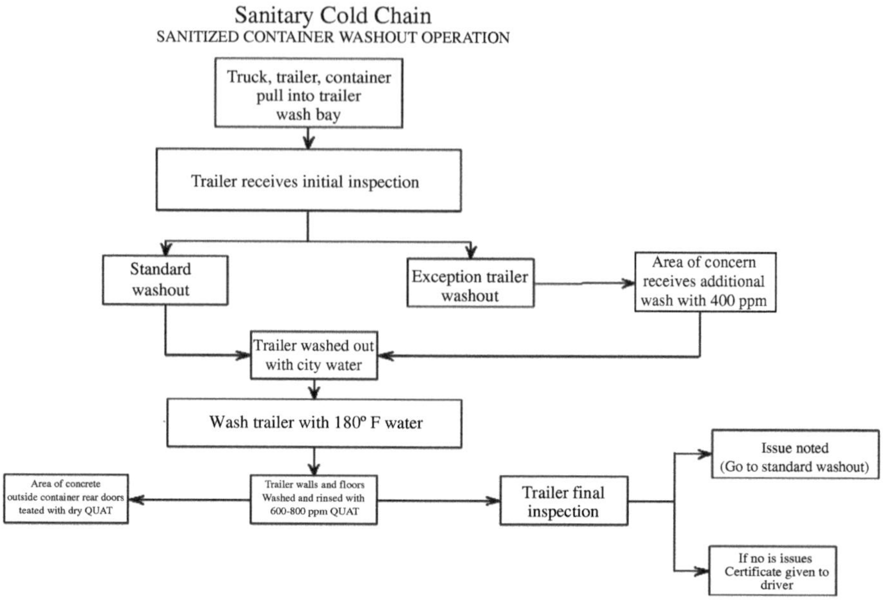

FIGURE 6.27

Basic trailer washout procedure.

OVERVIEW

A thorough washout of shipping containers is an operation that is recommended for all containers that ship or move perishables. This procedure should be followed whether a contaminant is monitored or not. The procedure will wash out debris as well as control potential sources of contamination on the floor and walls. Sources of debris can include, but are not limited to:

1. Wood, strapping material, parts of a carton, labels
2. Note: When a contaminate is noted the SOP (initial container inspector and contaminate washout) is followed

MATERIALS

High pressure municipal city water at tap temperature
High pressure municipal city water heated to 180°F
QUAT in a pressurized sprayer at 600–800 ppm
Brush to dean debris out of container (blue brush)
ATP Testing Kit
A certificate is given to the driver showing a successful washout procedure

The Sanitary Cold Chain Documentation Record

http://www.SanitaryColdChain.com PO Box 1290, Salinas, CA 93902
FAX (831) 769-0330 Cell: (831) 512 6267

PRE-INSPECTION AND POST-INSPECTION CONTAINER REPORT

TransCert Certified

			INITIAL INSPECTION RESULT			INSPECTOR	FINAL INSPECTION RESULT			INSPECTOR
DATE	TIME	CONTAINER ID	OK	ODOR YES/NO	CONTAMINANT IF YES, WHAT		OK	RE-WASH	ATP READING	

FIGURE 6.28

Sample standard pre-inspection and post-inspection trailer washout form.

PROCESS

The rear doors are partially opened and an odor check is done. This is done by an individual who sniffs the air. Any off odor and contaminate is recorded and will lead to the double cleaning of the container.

1. If no odor or contaminate is noted the following procedure is used.
2. Truck/container Information is recorded on the truck washout record.
3. A QUAT mixture of 600–800 ppm is made. City water is placed into a clean pressure sprayer and the concentration checked and recorded on the "QUAT Concentration Monitoring Form."
4. The container walls and floor are washed using city water at tap water temperature. Special attention is given to the floor to remove all debris.
5. The container walls and floor are washed using 180°F water that originated from the city water supply and run through a water heating unit.
6. The container walls and floor and then sprayed with a QUAT solution 600–800 ppm.

Record keeping is critical under preventive control rules. A sample pre-inspection and post-inspection record keeping form is shown in Fig. 6.28.

Of course, the need for procedures and appropriate record keeping includes many more procedures related to washout and sanitation. Listed below are a few of these needed procedures:

Color labeling and use guidelines for brooms, shovels, and other cleaning equipment
Procedure for cleaning tank sprayers
Mixing QUAT in sprayers and hand dip stations
Employee training
Use of hand and food dis
Worker hygiene
Maintaining MSDS sheets
OSHA requirements for washout personnel

REFERENCES

[1] Prevent Cross Contamination. http://www.health.state.mn.us/foodsafety/clean/xcontamination.html; June, 2016.
[2] Studies Find Reusable Produce Containers Often Contaminated. http://www.foodsafetynews.com/2014/11/studies-find-reusable-produce-containers-often-contaminated/#.VHyZCck3eM0; July, 2016.
[3] Rossen Reports: Some trucks carry unsafe food, authorities say. http://today.msnbc.msn.com/id/48691046/ns/today-today_rossen_reports/t/rossen-reports-some-trucks-carry-unsafe-food-authorities-say/#.UEY8yJaaJ8E; July 2016.
[4] Sysco Food Stored in Dirty Sheds Served to Bay Area Restaurants. http://www.nbcbayarea.com/news/local/Sysco-Food-Stored-in-Dirty-Sheds-Served-to-Bay-Area-Restaurants-215759351.html; July, 2016.
[5] General Guidelines for Use of the Term "HALAL" http://www.fao.org/docrep/005/y2770e/y2770e08.htm; July, 2016.
[6] Implementation of Sanitary Food Transportation Act of 2005. https://www.gpo.gov/fdsys/pkg/FR-2010-04-30/html/2010-10078.htm; July, 2016.
[7] Salmonella Poisoning Outbreak May Be Linked to Tanker Trucks. http://www.nytimes.com/1994/10/21/us/salmonella-poisoning-outbreak-may-be-linked-to-tanker-trucks.html; July, 2016.
[8] July 7, 2016 http://wwwnc.cdc.gov/eid/article/20/5/pdfs/13-1628.pdf.
[9] January 14, 2016 https://www.federalregister.gov/articles/2015/09/17/2015-21920/current-good-manufacturing-practice-hazard-analysis-and-risk-based-preventive-controls-for-human#h-415.
[10 August 11, 2016 https://www.federalregister.gov/articles/2015/09/17/2015-21920/current-good-manufacturing-practice-hazard-analysis-and-risk-based-preventive-controls-for-human#h-415.
[11] January 19, 2016 http://www.foodsafety.gov/recalls/recent/index.html.
[12] January 28, 2016 http://www.fooddrinkeurope.eu/uploads/press-releases_documents/temp_file_FINAL_Allergen_A4_web1.pdf.
[13] August 11, 2016 http://farrp.unl.edu/resources/gi-fas/informall.
[14] January 27, 2016 http://www.allergen.org/viewallergen.php?aid=754.
[15] August 3, 2016 http://www.fda.gov/Food/GuidanceRegulation/GuidanceDocuments RegulatoryInformation/Allergens/ucm106890.htm#q1.

CHAPTER

Supplier preventive controls and solutions

7

To a great extent, the part of the preventive controls rules is, perhaps, one of the most critical since it places significant responsibility on the company that hires, qualifies, and certifies food and service suppliers. In effect, it makes the receiving company liable for assuring that their suppliers establish and follow preventive controls. This is the U.S. food and drug administration (FDA) food safety modernization act (FSMA) requirements under what is called subpart G.

The reader should note that under the FSMA preventive controls validation rules, supplier validation controls do not need to be validated. However, careful tracking of supplier capabilities is critical and should be included in any preventive controls program.

The preventive control rules call for a risk-based preventive approach for all foods consumed in the United States whether imported or locally produced throughout the supply chain through the identification of risk and the application of appropriate food safety controls directed at prevention and elimination of adulterants through all processes.

Anyone who has been in business for any period of time knows that controlling suppliers and their products are fraught with danger to the receiving facilities operational stability. One bad ingredient or even a small quantity of bad product introduced into the receiving facility's processes can cause the receiving facility to face serious decisions regarding whether or not to scrap out a production run or to, perhaps, turn a blind eye to the problem and ship the final product on schedule. Such scenarios occur daily and create considerable internal turmoil between and among receiver functions. It is not unusual to hear the sales group and the operations personnel demanding to ship, whereas the food safety and quality groups stand steadfast against "meeting the schedule" under such circumstances. It is also not unusual for the operations group to ship product known to be contaminated.

The establishment of the U.S. FDA FSMA subpart G makes such activities a criminal act.

The overall rules, planning, and reporting systems for supplier preventive control rules comes under management responsibility and is therefore a topic to be addressed by common cause (CC) teams. Once ingredients or whole food reaches the incoming docks, the details involved in the analysis and throughput controls over the product come under the analysis and control of functional improvement teams (FIT) whose

Validating Preventive Food Safety and Quality Controls. DOI: http://dx.doi.org/10.1016/B978-0-12-810994-6.00007-9

responsibilities may go back to suppliers to assure that they establish acceptable preventive controls.

Assuming that a food company in the supply chain has its own valid preventive controls system on the basis of the ability to perform an accurate hazard analysis; controls risks in its processes; has excellent and valid procedures, practices, and products; knows how to take care of its sanitation issues; has a good local and federal compliance record along with an unblemished food safety history; controls temperatures as required; designs and performs excellent environmental sampling and test; and employs a good traceability system that gets on top of potential recalls quickly, the receiver must assure that company suppliers must also establish and manage an ongoing preventive controls system.

In short, liability, along the supply chain, becomes shared in a manner similar to what was previously reported as a result of the lawsuits that came from the Jack in the Box outbreak discussed earlier.

Some of the general requirements under subpart G are listed below:

- FDA FSMA preventive controls subpart G requirements are established to require food receivers to implement a supply-chain program that meets preventive control requirements.
- Liability is for received food shared by the receiver.
- Responsibilities of the receiving facility are defined.
- Using approved suppliers is a basic requirement.
- Conducting supplier verification activities for raw materials and other ingredients can also mean that the receiving company must assure that the verified systems are also meet requirements under the validation portion of the preventive controls requirements.
- Onsight audits of suppliers are required to assure compliance with preventive controls.
- Procedures for receiving of ingredients and records requirements are established [1].

Although many companies have already strengthened supply chain requirements, subpart G might be new for many other companies. Many industries have long ago established strong supplier control programs under standards such as the International Organization for Standardization has established.

There are at least three primary factors that cause food suppliers to adopt preventive supply chain controls. Market forces, from consumers and as a result of the publication of food outbreaks, drive customers and consumers to purchase from food safety certified forces. If a supplier cannot or will not establish valid preventive controls, the customer company, under subpart G, should not purchase from that supplier. If the customer company does purchase from an unapproved or un certified supplier, the customer company assumes the responsibilities and liabilities of the supplier. That's a dangerous game to play in terms of potential failure in the event of an FDA audit and in terms of financial losses such as those reported for the Chipotle case study.

In short, product liability laws establish the fact that a company is liable for what they buy and sell. Insurance costs may go up as suppliers are forced to pay for recall and food safety coverage and the opportunities for lawyers to get rich rises.

The third and probably least important factor that should drive customers to assure themselves that their suppliers are in preventive control is the FSMA subpart G rules themselves. On the heels of the passage of the FSMA, other governments are quickly adopting many of the rules that FSMA seeks to establish. Importers are particularly impacted on both sides of the borders since the receiving company must assure that food producers, packers, handlers, and processors outside of the United States must meet rules under subpart G.

CASE STUDIES

In September 2013, owners of the Colorado cantaloupe farm were arrested as a result of the 2011 listeria outbreak that killed 33 people. That outbreak was, at the time, one of the deadliest outbreaks ever recorded. The owners were arrested because they shipped contaminated food in interstate commerce and that it was likely that the listeria spread during the packing, storage, and cantaloupe shipment operations.

In this case, the owners and the quality manager were unaware of the listeria contamination and had changed company processes during the harvest period. Though it may seem that subpart G requirements would have been ignored by company personnel, the costs and impact of the outbreak would most assuredly have been shared by the companies that bought, distributed, and sold the cantaloupe.

Another important case to take a look at focuses on the salmonella impacted peanut shipments from the Peanut Corporation of America Virginia operation. In this case, the owner was found guilty of more than 70 criminal charges for knowingly shipping tainted food, obstruction of justice, conspiracy, and wire fraud. The owner received a 28-year sentence for intentionally ignoring internal testing that showed the product was contaminated. There were 72 counts of fraud, conspiracy, and introduction of adulterated food into interstate commerce charged. The owner's brother also received a 20-year sentence. The quality assurance manager received a 5-year prison sentence.

Some 360 companies were impacted with over 3900 different products impacted by the recall. ConAgra Foods, one of hundreds of customers, ended up paying over $11 million as a result of the outbreak. The peanuts were used in peanut butter, cookies, crackers, cereal ice cream, and other products causing a nation-wide outbreak that caused 33 deaths nation-wide.

The Chipotle case study illustrates how the FDA and the CDC will execute subpart G. Chipotle's problems seem to have originated on the farm although no published information confirms that fact. Because of this, authorities asked Chipotle to turn over information about its suppliers to conduct environmental sampling at each supplier. The search was for the types of bacterial hazards that caused the outbreaks and that might exist on one or more of the farms.

SUBPART G REQUIREMENTS

Under subpart G, there are new rule requirements that include 33 different sections intended to establish what food receivers "must" do to comply. The rules excluded food that is not intended for retail or distribution that might reach the United States consumer and food intended for use in research and evaluation (also that would not reach the United States consumer) [2].

The word "must" is significant and can be found in other preventive control final rules. Use of the word "must" indicates that this is a requirement under the law thus making violations illegal. Any time the word is used in a legal context, the statement and requirements become mandatory. This is a shift from the use of such words as "should" or "might" that are considered suggestions and carry no legal weight.

Under these rules the primary focus is on prevention. This is a significant shift and represents significant challenges to normal food purchasing operations focused on cost, delivery, service, and quality. Although most food buyers are generally restricted to use only approved suppliers, the new rules establish the fact that a company must only use approved suppliers.

To fulfill the requirements for using only approved suppliers, the rules require (must) that a buyer determine appropriate supplier verification activities and how often such verification activities must be conducted, conduct supplier verification activities and document the buying company's verification of the supplier's food safety system.

So, what is an approved supplier. Approved suppliers must have performed a hazard analysis for each food or ingredient being shipped to the receiver. They must also assure that hazard controls are implemented and that they verify their own performance, procedures, processes, and practices related to the food and ingredients. The suppliers must also meet applicable FDA food safety regulations and have a good compliance record. In other words, the supplier must have a good food safety history. Problems earlier found by the FDA or other audit agencies would be an indication that the supplier food safety history or compliance record were not satisfactory.

For a receiver to determine whether or not a receiver's list of suppliers (for each food or ingredient) was an approved supplier, there are several levels that could be implemented by receivers to establish a risk ranking for suppliers. Generally, suppliers are qualified based on one or more receiver business goals (cost, delivery, service, quality). Under the rules, preventive controls now take the top priority because the FDA does not investigate receiver records that rank suppliers on cost, delivery, service, or quality. First, suppliers must certainly be qualified. Under subpart G, qualification means that the supplier has a valid preventive controls system in place. Second, assuming that there is at least an assurance from the supplier that they do follow preventive control rules, a receiver could then certify that supplier as an "approved supplier."

If a rating system was employed for suppliers on each aspect of their preventive controls system, qualified suppliers would be easy to rate and rank according to a point system. The following simple stream is shown:

1. Qualify
2. Certify
3. Rate
4. Rank
5. Reward

By employing a point system, the supplier with the highest certification score would be ranked highest and should be receive product orders from the receiver more than other suppliers supplying the same product. In short, the supplier with the highest score for being able to establish valid preventive controls would earn the highest score meaning that they were the lowest risk supplier for that product.

Such systems are not new. Certainly, there will be times that a highly ranked supplier cannot fulfill receiver purchasing demands and buyers will be tempted to meet their own customer's needs by buying from unqualified suppliers. Such scenarios are exactly what subpart G rules are intended to undermine and eliminate because when buyers circumvent such rules, the opportunity for biological, chemical, and physical hazards to enter distribution channels increases, and the ability to trace back to outbreak sources diminishes.

Hence, the use of the word "must." Receiving company buyers who, as a matter of practice, circumvent food safety laws requiring the use of only approved suppliers are now subject to legal action. Indeed, the FDA has covered its bases well enough to be able to prosecute not only the buyer and food safety personnel for such violations but also others in the organization such as the owner.

The FDA leaves some doors ajar however with use of such words as "reasonable probability" which is not mathematically determined. In any case where there is a "reasonable probability" that hazards will result in health problems or death, only approved suppliers may be used after the receiving company determines how they will verify supplier preventive controls and conduct verification activities prior to using the raw material or ingredient. It is not likely that many perishables are without a reasonable probability that they could cause health problems or death.

If a supplier is a qualified supplier and the receiving facility receives written assurances, a reduced audit frequency may be established. This is a normal and, from a quality control perspective, standard practice for purchasing from certified suppliers.

With regard to the receiving facility, it must approve and use only approved suppliers and must have and use written receiving procedures for raw materials that are received only from approved suppliers. Further, the receiving facility must provide a written risk-based supply-chain program for received materials and ingredients for any product identified with hazards. The receiving facility must, if a nonsupplier is used, verify supply-chain-controls for that supplier. Apparently, that loophole allows the use of nonsuppliers as long as they do have a preventive control program in place.

In the case when the receiving facility receives product from a foreign supplier, both the receiving facility and the foreign supplier must be in compliance with the Foreign Supplier Verification Program requirements.

Receiving facilities must document and provide records for the list in Table 7.1.

Table 7.1 Receiving Facility Records Requirements

Written supply-chain program
Importers
Supplier approval
Receiving procedures
Supplier verification activities
Onsite audits (supplier, auditor, procedures, dates, conclusions)
Sampling and testing (dates, results, actions, lab, etc.)
Supplier's relevant food safety records (dates, names, conclusions)
Alternative verification activities
Written assurances ("not a covered farm," "food is covered by.")
Written results of an FDA or government audit
Actions taken for nonconformances
Documentation showing written procedures are followed
Applicable documentation from "other than receiving facility"
Third party audit/auditor records
Records from others providing supply chain control services

The receiving facility must document that the supplier has a written supply-chain program and conform to importer and supplier approval procedures. As part of the preventive controls requirements, onsite audit, sampling and test data, food safety records, and other supplier FDA and food safety records must be available. The receiving facility must also be able to provide documentation (internal audits) that procedures are followed and must have copies of any third party audits of the supplier that have been conducted on their behalf. In additon in the event when the supplier or others provide supply chain control services, there must be records showing what services were delivered, where they were delivered, and when they were delivered.

The receiving facility may not accept or use as verification any verification or audit performed by the supplier themselves. Nor can the receiving facility accept verification activity records from the supplier for product risk or performance related to validation of the preventive controls.

SUPPLY CHAIN INTEGRATED DATA SYSTEMS

Included here is a set of potential record keeping solutions for the receiving facility. Assuming that the receiving facility has numerous (sometimes hundreds) of suppliers, record keeping can become onerous if a system for such record keeping is not established early in the game.

Fig. 7.1 illustrates the integration of risk, operational improvement, inspection, sampling, traceability, and recall data that can help receiving facilities to control records.

The FDA is in the process of establishing and integrated approach to food safety by standardizing data and formats from federal state and local food safety agencies.

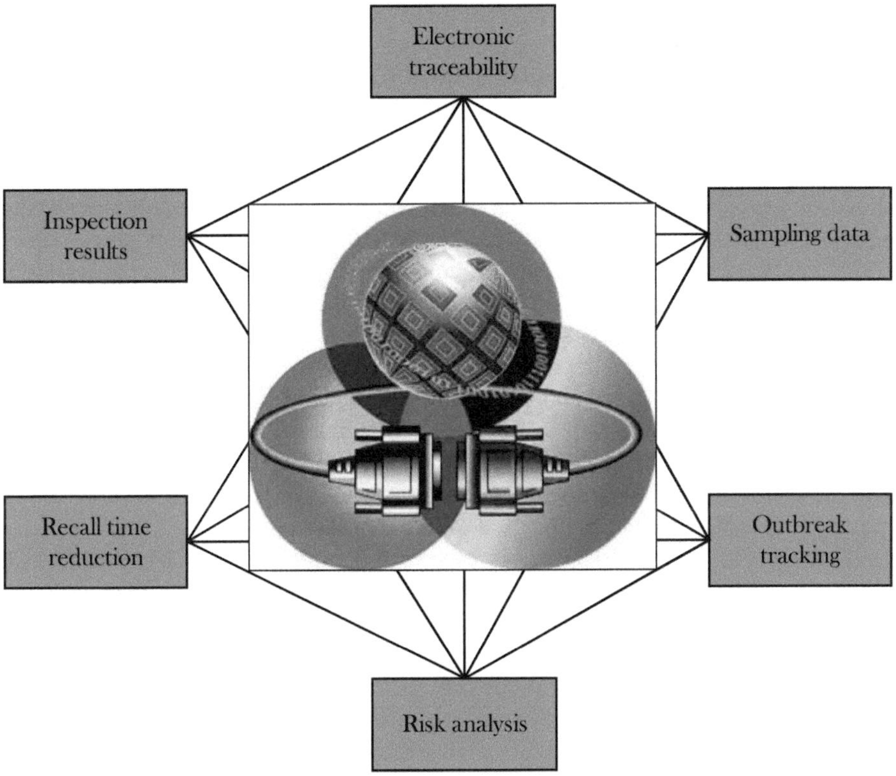

FIGURE 7.1

An integrated data system.

The intent is to allow all three levels of government to be able to identify, record, and analyze data from all levels. This attempt to integrate food safety data is primarily intended for enforcement purposes. Recall that above, the issue regarding supplier FDA and violation data was highlighted as a requirement for receiving facilities. In that case, the receiving facility was supposed to know through records, the status of their suppliers. The FDA along with state and local agencies intend to share inspection, test, audit, and other report data to help them rate and rank suppliers in terms of risk based on their compliance histories at all levels of government.

The FDA system is similar to what should be established for any receiving facility. As the receiving facility must assume record retention (Table 7.1) for many supplier features, the receiving facility is obligated to formalize a record keeping system to be able to answer question regarding their suppliers.

Historically, much of the food safety information for any facility or operation has come from on-site audits focused primarily on auditor reviews of existing records.

For some companies, a file drawer, if properly organized, allows the receiving facility to collect and manage paper-based systems. However, the use of paper-based systems leaves data basically unusable for most management purposes, especially food safety and quality system purposes. A receiving facility that chooses to maintain the data in an electronic, computer format has a significant advantage when it comes to locating contaminated foods (recall), assessing supplier risks, looking at the likelihood of who might have caused the recall and ranking, qualifying and certifying suppliers to quickly locate impacted product with the intent of reducing recall times to stop extended illnesses and death. Of equal importance here is that rapid control and recall helps significantly to protect innocent supply chain members caught up in the public's fear of impacted products.

Assume a farm is shipping produce into a distribution center. Under new environmental sampling rules, plants and water may be sampled for biological and chemical contaminants. These samples provide data for a database. Assume also that the farm is food safety certified through standard third party audits and the farm, in agreement with the distribution center, has established a barcode type of case level traceability system. This is all data that can be used to risk rank suppliers.

If the receiving facility's staff assigns potential points (based on hazards) to each type of data they need to qualify and approve a supplier, a system is easy to envision. Table 7.2 shows points awarded to a single supplier for testing, audit, and traceability fulfillment.

For this supplier farm with a total score of 36 points, it is easy to see how they might improve their ranking. Improvement of water testing for chemicals and buying into the electronic traceability system will increase their scores nicely.

It should be noted that traceability is not a preventive control requirement. However, temperature monitoring and data collection are required by the FDA FSMA Sanitary Rules on the Transportation of Human and Animal Foods. Temperature monitoring is a requirement under those rules and, more importantly, when coupled with traceability (where, date, time) data that can easily be collected using today's technology provides a more complete food safety system.

The receiving facility's traceability system requirements are shown in Fig. 7.2.

Table 7.2 Sample Farm Supplier Scoring

8	Plant biological
6	Plant chemical
9	Water biological
3	Water chemical
10	Certification audits
0	Electronic traceability
36	Total score

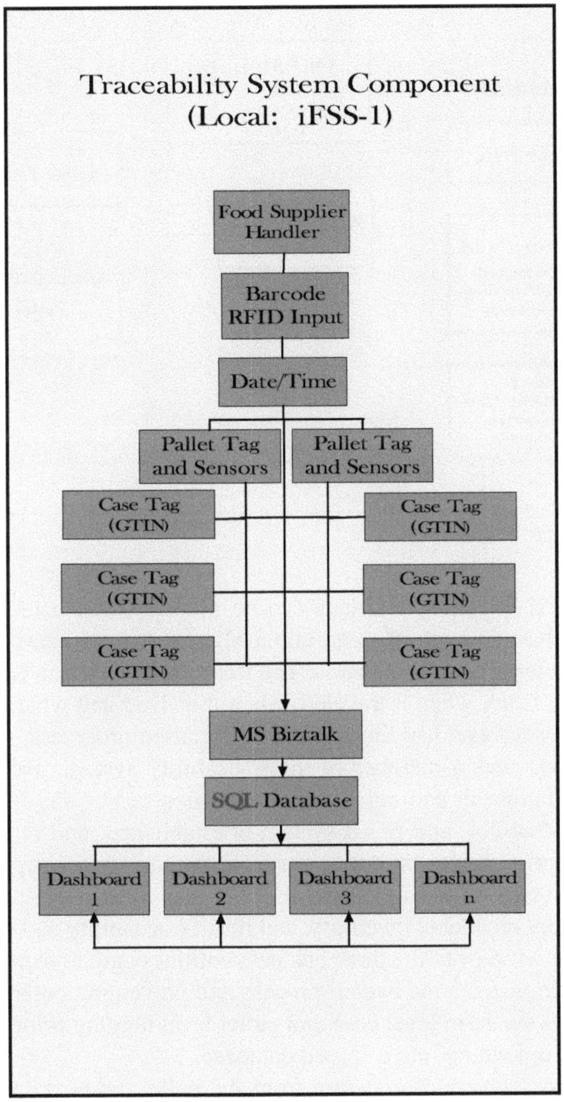

FIGURE 7.2

Distributor's traceability system.

SUPPLIER APPROVAL

The figure shows that barcode case level tags using global trade identification numbers from global systems 1 (GS1) are used in conjunction with radio frequency identification (RFID) temperature monitoring pallet tags. Using barcode scanners

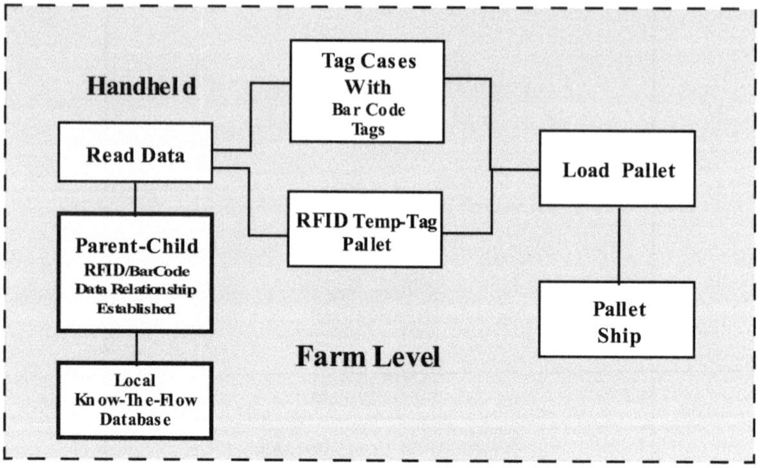

FIGURE 7.3

Traceability at the farm level.

and RFID readers, the case level tags can be associated with the RFID temperature records. Both sets of data then go into a Microsoft database and results may be viewed on computer screen dashboards. The traceability data can easily show where the product came from, when it traveled, when it arrived and what temperature was maintained during storage, handling, and transportation processes.

If the farm becomes a member of the traceability system, and food is tracked through transportation, in and out of the distribution center and into the retailer, a farm to retail traceability and recall system is established, and the farm (as a supplier), the distribution center (as a receiver from the farm and a supplier to the retail outlet), and the retail outlet as the final receiver can collectively control inventory, locate and intercept recallable inventory, and fulfill traceability and temperature control requirements. Moreover, the three business entities begin to work as a food safety team capable of improving the overall process and preventing outbreaks.

Fig. 7.3 shows the farm level case and pallet level tagging prior to shipment and data reading and uploading into a shared database.

Fig. 7.4 shows temperature reading from the pallet temperature monitoring tag and product movement through the distribution center along with data collection using both barcode and RFID systems.

Fig. 7.5 shows data reading using barcode scanners as the pallet and cases are received at retail the incoming area.

Assuming all collected data is now in a computer and is available to shippers, carriers, and receivers in a dashboard format, management is not only armed with information regarding food safety issues but can also use such data to manage inventory flows through all three operations.

Fig. 7.6 shows a typical dashboard receipt at the distribution center for lettuce, mushrooms, and tomatoes as they were stored in different coolers to maintain different temperature requirements.

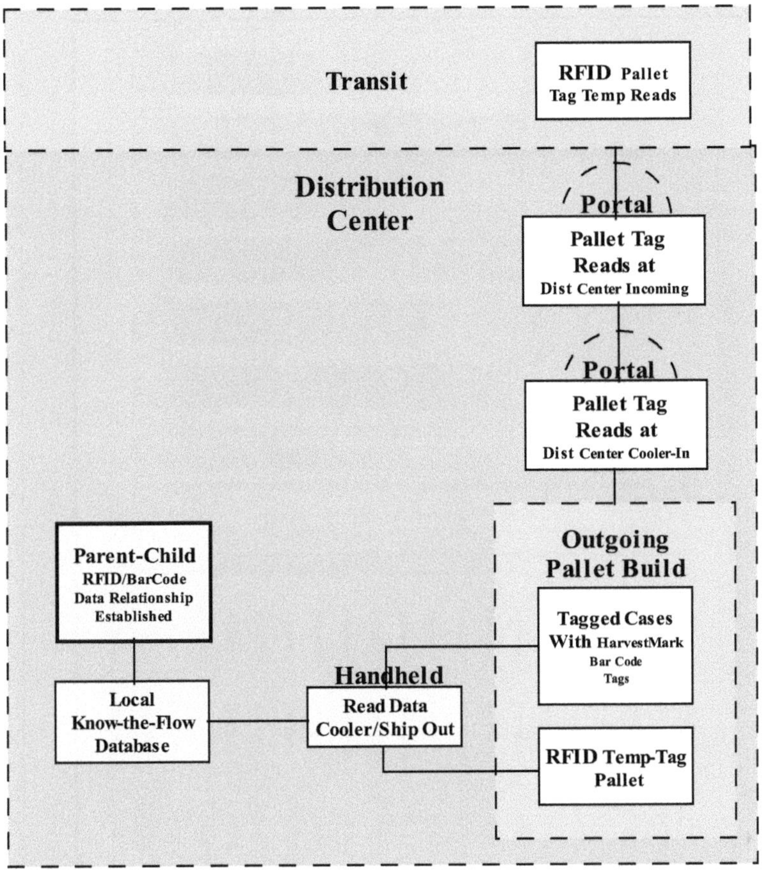

FIGURE 7.4

In transit and distribution center traceability.

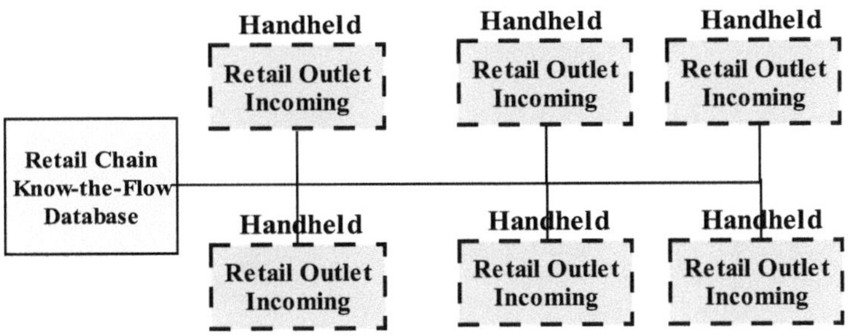

FIGURE 7.5

Traceability at receiver incoming.

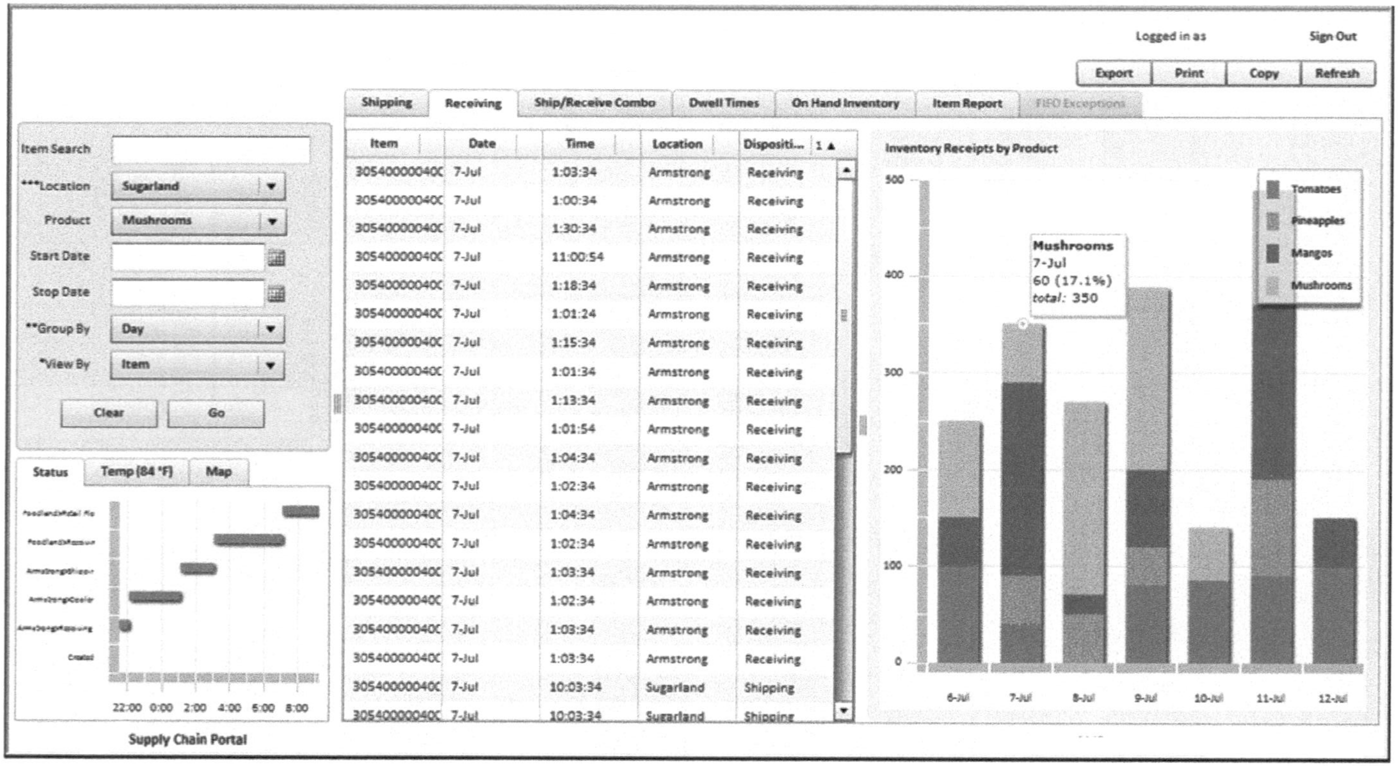

FIGURE 7.6

Distribution center inventory dashboard.

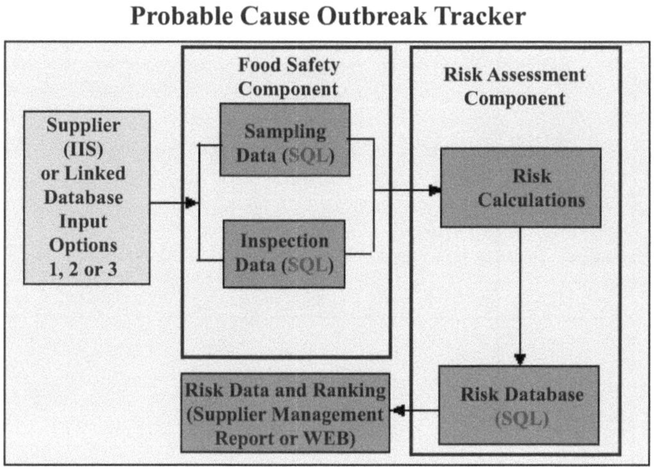

FIGURE 7.7

Assigning ranks based on probability of causes for outbreaks.

We can take this system even further. As the receiver is responsible for assuring that the supplier meets a list of FDA requirements under subpart G, and as the receiver is responsible for assuring that they have records to prove compliance, an integrated electronic system can combine traceability, temperature, sampling, inspection, and other data listed in Table 7.2, to risk rank suppliers thus establishing a system to control approved suppliers.

Fig. 7.7 shows the integration of supplier sampling and inspection data into a system that allows for risk calculations and supplier ranking for product purchases. As a ranking system based on supplier data, the receiver can perform an analysis of probable causes or causers in the event of a recall. Lower ranking suppliers are more likely (because of missing food safety components) to have caused an outbreak and should be first to be investigated as sources of the outbreak.

It seems reasonable to assume that farms using clean water that test for and maintain control of biological and chemical contaminants on product and have passed standardized inspections and control temperatures during transportation processes are less likely or are at lower risk to cause illness and death than those not employing such generic food safety practices.

If the likelihood of recall is a function of a supplier's ability to provide traceability data, be certified by audit for food safety, tests, and reports biological and chemical contaminants in the produce and in the water and has appropriate temperature controls during transportation processes, data from that supplier can be used to provide the scoring shown in Table 7.2. With multiple suppliers for the same product, each supplier will fall into a ranking system and be placed in order of likelihood of causing problems. Fig. 7.8 illustrates such risk ranking with the top five lowest scoring suppliers (the weakest suppliers) shown at the top.

Outbreak Risk Report: California

Organizational Level: All Product: Melon Suppliers

Risk Ranking is High to Low

	Risk Rank	Production and Harvest	Risk Rank	Post Harvest	Risk Rank	Fresh Cut/Value Added	Risk Rank	Distribution	Risk Rank	Restaurant or Retail
Top 5	1	82222	1	82222	1	82222	1	50162	1	47777
	2	99901	2	99901	2	99901	2	20413	2	24560
	3	00098	3	00098	3	13990	3	12906	3	20991
	4	53110	4	53110	4	73772	4	96952	4	30927
	5	14471	5	14471	5	00909			5	48937
	6	45425	6	21457	6	24444			6	76483
	7	21457	7	45425	7	76555			7	39028
	8	08263	8	08263	8	39393			8	49403
	9	89121	9	66157	9	43217			9	47363
	10	29582	10	29582	10	10999			10	09090
	11	29078	11	29078					11	11218
	12	66157	12	59368					12	98763
	13	23953	13	89121					13	09856
	14	59368	14	34881					14	74647
	15	91444	15	23953					15	29029
	16	37894	16	91444					16	30938
	17	34881	17	37894					17	40948
			18	98431					18	29827
									19	10198
									20	10199
									21	20999
									22	30876
									23	35555
									24	09076
									25	87392

Click on highlighted operation numbers to look at supply chain and operation name/locations.

FIGURE 7.8

Outbreak risk ranking report.

A couple of important issues arise with this system. First, those suppliers ranked at the top as the weakest suppliers can be isolated for receiver attention and management in an effort to help them improve their ranking. Second, as previously mentioned, these suppliers are the most likely causes in the event of a recall and should be investigated using on-site sampling. They should be the first to be investigated.

If the system is designed to quickly identify and locate all impacted cases of product associated with the outbreak, the system recall component can quickly locate and be used to recall or isolate brother and sister impacted product in an effort to quell improper distribution into public channels. This search capability is shown in Fig. 7.9.

With agreement among all suppliers, all data can be uploaded to cloud services that will enable, with appropriate logins, all impacted supply chain members (suppliers, distributor receivers, and retail receivers) to perform whatever investigations and product isolation and recall actions needed. Such vision is shown in Fig. 7.10.

It is not difficult to envision a single unit that includes the software for electronic traceability, supplier compliance, risk analysis, and recall controls into a single system as shown in Fig. 7.11.

When networked among suppliers, distributors, processors, packers, restaurants, and retailers, all with permission controlled access, a supply-chain Intranet is established as shown in Fig. 7.12.

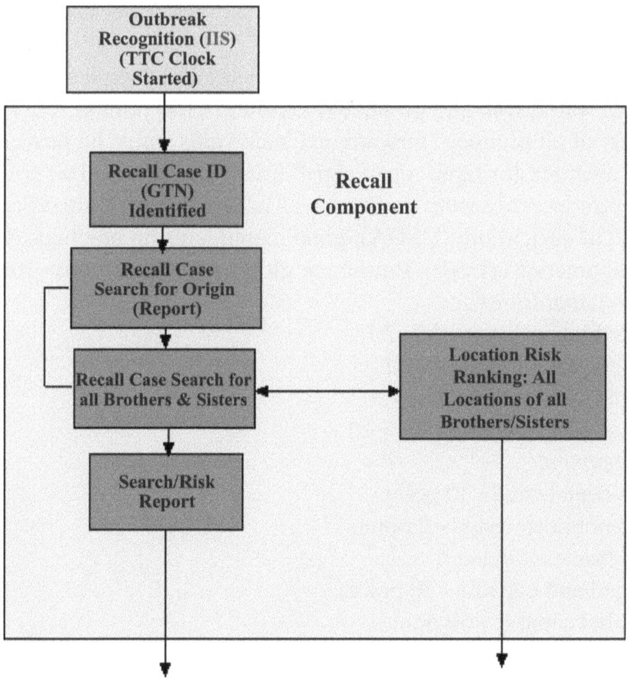

FIGURE 7.9

Recall component.

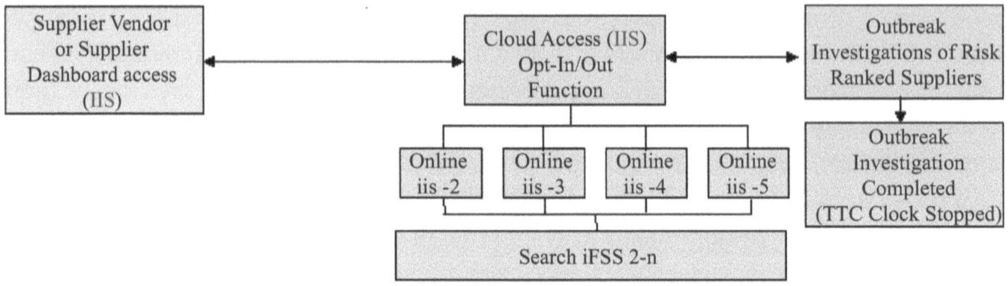

FIGURE 7.10

Cloud storage and access using dashboards to support outbreak investigations.

APPROVED AND CERTIFIED SUPPLIER RECORD KEEPING AND TRACKING

In order for such a system to work, a standardized point award system for measurable and reportable data is required. For instance, room for and a collection of water and product chemical and biological test data is required to meet preventive control environmental sampling requirements. The frequency of such testing can be used to establish a point award system as shown in Table 7.3.

Other point structures can be established such as:

1. *Risk assessment* consists of a walk-through audit and chemical and biological sampling of water, soil, and produce (maximum = 160 points).
2. *Traceability* of all produce (forward and backwards) must be proven. Higher points are awarded for rapid recall capabilities (maximum = 100 points).
3. *Full food safety certification audit* such as is awarded by United States department of agriculture (USDA), good manufacturing practices (GMP), good agricultural practices (GAP), Primus, or global gap (maximum = 100 points).
4. *Cold chain capabilities*
   Refrigerated incoming trucks = 20
   Refrigerated receiving floor = 20
   Refrigerated storage (coolers) = 20
   Refrigerated outgoing shipping = 20
5. *Recall component*
   Recall has been tested = 30 points
   Recall has not been tested = 0 points
6. *Track and trace component*
   RFID tagged and capable = 70 points
   Barcode label capable = 60 points
   Manual data entry to a centralized system = 50 points
   COOL identification only = 20 points
   GS1 or USHI numbering only = 20 points
   No formal traceability system = 0 points

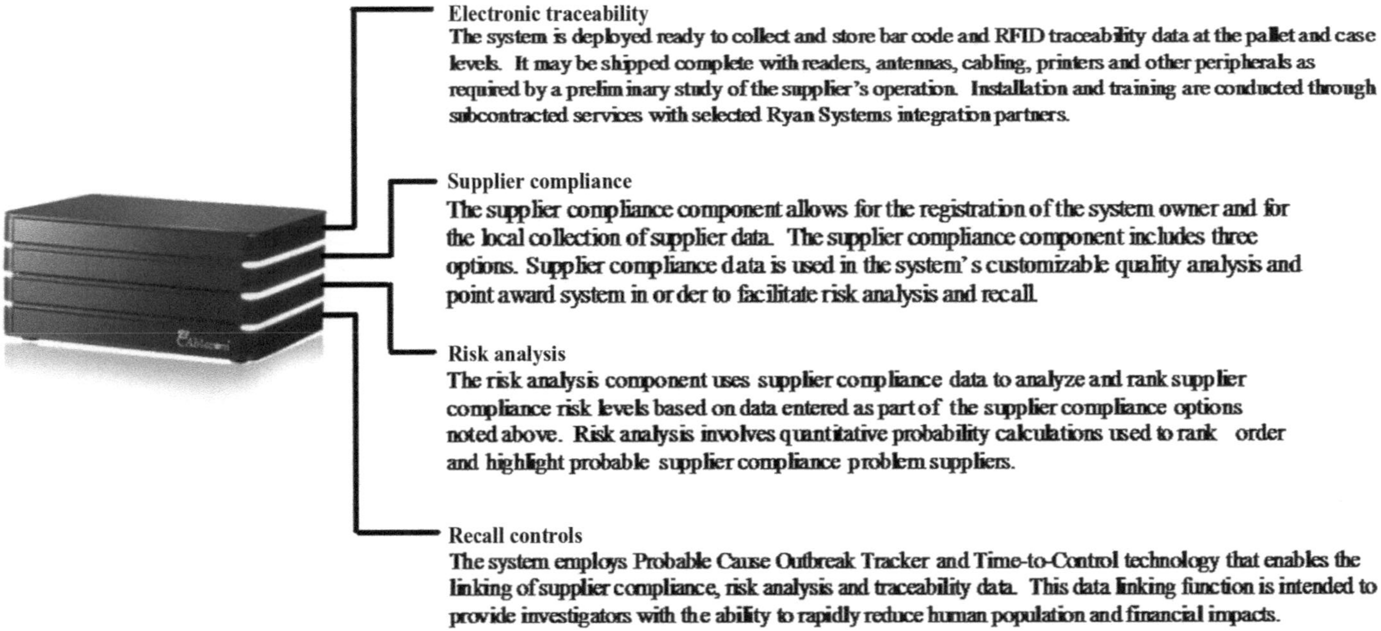

FIGURE 7.11

The integrated food safety system.

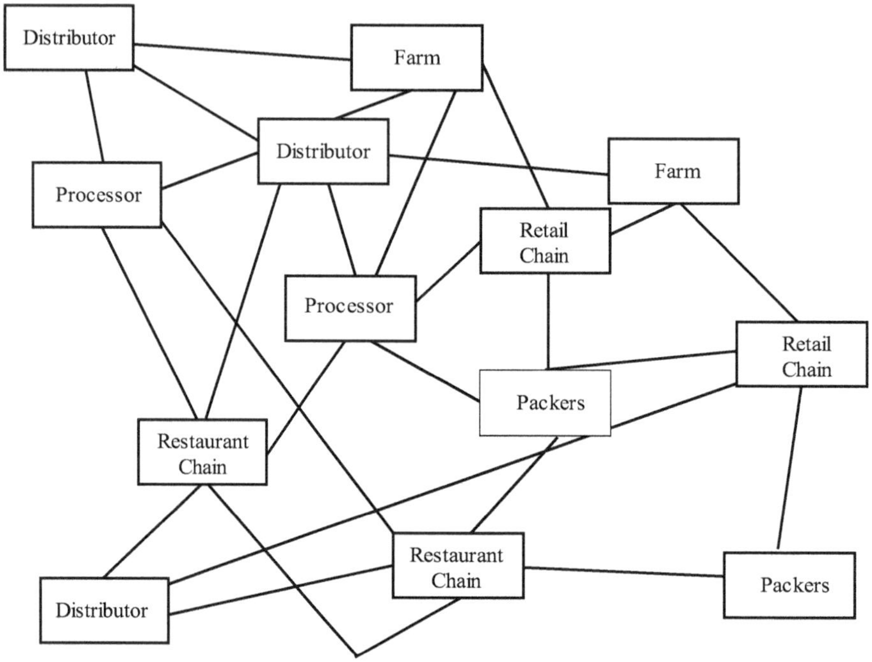

FIGURE 7.12

Integrating users for the integrated food safety system.

Table 7.3 Test Frequency Point Award Structure

Water Tests (Chemicals)		Water Tests (Biological)	
Annual test	5	Annual test	5
Quarterly test	10	Quarterly test	10
Monthly test	20	Monthly test	20
No testing done	0	No testing done	0
Produce Tests (Chemicals)		**Produce Tests (Biological)**	
Annual test	5	Annual test	5
Quarterly test	10	Quarterly test	10
Monthly test	20	Monthly test	20
No testing done	0	No testing done	0

7. *Tracking the use of chemicals (pesticides, fertilizers, fungicides, herbicides)*
   Chemical use data entered electronically = 60 points
   Chemical use data entered on forms checked annually by state department of agriculture inspectors = 40 points
8. *Food safety audits passed*
   HACCP
   GMP
   USDA
   Global gap
   GFSI
   NSF
   State/city
   Primus

ADVANTAGES

There are a few advantages to both the supply base and receivers for integrating such data. These include:

1. Suppliers can increase sales through food safety certification ranking and status
2. Suppliers can work to improve ranking on the website listings
3. A supplier can check competition to find out how their company compares
4. Suppliers can contact product and service companies to help them improve

Fig. 7.13 illustrates a quick visual check for any receiver buyer to determine supplier status and points awarded.

In this case, the supplier is obviously lacking in overall points for food safety. Buying from the supplier transfers the risk to the receiver or, on a more positive side, allows the buying company to drive supplier improvement or to avoid the supplier all together.

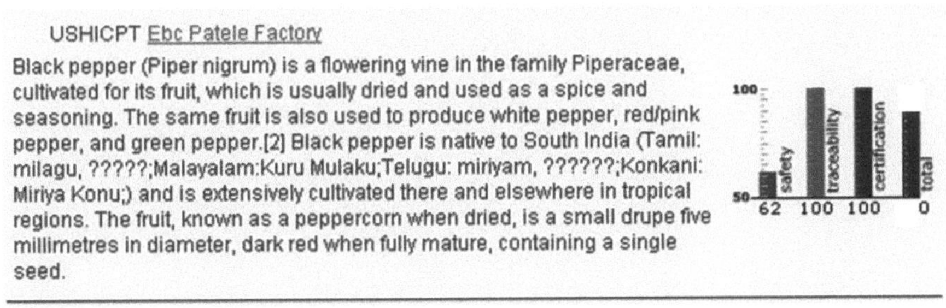

FIGURE 7.13

Visual presentation of supplier status.

REFERENCES

[1] FSMA Final Rule for Preventive Controls of Human Food <http://www.fda.gov/Food/GuidanceRegulation/FSMA/ucm334115.htm> March 22, 2016.
[2] <http://www.fda.gov/Food/GuidanceRegulation/FSMA/ucm334115.htm> ibid 1; May 9, 2016.

CHAPTER

Cycle time analysis in preventive food safety and quality control practices

8

The food industry is perhaps the single industry that is on top of trying to assure that food is delivered well within shelf life or expiration limits. Generally speaking, inventory turns are very high and the time from the farm to the store is minimal.

While not required under the Food Safety Modernization Act (FSMA) validation rules, cycle time analysis can be used to validate food through-put speeds. Reduction of handling and food times-in-process is critical to establishing valid preventive process controls since both are associated with hazard control.

Regardless, the Food and Agriculture Organization of the United Nations (May 11, 2011) estimates the following:

- "Roughly one-third of the food produced in the world for human consumption every year—Approximately 1.3 billion tonnes—Gets lost or wasted, according to an FAO-commissioned study.
- The industrialized and developing countries dissipate roughly the same quantities of food—Respectively, 670 and 630 million tonnes.
- Every year, consumers in rich countries waste almost as much food (222 million tonnes) as the entire net food production of sub-Saharan Africa (230 million tonnes).
- Fruits and vegetables plus roots and tubers have the highest wastage rates of any food.
- The amount of food lost or wasted every year is equivalent to more than half of the world's annual cereals crop (2.3 billion tonnes in 2009/2010) [1]."

Fig. 8.1 illustrates piles of excess or obsolete inventory that go unsold as a result of such waste.

A LOOK AT SOME ASSOCIATED COSTS

Of equal importance are the wasted resources that go along with wasted food. Assuming we use 30% to estimate wasted food. The water pesticides, herbicides, fertilizers, transportation, distribution, processing, handling, and other associated costs went into the landfill along with the food. Companies worrying about slim profit margins need to take a very close look at handling and inventory wastes to figure out why such margins are so low.

Validating Preventive Food Safety and Quality Controls. DOI: http://dx.doi.org/10.1016/B978-0-12-810994-6.00008-0

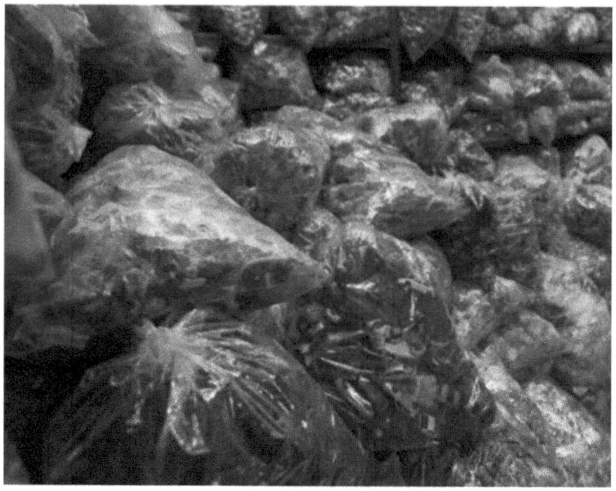

FIGURE 8.1

Unsold product.

					1		Costs				
Incoming							Yield	Inspection	Overhead	Transport	Total Loss
Farm Operation # 1	Yield Loss %	Yield Loss #	New Shipout Weight	Reason	Per lb Sales Price	Shipout Value	Losses Shipout $ Loss	At $8 per hour	at .05 per Lb	at $.15 per Lb	
100	30	30	70	Packout	$1	$70	$30.00	$2.00	$3.50	$10.50	$46.00

FIGURE 8.2

Farm level loss calculations.

If we apply some basic cost analyses to each operational supply chain step, we can begin to see the potential for some serious cost savings.

The questions quickly become "where is the inventory" and "what can we do?"

Starting at a farm, Fig. 8.2 illustrates potential losses. Beginning on the left, if a farm has a 30% or 30-lb loss for a 100-lb harvest and the sale of fresh tomatoes is set at about $1/lb, the ship out loss is 30 lb, and the ship out weight is now 70 lb or $70 with a loss of $30. Add to that the cost of inspection ($8/h), overhead at $.05/lb and transportation costs at $0.15/lb, the supply chain losses add up quickly.

The total yield and sales losses on the initial 100 lb is $46.

Following the same logic through distribution (Fig. 8.3 at $25.10), processing (Fig. 8.4 at $40.59), and retail (Fig. 8.5 at $39.22), the losses roll up through the supply chain.

Fig. 8.6 adds up the costs across all four supply chain phases. The overall loss as a percentage of the initial 100-lb harvest ends up showing a total loss of $895 or a whopping 16.86%.

2											
							Co sts				Total Loss
Incoming							Yield	Inspection	Overhead	Transport	
Distribution			New		Per Lb		Loss				
Operation # 2	Yield Loss %	Yield Loss #	Shipout Weight	Reason	Sales Price	Shipout Value	Shipout $ Loss	At $8 per hour	at .05 per Lb	at $.15 per Lb	
70	10	7	63	Culling	$1.50	$95	$10.50	$2.00	$3.15	$9.45	$25.10

FIGURE 8.3

Distribution loss calculations.

3											
							Co sts				Total Loss
Incoming							Yield	Inspection	Overhead	Transport	
Process			New		Per lb		Losses				
Operation # 2	Yield Loss %	Yield Loss #	Shipout Weight	Reason	Sales Price	Shipout Value	Shipout $ Loss	At $8 per hour	at .05 per Lb	at $.15 per Lb	
63	15	9.45	53.55	Rejected	2.95	$157.97	$27.88	$2.00	$2.68	$8.03	$40.59

FIGURE 8.4

Processing loss calculations.

4											
							Co sts				Total Loss
Incoming							Yield	Inspection	Overhead	Transport	
Retail			New		Per Lb		Loss				
Operation # 2	Yield Loss %	Yield Loss #	Shipout Weight	Reason	Sales Price	Shipout Value	Shipout $ Loss	At $8 per hour	at .05 per Lb	at $.15 per Lb	
53.55	15	8.03	45.52	Albert	3.5	$159.31	$28.11	$2.00	$2.28	$6.83	$39.22

FIGURE 8.5

Retail loss calculations.

	Loss	Summary
	Yield/Wt	$96.49
	Inspection	$8.00
	Ohead	$11.60
	Transport	$34.81
Loss Summary		$150.90
Sales Potential @ 100lbs		$895.00
Loss as % of 100 lb Sales		16.86

FIGURE 8.6

Rolled up supply chain costs.

Inventory is a critical issue and as far as controlling such costs is concerned can become the difference between companies able to control such costs and those unable to control such costs.

Although the analysis is a bit simplistic, consider the factors noted in Fig. 8.7 that can accrue based on food and drug administration (FDA) rejected shipments.

Added	Costs from	FDA international rejected shipments						
	Relabeled	Recondition	Refusal	Detained	Seized	Destruction	Examination	
	Documentati	on	Registrati	on w/FDA		Holding	GMP/GAP In	spections
	Traceability							

FIGURE 8.7

FDA-rejected shipment information.

When relabeling, reconditioning, detention, seizures, destruction, examination, inspection, testing, lack of proper documentation, and other such expenses are potentially added moving the right inventory in the right condition becomes a critical market issue.

From a business perspective, regardless of food safety or food security, inventory is money.

Any person in any company can take a walk around the company and look at different piles of inventory. When you look at raw materials, WIP, and outgoing inventory, pretend you are standing in a bank vault looking at heaps and piles of money. Money that could be used to pay better benefits or salaries, invest in new products, better control systems, or other investments that would help to improve the company's operations or longevity.

For both vegetable commodities and products and animal commodities and products, the report outlines the following areas noting that causes and preventive practices must be applied throughout the entire supply chain from origin to consumer:

1. Agricultural production
2. Post-harvest handling and storage
3. Processing
4. Distribution
5. Consumption

The report notes that the overall supply chain (production to retailing) is significantly more wasteful worldwide than consumers, industrialized nations lead in wasting foods, agriculture, and food processing lead in food losses.

The report also notes several contributing causes:

- "In industrialized countries foods gets lost when production exceeds demand"
- "High 'appearance quality standards' from supermarkets"
- "Poor storage facilities and lack of infrastructure cause post-harvest losses in developing countries"
- "Unsafe food is not fit for human consumption and therefore is wasted"
- "Disposing is cheaper than using or re-using attitude in the industrialized countries"
- "Lack of processing facilities causes high food losses in the developing countries"
- "Large quantities on display and a wide range of products/brands in supply lead to food waste in the industrialized countries"

- "Inadequate market systems cause high food losses in the developing countries"
- "Food wasted at consumer level is minimal in the developing countries"
- "Abundance and consumer attitudes lead to high food waste in the industrialized countries"

The report offers a number of preventive suggestions including communication, cooperation, and organization among farmers, consumer surveys (to forecast needs and wants), increased investment in infrastructure and transportation, educating food chain operators in food handling, establishing and educating food chain operators in safe food handling practices, establishing markets for sub-standard (but safe) foods, improving market systems, and increasing public awareness of the problem.

While the problem of wasted food is not new, some assumptions are clear:

1. All food ages
2. All food has an expiration date (regardless of label information)
3. All food sits in inventory at different times and in different places
4. As food ages, the likelihood that it will be subject to spoilage or contamination increases
5. Preventing aging, spoilage or contamination (under the right controls) means that food must move from production or processing to the customer in the shortest time possible
6. Controlling food cycle times is a critical preventive strategy for both food safety and food security

In this section, the power of cycle time analysis is explored as a quantitative tool for reducing the time it takes food to go from a farm to the consumer or reducing the time it takes the food to go through any single food process.

In the case of the food supply stream, cycle time analysis can be said to have at least two goals:

1. Reduce the time it takes to preserve food quality and establish improved food security
2. Prevent food safety problems from excessive and obsolete food items
3. Establish an ideal cycle time for the process
4. Reduce wait times to zero

Inventory turns is a common strategy for financial analysts to determine company health. Fig. 8.8 summarizes how to calculate inventory turns.

The calculations are simple. The cost of goods sold is found on the company income statement and is divided by the average inventory figure that can be found on the company balance sheet. In Fig. 8.8, the company exhibits 3.65 turns per year which can be interpreted to mean that from the time the product is ordered to the time the product has gone through all company processes and been paid for, the company receives payment on their expenses about every 3.3 months.

Fig. 8.9 illustrates a basic cycle time analysis. In a process that takes 11 hours, the analysis shows that about 4 hours (36.4%) waiting while the actual time it takes to

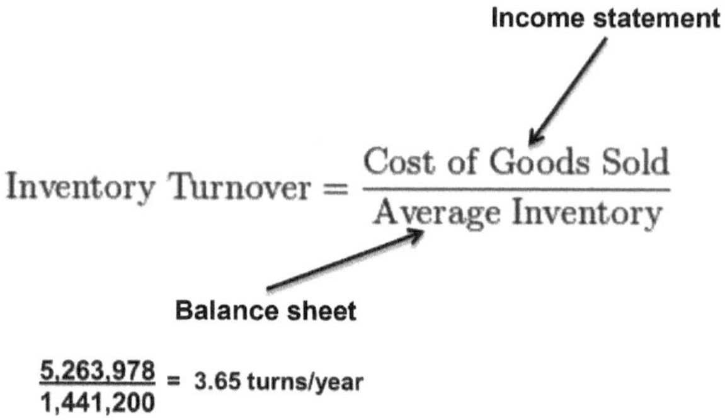

FIGURE 8.8

Inventory turns analysis.

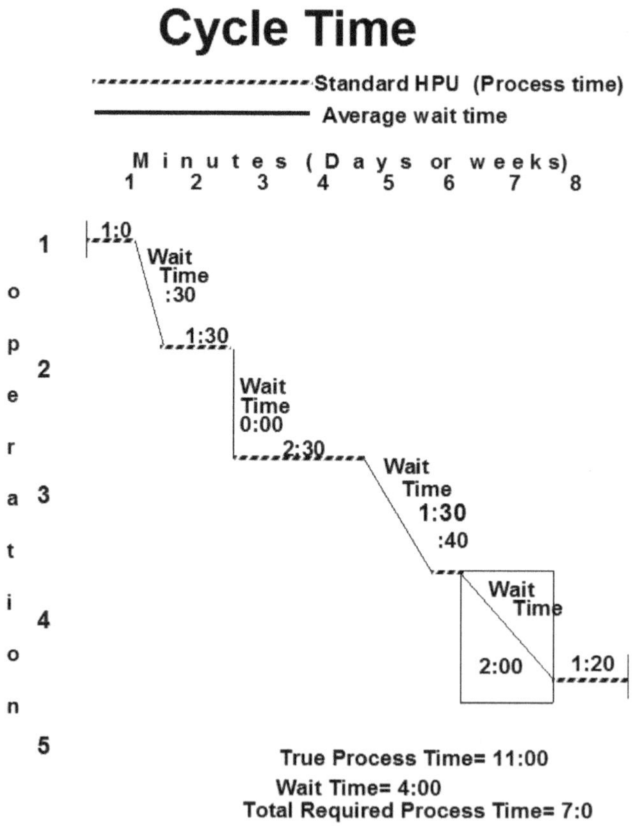

FIGURE 8.9

Illustrated cycle time analysis.

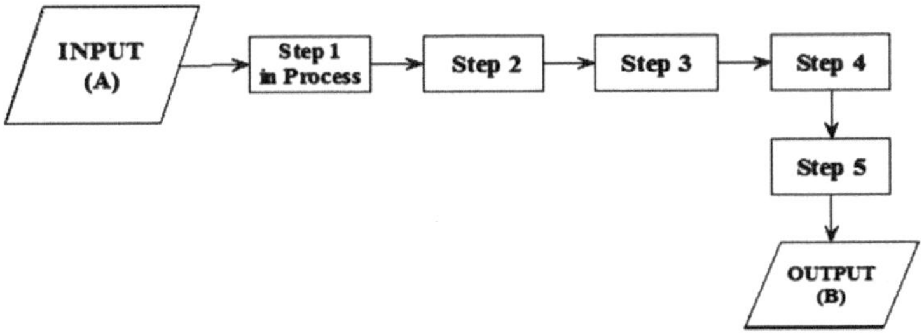

FIGURE 8.10

Simple input to output process (steps 1 through 5).

handle and process the product is 7 hours (64%). The processing time stand is shown as a dotted line while the average wait time is depicted as a solid line.

The process begins with a simple process flowchart showing each process step from input to process output as shown in Fig. 8.10.

The illustration shows that the product goes through five processes. For example, the time taken by process 1 is 1.0 hours, but the product waits for the next process approximately 30 minutes. Inspection of the analysis shows that the wait time between process step 3 and process step 3 is 2 hours. That wait time has a square drawn around it to highlight it as the longest wait time established in the process.

Note that the analysis can be set up for any time period (hours, days, or months) allowing cycle time analysis to be used for any just about type of process.

DATA COLLECTION

For cycle time analysis, the time for each process step and each wait time must be measured. This is done with a stopwatch by measuring the process and wait times over between 20 and 30 batches of product going through the process. A batch could be a bin, or pallet or a larger quantity of product. A process tracking (Fig. 8.11) sheet is attached to each batch that allows the person receiving the batch to record the time received and the time finished at each process step. Once 20 or 30 batches have gone through the process, the process step entry and exit times is used to determine the average or mean time taken in the process step or while waiting.

The process tracking sheets has a box to include notes taken for each tracking sheet. The individual managing the process tracking sheet is expected to include any observations of the process that might be important for team members to know.

Assume that 30 process timing sheets are collected from 30 batches. An Excel spreadsheet is used to record times from all 30 sheets (Fig. 8.12).

Using each data sheet, enter the time in and time out for each process step. Subtract the time in from the time out to determine the process time. As the batch arrives at step 2 through n, calculate the wait time by determining the difference between the ending time out from the previous step and the time in from the current step.

Process Tracking Sheet

Team Name__________ **Measurement Number** __________

Date __________ **Process Name** __________

Name of Person Doing the Measurement __________

Process Step 1
Process Time ______
Wait Time ______

Process Step 2
Process Time ______
Wait Time ______

Process Step 3
Process Time ______
Wait Time ______

Process Step 4
Process Time ______
Wait Time ______

Process Step 5
Process Time ______
Wait Time ______

Observation Notes

All Process Steps (Total)
Total Process Times ______
Total Wait Times ______

All Process Steps (Total)
Average Process Times ______
Average Wait Times ______

FIGURE 8.11

Process cycle time process tracking data collection sheet.

There are a number of potential issues to be investigated. These include the following:

- Bottlenecks (in processes)
- Administrative redo's (paperwork)
- Inventory pileups
- "Not enough time"
- Takes too long!
- Late deliveries
- "I need more people!"
- Working long days?

Data Sheet Number	Step 1				Step n			
	In Time	Out Time	Process Time	Wait Time	In Time	Out Time	Process Time	Wait Time
1								
2								
3								
4								
5								
.								
.								
.								
.								
n								

FIGURE 8.12

Recording data on the Excel spreadsheet.

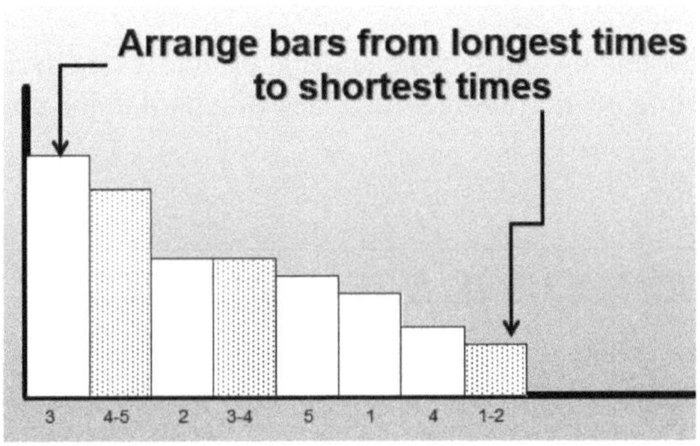

FIGURE 8.13

Cycle time Pareto analysis.

We can take the data from the illustrated analysis and create a Pareto analysis similar to what we do on the solution tracking sheet (STS). Fig. 8.13 illustrates the cycle time analysis for this illustration. The figure shows, as usual, that the wait and process times are arranged from left to right in terms of the time each process stem and wait time take on the basis of process time measurements. The Pareto analysis is transferred to the STS.

The next step becomes one of measuring cycle times and plotting inventory trends over time as shown in Fig. 8.14. Fig. 8.14 illustrates a breakdown of total inventory (top line) raw materials (line with steep upwards slope below the total line), work in process, and finished goods. These trends show a company with increasing total inventory over a 4-year period.

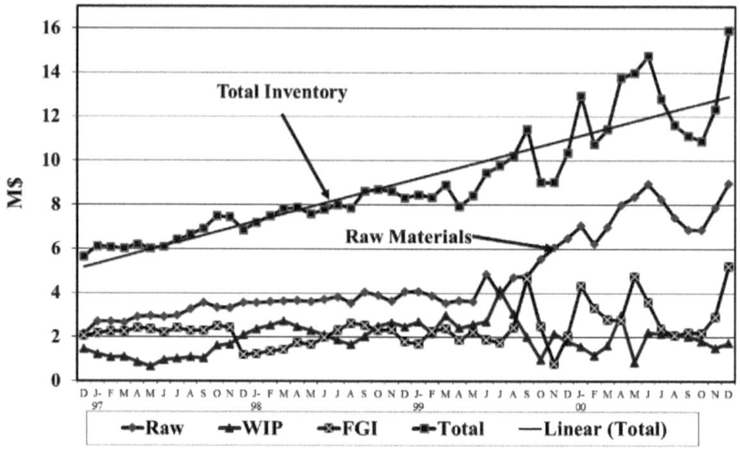

FIGURE 8.14

Analyzing inventory with a simple trend analysis.

The trends show that inventory is increasing, primarily due to raw materials. This may be contributed to over ordering with a lack of regard to the company's ability to process WIP.

CYCLE TIME ANALYSIS IS A TEAM ACTIVITY

The team approach can be used to establish trends, target improvements, the Pareto analysis, causal analyses, and team action items in an effort to get control over the inventory trends. Usually, a common cause (CC) team is established among functional managers who work together to reverse inventory trends using the solution tracking sheet (STS) as shown in Fig. 8.15.

The corrective action team (CAT) can consider the following list of potential causes:

- Line bottlenecks
- Reduce steps in the process
- Reduce movement and handling
- Synchronization (line balance)
- Simplify process operations
- Combine steps or operations
- Eliminate steps or operations
- Identify and eliminate wasted movements
- Reduce overproduction
- Eliminate unnecessary production steps such as inspection and test
- Reduce transportation and handling

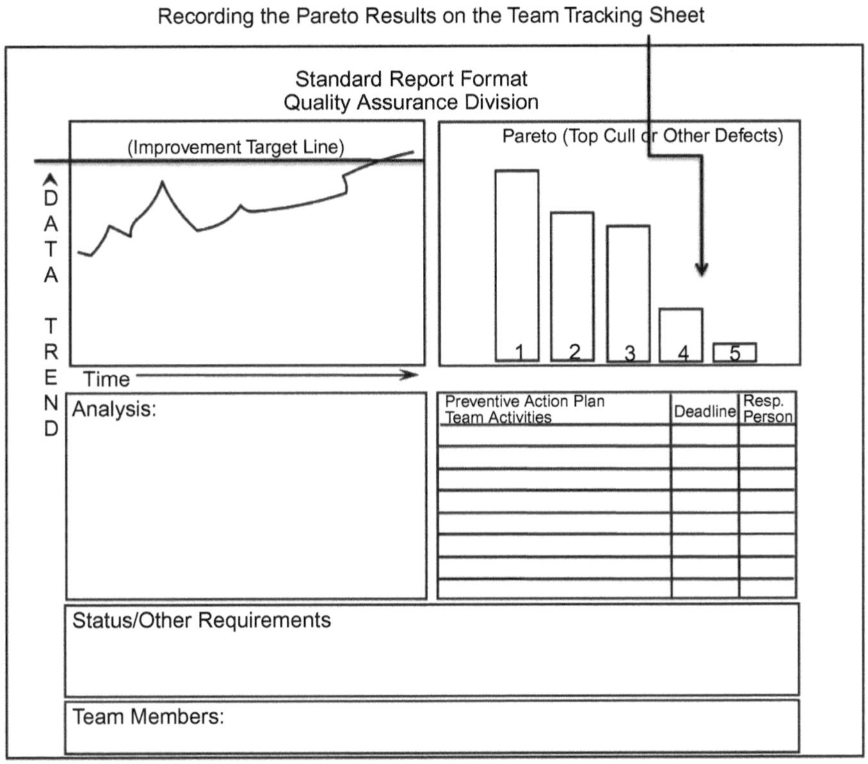

FIGURE 8.15

The STS.

- Reduce excessive inventory
- Reduce excessive motion

System or assignable causes can be team analyzed using the fishbone diagram found on the STS as shown in Fig. 8.16.

Fig. 8.17 is an illustration of one team's success over time to continually improve the overall inventory trend that is transferred to the STS.

THE IDEAL CYCLE TIME

The ideal cycle time is the time it takes to process one unit with no wait times between process step. In other words, a continuous flow similar to what might be observed in automated processing.

Fig. 8.18 shows one team's cycle time analysis with an ideal cycle time established as an average process time for each operation step.

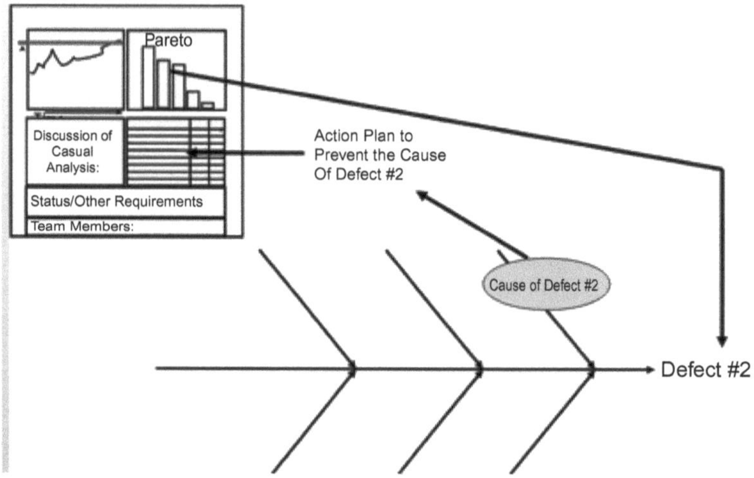

FIGURE 8.16

Fishbone analysis.

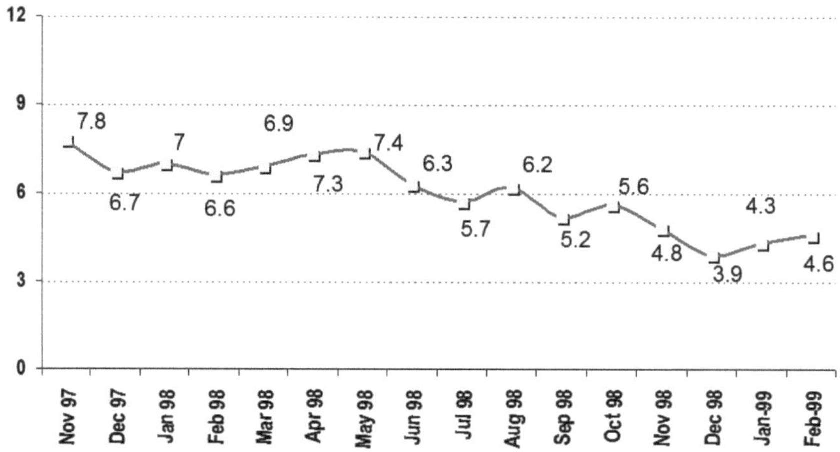

FIGURE 8.17

Sample CC team inventory control continuous improvement trend.

The cycle time analysis steps can be summarized as follows:

1. Calculate inventory turns
2. Establish cycle time teams (both CC and FIT teams may be involved) for the process
3. Make sure management supports the teams

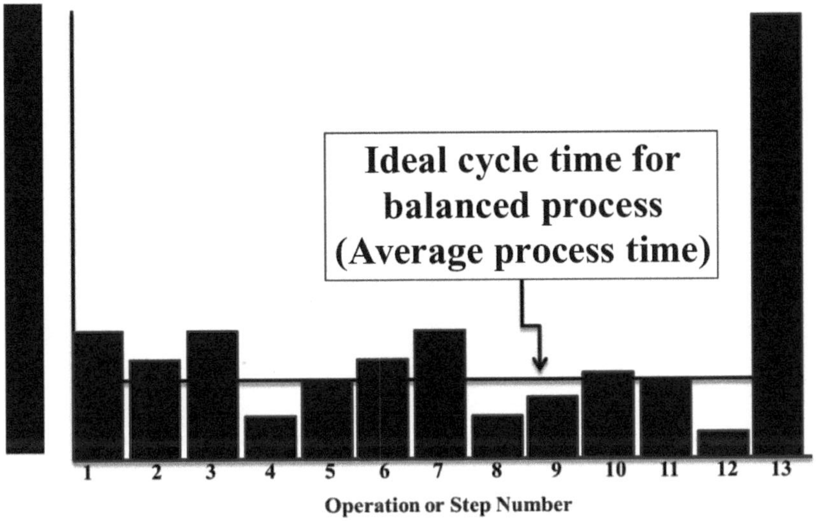

FIGURE 8.18

Establishing an ideal process time for each process step.

4. Flowchart the process
5. Identify process and wait areas in the process
6. Measure the process times and the wait times
7. Perform calculations using an Excel spreadsheet
8. Plot the process and wait times on the STS
9. Set up the Pareto analysis on the STS
10. If possible, determine causes for the longest wait time
11. Have the team work on eliminating the cause using the STS
12. When the longest wait time in the process has been eliminated, work on the next longest wait time
13. Re-measure the process times and the wait times in the new process
14. Re-do steps 6–11 until wait time is equal to the target hours per unit (wait time = 0).

REFERENCE

[1] Global Food Losses and Food Waste. <http://www.fao.org/docrep/014/mb060e/mb060e00.pdf> June, 2016.

CHAPTER

Other critical preventive control issues, concepts and validation concerns

9

The chapter addresses a number of issues often left out of preventive control training under food and drug administration (FDA) rules. Unfortunately, from a food safety and food quality position, these issues cannot be ignored or put on the back burner. As critical business and food safety issues, these issues should be of critical concern to both common cause (CC) and functional improvement team (FIT) teams and any preventive control program validation effort. Common cause or management teams need to be established to take responsibility for each topic and to begin outlining basic validation strategies or plans to work on each. Under CC team guidance, details of the CC plan can then be assigned to functional improvement or specialized teams, and the improvement and close control of each issue can be managed by the assigned cause team when required.

The topics addressed in this chapter include the following:

1. Recall basics
2. Traceability
3. Temperature monitoring
4. Packaging
5. Food fraud
6. Food cargo theft

Regardless of FDA requirements, traceability and recall systems should be tested, managed and undergo validation studies.

RECALL BASICS

In the United States, the FDA under food safety modernization act (FSMA) requirements has left traceability out of the rules, whereas in many other countries, traceability systems capable of basic track and trace capabilities have been established as a basic food safety need. Traceability concepts related to supplier risk ranking have been previously covered in Chapter 6, Cross Contamination, supplier controls. In that chapter, the concept of contaminant flow was also addressed because of the likelihood that contaminants flow through all supply chain processes in a manner not dissimilar to the picture of contaminants flowing down a river as shown in Fig. 9.1.

Although the river contaminants are clearly visible, chemical, biological, and physical hazards are not visible unless monitoring samples are taken at different points throughout the supply chain.

Validating Preventive Food Safety and Quality Controls. DOI: http://dx.doi.org/10.1016/B978-0-12-810994-6.00009-2

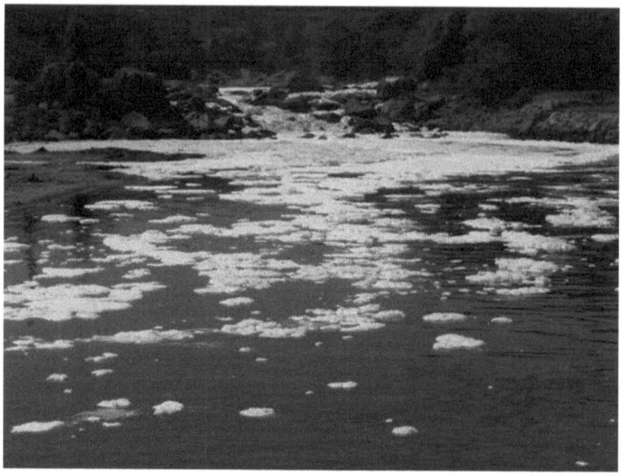

FIGURE 9.1

Visible contaminant flow through a river distribution system.

With modern food supply chains, if readers live in the United States and open their refrigerator doors, the food inside, on an average, has traveled over 2000 mi to reach the home. Of equal importance, legal issues covering product liability demand that a company be responsible for their suppliers (including transporters) abilities to deliver temperature controlled, safe, sanitary food. In short, supply chain visibility takes its place as a preventive control mechanism.

Furthermore, if, as most countries' laws require, recall is a significant requirement, how can a company do a rapid and complete food recall without a competent and standardized traceability system?

Though it has been previously discussed, recall is not a preventive control mechanism since prevention would mean to determine the cause and to modify system attributes to validly prevent their occurrence. Recall is, of course, evidence of the lack of the existence of a valid preventive control system and represents an external failure and, as such, wastes huge sums of company and supply chain money. Recalls are the opposite of preventive controls.

Regardless of any country's legal requirements for competent and rapid recall systems, we know that market forces, product liability issues, and food safety laws are all driving forces behind the movement by different market segments and company to implement traceability systems.

Preventive controls run from farm to retail and for local and imported foods with heavy fines for shipments stopped as suspect. Documentation requirements covering all supply chain members are now established to provide some evidence of whether or not suppliers do or do not comply with good practices.

Consumers and food suppliers are now capable of reviewing daily online recall notices such as those posted by the U.S. Food Safety Inspection Service (FSIS) and the FDA.

Here is a very short list posted by FSIS in the mid of August 2016.

071-2016 Sam Kane Beef Processors, LLC recalls ground beef products due to possible foreign material contamination | En Español	Aug 10, 2016	N/A (class II recall)
070-2016 EXP Al Shabrawy Incorporated recalls meat and poultry products due to misbranding and undeclared allergens | En Español	Aug 10, 2016	
070-2016 Al Shabrawy Meat Incorporated recalls meat and poultry products due to misbranding and undeclared allergens | En Español	Aug 06, 2016	
069-2016 Grossglockner Inc. recalls pork products due to misbranding | En Español	Aug 03, 2016	N/A (class II recall)
059-2016 EXP Michael Angelo's Gourmet Foods, Inc. recalls shrimp scampi and meat lasagna products due to misbranding and undeclared allergens | En Español	Aug 01, 2016	Aug 09, 2016
068-2016 Santana's Black Label Gourmet Beef Jerky recalls beef jerky products produced without benefit of inspection | En Español	Jul 29, 2016	Aug 04, 2016
067-2016 Casa Di Trevi recalls meat pasta products produced without benefit of inspection and due to misbranding and undeclared allergens | En Español	Jul 28, 2016	Jul 29, 2016

The FDA defines recall as "are actions taken by a firm to remove a product from the market" [1,2].

A trade recall involves recovery of the food product from food premises not controlled by the business having primary responsibility for supplying the food product. This means that the food has left the premises of the processor, distributor, wholesaler or carrier. On the other hand, a consumer recall more extensive than a trade recall. It involves recovery of the food product from all points in the production and distribution supply chains and includes any affected food product in the possession of consumers. Distribution networks/chains include, but are not limited to, trade outlets, retail outlets, supermarkets, grocery stores, health food stores, and any other places that sell food.

In the United States, if a company is caught in a recall, the entire supply chain is suspect. The FDA will ignore any and all food safety certificates issued by external or internal auditors and will take samples to be analyzed by labs. Samples are the FDA's single source of objective analysis and provide evidence of guilt or innocence. In terms of preventive control environmental monitoring and preventive control validity, a company with no such records whose product show evidence of the contaminant in question are considered guilty. In other words, having no records indicates you have no proof and are guilty on multiple counts [3].

In the United States, both the FDA and the United States department of agriculture (USDA) require registered companies to notify them of a recall if the company suspects they have handled or shipped food products that might be contaminated.

In such cases, the recall is known as "voluntary" recall and requires initiation of the recall through notification that involves issuing a recall alert, collecting relevant recall information, submitting a recall recommendation to various product centers, offering guidance, monitoring the recall, and terminating classes II and III recalls. The FDA, as an example, classifies recalls into three primary categories: Class I ("a reasonable probability that the use of or exposure to a violative product will cause serious adverse health consequences or death"), class II ("use of or exposure to a violative product may cause temporary or medically reversible adverse health consequences or where the probability of serious adverse health consequences is remote"), or class III ("use of or exposure to a violative product is not likely to cause adverse health consequences"). Each type of recall requires that a different set of procedures is followed [4].

A normal recall scenario is illustrated in Fig. 9.2. Beginning at the farm shipping to packers, processors, restaurants, retail outlets or farmer's markets from the bottom of the figure, at some point, the food ends up in the hands of the consumer who, if the food is contaminated, begins to feel ill anytime between 12 hours or 2 weeks later. Obviously, if a person experiences illness after 2 weeks have passed, tracking back to the source becomes nearly impossible.

If the impacted individual visits a doctor after the onset of the illness and either provides a stool sample to the doctor or goes to the hospital and is admitted, the stool sample ends up in a laboratory for analysis. On the basis of analysis and identification of the guilty bacteria or chemical, the data resulting from the analysis goes into the lab's computer where it is, if the lab is a registered lab, likely to be identified by a robotic computer system owned by the government at some level. The lab's results then become part of the government database, and the robotic system looks for matches. If a number of matching causal factors are found in these databases, a recall outbreak investigation may be launched, the public notified and potential supply chain members notified that the investigation is underway.

For supply chain members, it is time to participate in the investigation and to assure that their monitoring documentation is in proper order.

The USDA Food and Nutrition Service working with the National Food Service Management Institute at the University of Mississippi provides a good example and discussion of "Responding to a Food Recall: Procedures for Recalls of USDA Foods" [5].

Although there are many steps for a company to take to initiate and fulfill recall requirements, recall food safety standards require that all companies have a recall plan and that plan must be tested. Complete documentation is required as evidence of procedural effectiveness. Most companies establish recall teams responsible for handling the recall and for determining causes of the recall. In other industries, the team consists of personnel from various departments within the organization to evaluate impact and associated costs. The team must notify all upstream and downstream parties, establish, and implement clear recall documentation systems, issue reports, monitor recall effectiveness, notify the public when required, dispose of or otherwise get control of the product, and dispose of products (e.g., donate, recondition, cull, destroy, repackage, clean, reprocess, relabel, sort, segregate).

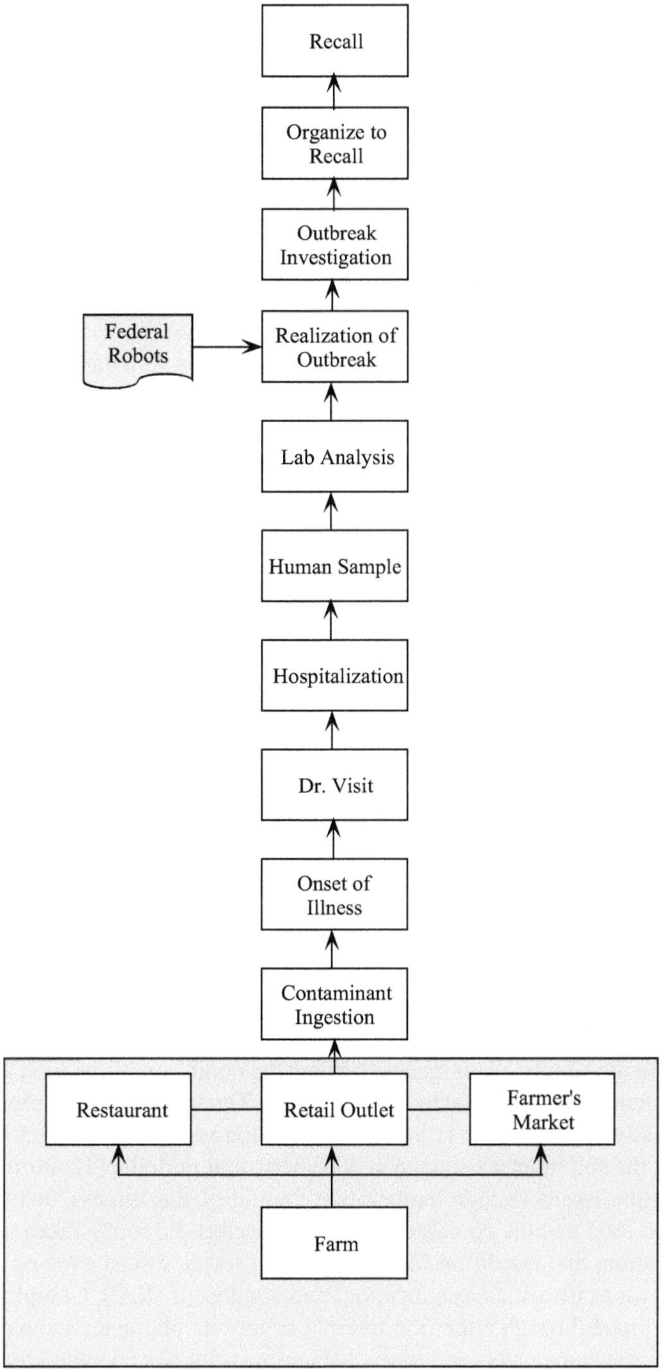

FIGURE 9.2

A basic recall scenario.

The "Food Recall Manual" department of food safety and human nutrition (FSHN) 04-10 updated in February 2014 provides excellent information for those facing recalls [6].

Of course, the potential for criminal or civil legal issues may remain for months or years after the recall as a result of who and how people were impacted. It is not uncommon for human problems to remain for years as a result of some bacterial and chemical hazards.

It is basic to all recalls that supply chain communication is key and that appropriate government agencies are notified and involved when required. In most recall, insurance is purchased (expensive) or established by companies that can self-insure their operations.

The greatest recall challenges come from situations where the public is impacted because the product has been distributed into retail or restaurant operations and has escaped the supply chain. In other complex cases, recalls involving ingredients can be difficult because all ingredients are suspect, the source becomes blurred (see chapter: Chipotle Case Study), and the outlets are far-flung.

TRACEABILITY

Traceability and traceability systems are another significant issue all food supply chain members must face regardless of the fact that in the United States. The FDA has issued no legal basis for traceability. Fully capable traceability systems can provide significant food protection that allows shipper, carrier, and receiver management to prevent potential hazards as a result of temperature loss, accidents, spills, fraud, and theft.

There are at least four levels that may be established for traceability system capabilities: Item, case, pallet, and container levels.

The technology to track and trace through the entire food chain is available at a variety of price levels today so there are really no excuses for establishing a traceability system at one or more levels. Companies must get over the "one up and one down" traceability system planning and response attitudes due to today's vicarious supply chain liabilities.

In short, the supply chain is a process; it can be defined, monitored and measured. Visibility into the supply chain means to know the condition of the food anywhere in the supply chain at any time including in-transit. The identity of the product should indicate exactly what product is involved. Location issues require that latitude and longitude of the shipment are known at all times (or at periodic (15–30-minute intervals). Condition issues include temperature, humidity, cleanliness, and other issues related to the food and the containers used to transport the food. Taken together, the identity, location, and condition factors represent today's most evolved traceability systems known as identification, location, and conditions (ILC). Complete ILC data is generally piped through either the Internet or mobile phone technology into databases into massive data storage servers located in what has become known as "The Cloud." The cloud is really established by huge data centers (often hidden in remote locations) where massive sets of servers must be kept operational at controlled temperatures at all times. These centers also provide what are called redundant systems which refer to the fact that there are backup power and storage systems established in case of some type of failure.

Electronic data collection and record keeping are commonly established to help companies meet various food safety and quality standards, achieve food safety certification, and to serve as proof for third party, federal, state, or local governmental auditors.

Fig. 9.3 illustrates the data that is commonly available when ILC systems are used. Such data can be viewed by shippers, receivers, and carriers and includes maps that show trucking routes with temperature and data collection points (squares on the map), data details, temperature and humidity profiles, and device settings.

Trace forward and trace back are commonly defined as follows:

Trace forward: To identify the physical location of the affected product in the food chain.
Trace back: To determine whether there are other products on the market or in the food supply chain that may have been affected by the same hazard as the food subjected to the recall.

A simple sketch of an overall process that ties traceability data to other food safety data from the farm level through to distributors, restaurants, packers, processors, and retailers is shown in Fig. 9.4. The farm in the upper left hand corner is shown collecting water, soil, and product samples as part of its overall food safety preventive control system. In the left hand flow, samples are submitted to labs and food safety audits are conducted resulting in movement of the data into some type of data repository (in this case a state hosted system) where management reports can be generated.

On the right hand side of the illustration, traceability of the product from the farm into the restaurants and other customers is shown with a tracking system that includes ILC as well as other information regarding the product. Such other information should include the specific product being shipped, the specific name/location of the grower/shipper and, in a unique number representing the case or package being shipped. When temperature, humidity, and other monitors are also included in device capabilities, a near real-time monitoring system is established that provides system users with the opportunity for tight management control over transportation processes.

According to the produce traceability initiative (PTI), the system should include standardized global systems 1 (GS1) information on barcodes for each case. GS1 barcodes are a means of electronically tracking cases and require GS1-enabled bar code tags on each case, a bar code reader at each shipping, receiving, and storage point. Such systems require data collection and storage software that can be tied to local inventory systems thus allowing for a more complete and manageable system designed to maintain established controls and to prevent the growth and distribution of hazards through the supply chain. These systems are also recommended for

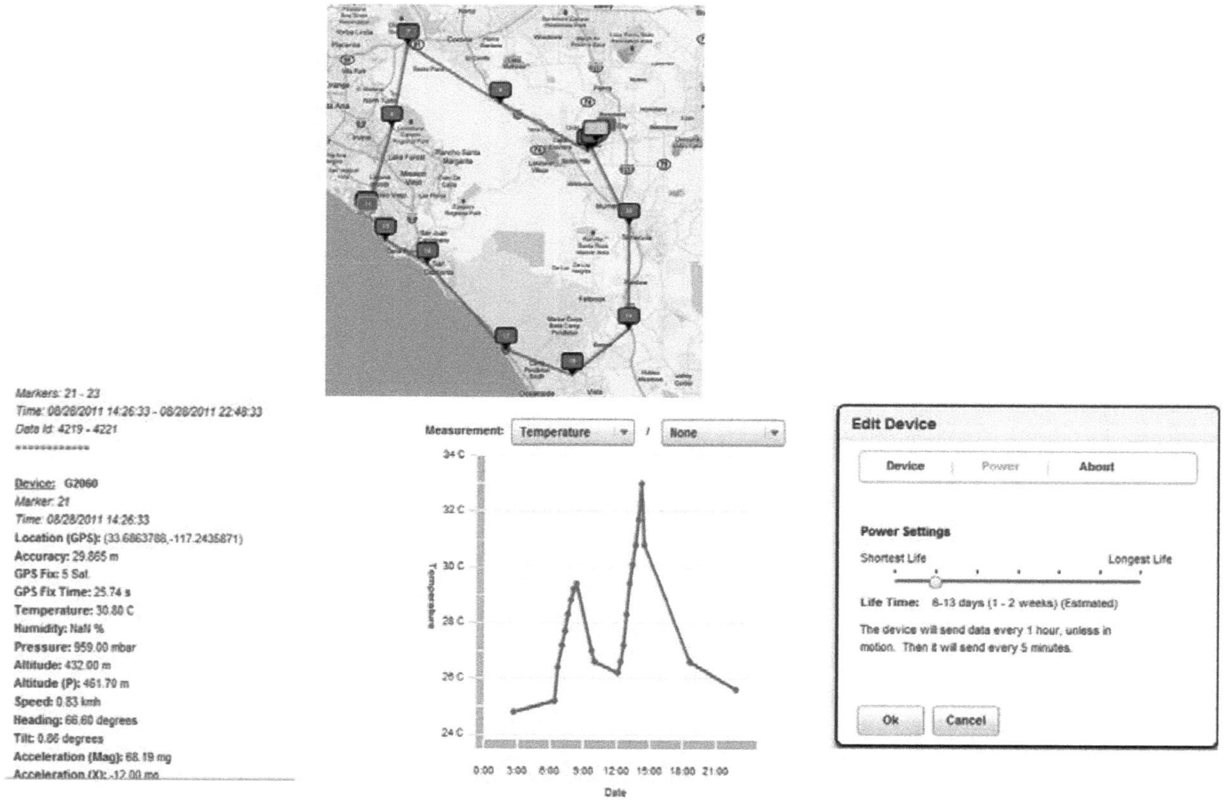

FIGURE 9.3

Near real-time visibility data.

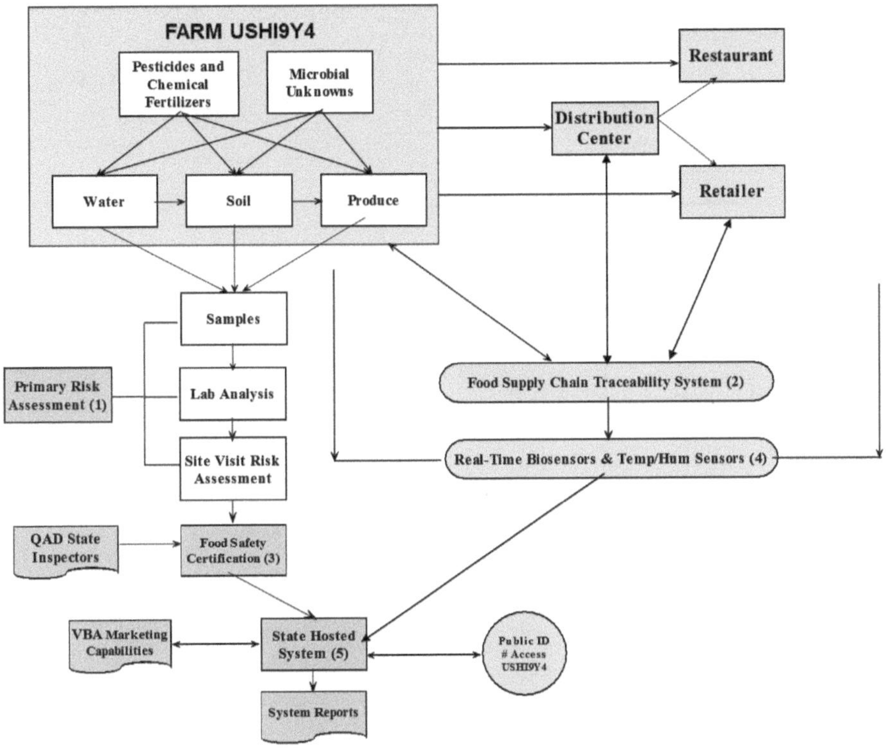

FIGURE 9.4

Traceability from the farm to various customers.

improving recall capabilities as the data is available to pinpoint when and where any controls were not properly managed.

A basic PTI-enabled barcode system is shown in Figs. 9.5–9.7.

In Fig. 9.5, the farm is shown tagging of individual cases of product with GS1 labels, the loading and shipping of the pallet, adding radio frequency identification (RFID) temperature monitoring tags to the pallet, reading the case barcode tags with a barcode reader, and the pallet RFID temperature monitoring tag with a RFID reader. On the left hand side of the figure, the data that has been read is electronically transmitted into a data repository where the case tag data is paired up with the RFID tag data, thus establishing temperature monitoring for the cases on the pallet. All data is uploaded into the system database.

In Fig. 9.6, the pallet laden cases are transported (with temperatures being read by the RFID system in the truck trailer) and offloaded into the distribution center where temperatures and barcode tags are read when the product enters the distribution center, into cooler storage, during specified customer pallet builds (smaller quantities of many products are loaded onto new temperature monitored pallets in preparation for retail outlet delivery).

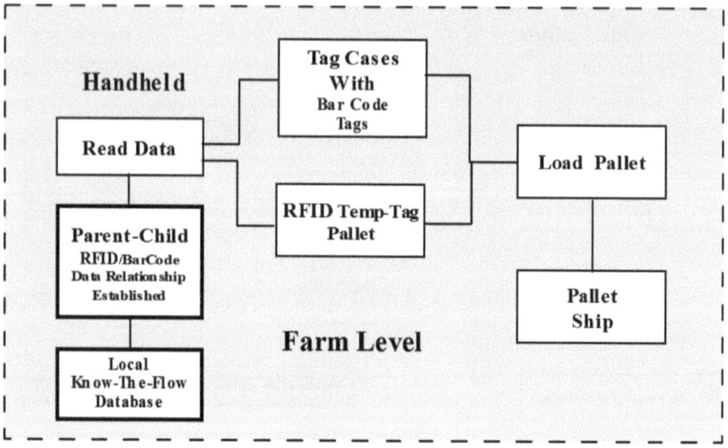

FIGURE 9.5

Tagging at the farm level.

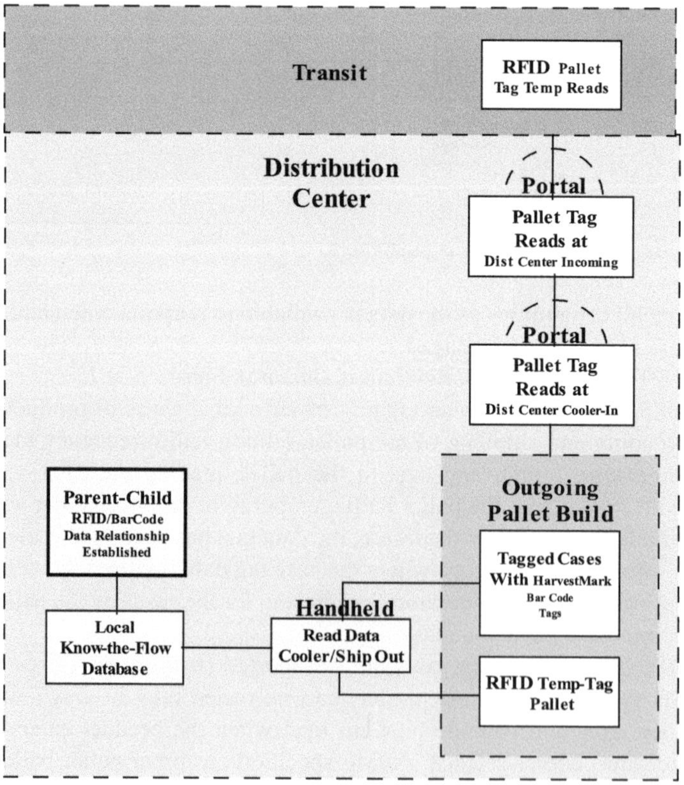

FIGURE 9.6

Distribution center tracking in, into coolers, reconfiguration, and shipment out.

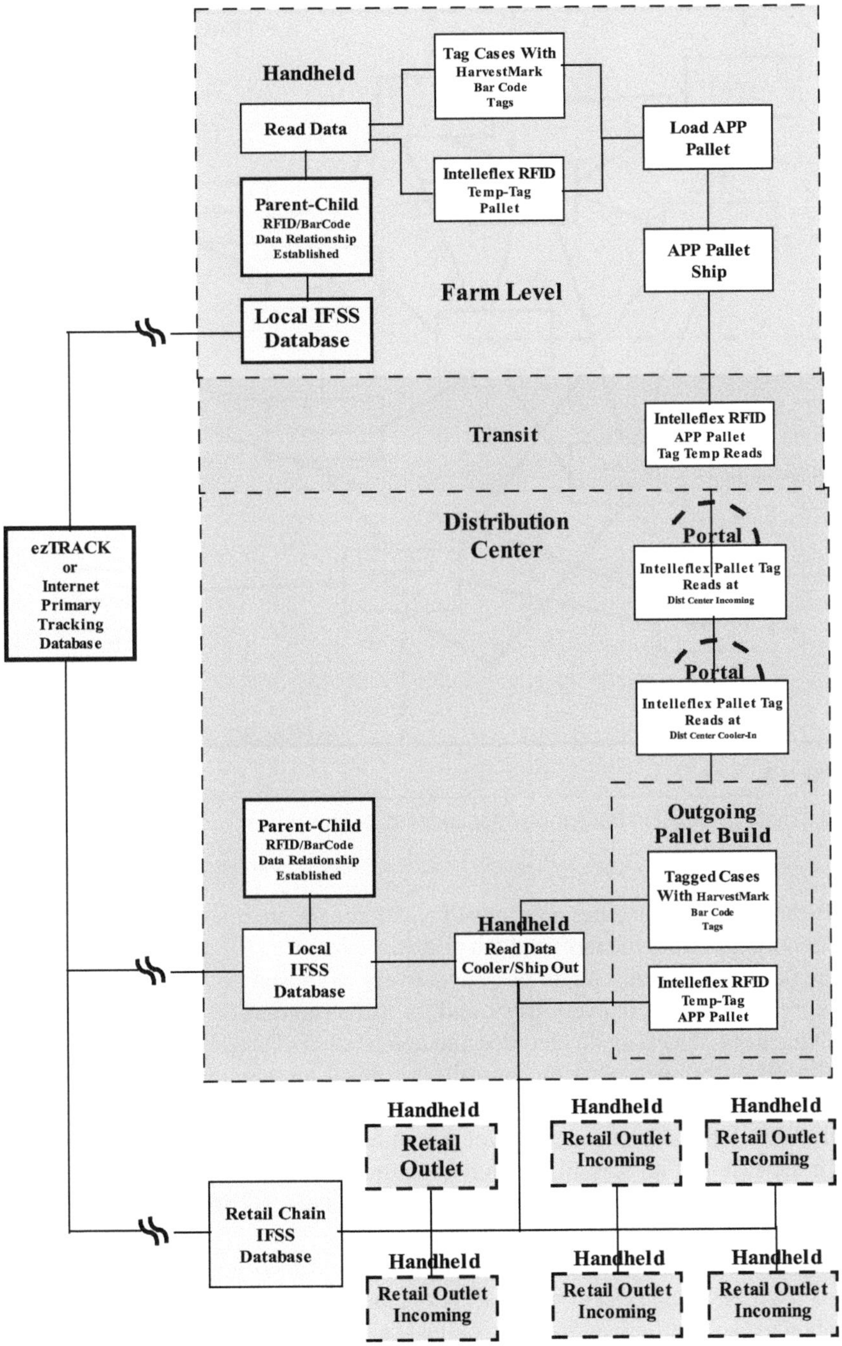

FIGURE 9.7

GS1 and RFID temperature monitoring traceability system.

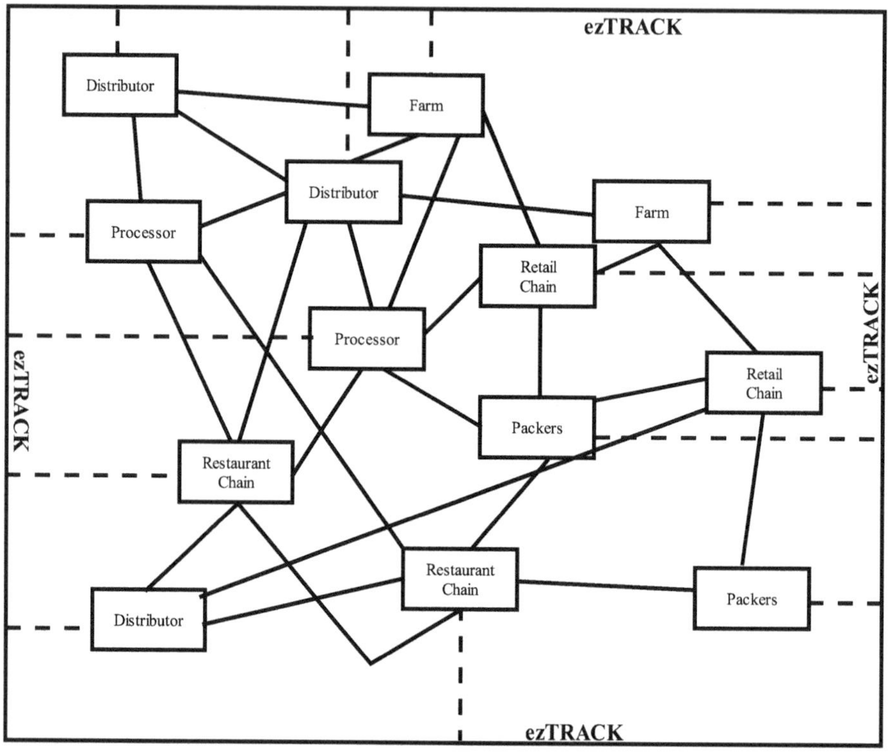

FIGURE 9.8

Food handling operation traceability/monitoring data sharing.

In this example, food has now moved with temperature monitoring and GS1 product identity tags from the farm and out of distribution. Fig. 9.7 shows the basic receipt by the retail outlet or restaurant prior to delivery to consumers. Temperature tracking has continued on the delivery truck and, at the restaurant or retail outlet rear door receiving dock, data is again recorded and uploaded to a centralized inventory system.

Fig. 9.7 illustrates what the overall case level temperature monitoring system would look like when all parts are connected to establish a system flow that can be used to develop and implement preventive control plans.

In the case of Fig. 9.8, all data has been uploaded into a centralized system that allows all supply chain parties (farm, distribution center, carrier, receiver) to monitor, share data, and manage the system.

Fig. 9.8 shows all data being uploaded into a cloud system such as that shown as the ezTRACK, cloud system which serves as the central data repository. In the example shown, each participant in the tracking scenario can keep internal data protected and share only selected data with supply chain partners based on what permissions are granted to each shipper, carrier, and receiver. In this way, all data held in local

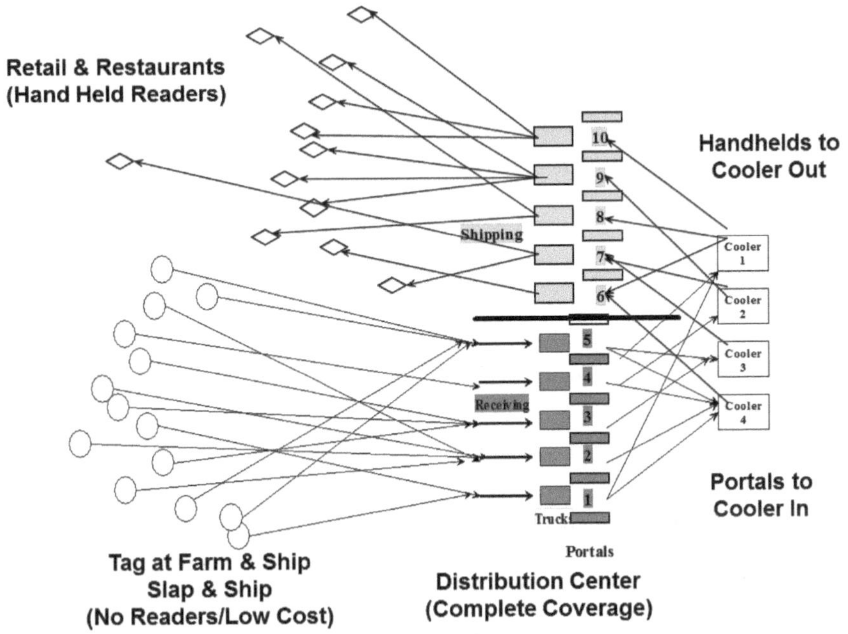

FIGURE 9.9

Some traceability system details at the distribution center.

computers can be kept private and under local protection, whereas any data uploaded to a cloud system can be controlled by data owners. It is also important to note that in the event of a recall, other permissions such as those that might be demanded by government officials can be granted.

A closer look at the distribution product flow is shown in Fig. 9.9. At the bottom of the illustration, tagged product can be seen entering the distribution center incoming receiving docks, moving into one of the four coolers, and, after pallet reconfiguration, moving out through shipping docks for transportation to retail and restaurants. Temperatures are collected throughout the process and paired with specific case GS1 tag information.

INTEGRATED FOOD SAFETY AND QUALITY DATA SYSTEMS

From a preventive controls perspective, the ability to integrate food safety and quality data from various sources and into various databases becomes an issue to be reckoned with. The objectives of such integrated systems include standardized data across all players and supply chain levels to share control and reduce risk, to speed recall processes to control escaped products, and to eliminate later health hazards.

To establish integrated food safety and quality data systems, it is important to look at the differences between business and governmental data requirements and needs.

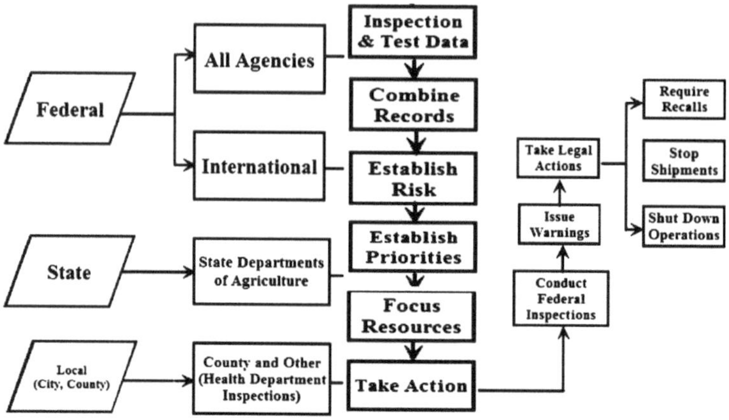
Federal
State
Local
(City, County)
All Agencies
International
State Departments
of Agriculture
County and Other
(Health Department
Inspections)
Inspection
& Test Data
Combine
Records
Establish
Risk
Establish
Priorities
Focus
Resources
Take Action
Conduct
Federal
Inspections
Issue
Warnings
Take Legal
Actions
Require
Recalls
Stop
Shipments
Shut Down
Operations

FIGURE 9.10

Government level integrated food safety systems.

As the government operates on the federal, state, and local levels, current government food safety and quality databases are separate and collect different data in different formats and with different systems; the inspection and test data existing in those systems represents a significant challenge when it comes to enforcement activities (the primary purpose of government agencies).

On the left side of Fig. 9.10, federal, state, and local agencies currently collect food safety inspection data from various federal, international, state, and local cities and county agencies. The goal of the government efforts to integrate food safety data mean that data from all sources must be standardized and combined into a company's database. The combined records allow the federal government to establish risk levels for the company, its products and its processes. Using this risk level data, inspection priorities may be set. High-risk companies and products float to the top of the data, and the government is able to establish audit priorities from these risk rankings. Once the prioritized list is established, officials will focus resources to visit and inspect high risk facilities where, when required, they will provide a list of needed corrective actions for the audited facilities. If required, warnings will be issued. If warnings are not heeded and actions not taken, the government is empowered to take recall, stop shipment or shut down action.

So, from the government perspective, the issues of concern are primarily that of driving improvement and enforcement.

As an alternative, businesses should have a vested interest in integrated food safety and quality systems as a means of protecting their businesses and their supply chain, knowing what product is where and knowing the condition of that product at any single moment in time. Of course, businesses often want to avoid responsibility for hazardous products and to assure that the guilty party is identified as a means of clearing their own reputations.

From the business side, the standardization of traceability and monitoring data through the supply chain is an important issue to consider if the supply chain as a whole desires to protect its members.

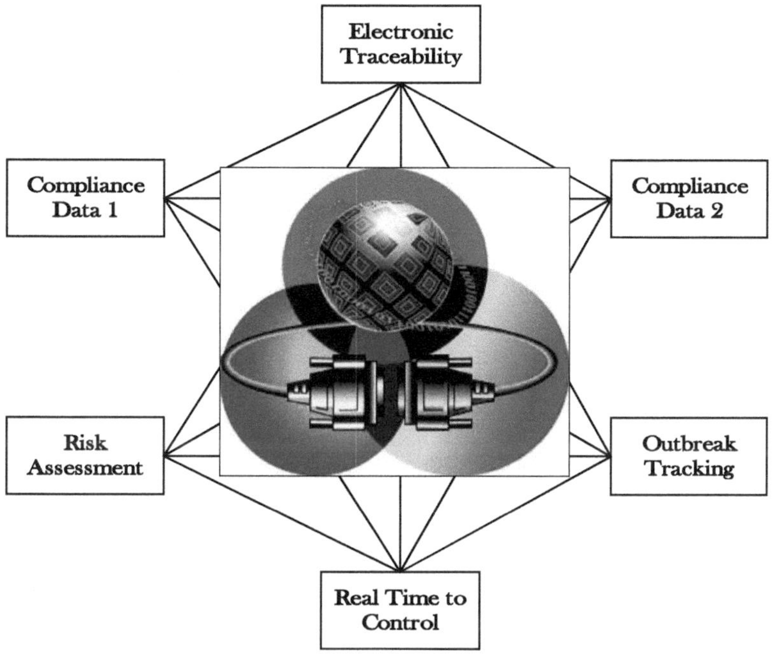

FIGURE 9.11

Supply chain food safety, quality, and traceability data integration.

This integration of food safety and quality data can also be accomplished systematically. Fig. 9.11 shows how traceability, compliance, inspection, test, and outbreak data can be used collectively to identify and drive high risk operations towards better preventive controls as a means of protecting not only their own businesses, but also their customers and the public.

At the bottom of Fig. 9.11, the "Real Time to Control" aspect of the system is designed to use risk rankings from all collected data to reduce recall times by directing investigative efforts towards those companies whose systems are at higher risk based on quantified risk ranking.

Fig. 9.12 is a system diagram for how the system can be operationalized.

Figs. 9.13–9.16 provide system breakdowns for easier understanding.

Beginning with the traceability system component (Fig. 9.13), suppliers are seen to apply GS1 barcode labels to all cases, and the cases are loaded onto RFID temperature monitoring pallets. Both barcode and temperature data are loaded into the overall data system to be analyzed and displayed on computers as dashboards. Dashboards are simply single screen displays showing summaries, trends, and other information as a result of data analysis. Dashboards provide a quick visual display of what is going on for any set of products during transportation, handling, and other processes.

Fig. 9.14 illustrates how food safety inspection and environmental sampling data from linked supplier databases or manual input can be used to quantitatively establish

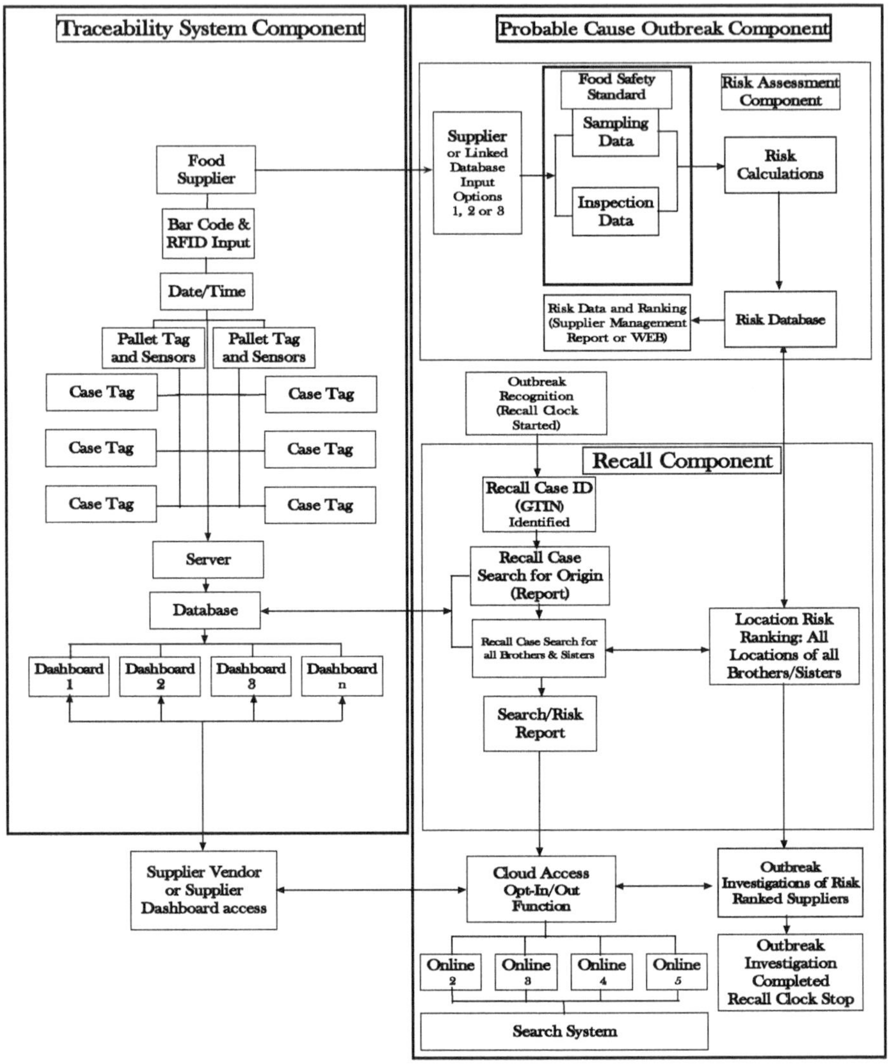

FIGURE 9.12

Integrated food safety and quality system diagram.

operational risk scores that are then used to calculate risk levels and to rank suppliers based on their scores. In this case, as an example, a supplier (A) who is not providing adequate environmental sampling or does not establish a preventive control plan will receive a low score on those characteristics. The low score then means that supplier (A) is at higher risk than a supplier (B) that has established a good environmental monitoring and preventive control system. Theoretically, when there is a food safety outbreak, the higher risk supplier should be the first one to investigate. If high risk

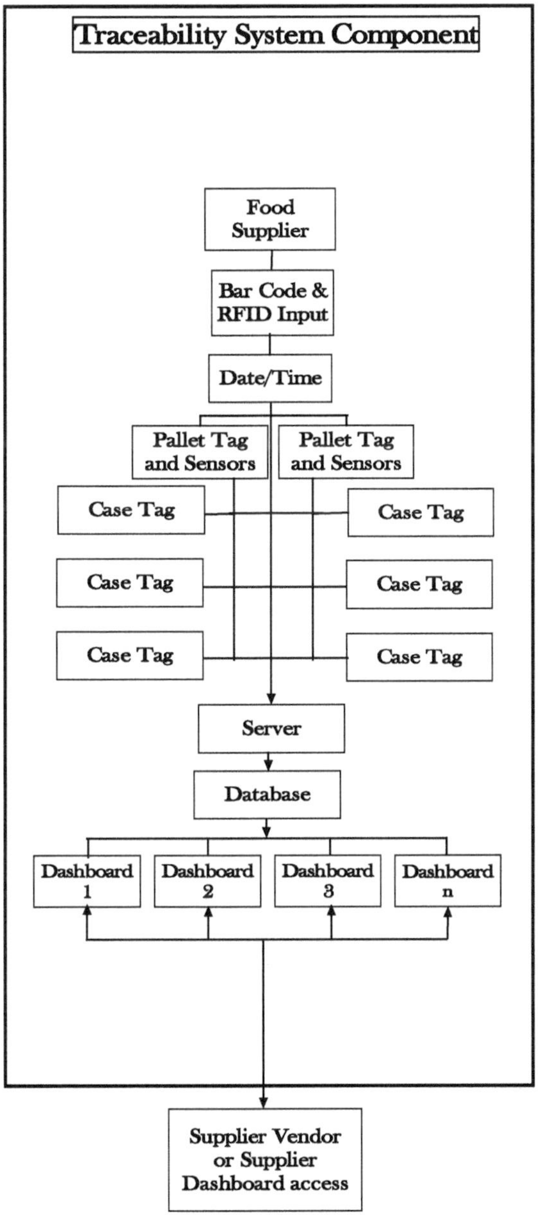

FIGURE 9.13

IFSS traceability component.

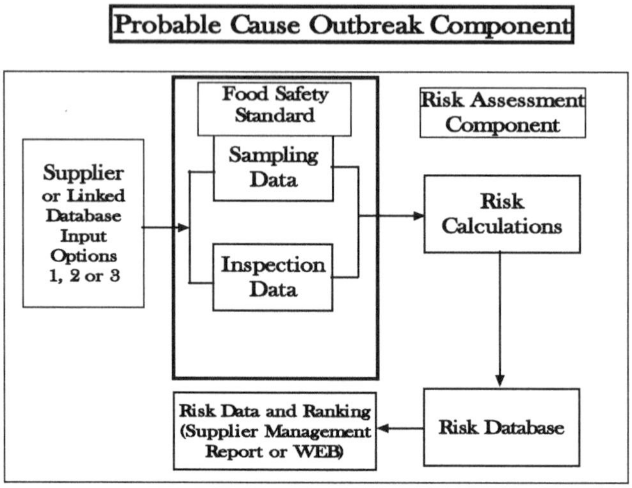

FIGURE 9.14

Establishing a probable outbreak cause in minimal time.

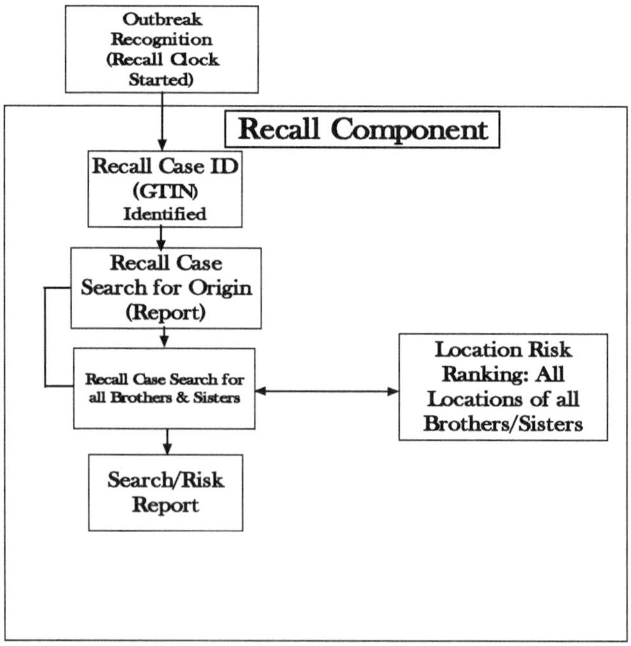

FIGURE 9.15

The traceability/recall component.

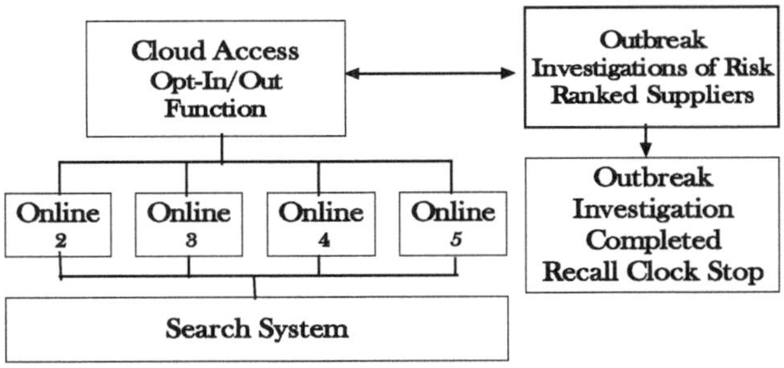

FIGURE 9.16

Establishing time to recall as a measure of recall success.

suppliers are found to be the cause of the outbreak or at least a contributor (through inadequate food safety practices), the time to identify and eliminate the cause of the outbreak would be greatly reduced. Reducing outbreak time is a primary objective of recall professionals aiming to protect human health.

The lag time between discovery of the outbreak and finding and eliminating the source (cause) of the outbreak is perhaps the most elusive aspect of successful outbreak management.

This is the same type of thinking used by governmental agencies to establish audit priorities.

Even if the source is quickly identified, the problem of locating all impacted product in all places confounds reducing the lag time mentioned above. Traceability systems and the system's traceability component (Fig. 9.15) are designed to establish standards, collect traceability data, and support the risk assessment rankings. By knowing the specific location of all goods that have not escaped the supply chain into the public at large, the traceability system, if competent, can be used to provide rapid location identification.

In a manner similar to the probable cause ranking system as in Fig. 9.14, companies with good, adequate, poor, or no traceability systems are ranked by the system, and this ranking data is used conjointly with food safety readiness results to provide a combined ranking system: Inspection, test, traceability data (and others) may all be used in the ranking and recall processes.

Of course all raw system, input data must be collected, stored, and reduced to dashboard level analyses to establish a basis for preventive management actions and control.

Fig. 9.16 shows data flowing into the cloud databases so that the online screens can function based on management searches.

In the event of a recall, the system clock can be quickly enabled to provide up to date rankings. Once the recall event is activated in the system, humans take over and follow leads provided by the system. When the cause of the event is clearly identified and preventive causal analysis actions are completed, the clock can be stopped. The resulting start and stop times provide participants and the government with what is called "Time to Recall" which is a measure of the overall success of any recall system.

TEMPERATURE MONITORING

Temperature monitoring during transportation operations is a critical issue impacting all transportations operations focused on perishables. Generally speaking, the plan for how temperatures will be monitored throughout all food transportation processes should come from a specialized CC team, whereas implementation, testing, and maintenance of the monitoring system falls within the assignable cause requirements that are the responsibility of FIT teams.

The questions involved with temperature monitoring tend to focus on how can a company employ preventive food safety and quality practices, increase security, provide traceability and recall, meet legal requirements, reduce liabilities, and increase return on investment while solving costly and wasteful practices?

Many companies have developed the needed technology. Supply chain members just need to select and put the correct technology together.

INTELLIGENT DELIVERY CONTROL SYSTEMS

There are some systems on the horizon that are being designed as intelligent delivery control systems. The list below shows some advantages of real-time GPS and sensor-enabled tracking and detection for temperatures, humidity, explosives, and, coming soon, bacterial contamination.

- Sensor supplied data
- Improve delivered product food safety and quality
- Reduce culls, rejects, returns
- Comply with Department of Homeland Security (DHS), customs and border protection (CBP), international foundation for science (IFS), and other reporting requirements
- View data live anytime, anywhere
- Control over international shipments using GS1 international standards
- Establish shipping priorities
- Improve routing procedures
- Eliminate mixed shelf life pallet loading
- Manage imports and exports

An example of using intelligent food routing systems is shown in Fig. 9.17 depicting distribution center loading using multiple types of electronic monitoring tags. In the upper left hand corner of the figure, inbound pallets are shown with temperature monitoring tags attached. As these pallets enter the distribution center, supply chain temperatures are downloaded at the receiving dock, into coolers, at pallet reconfiguration and out through the shipping dock where the truck trailer or container records and reports global positioning system (GPS), temperature, and other sensor data en-route.

Fig. 9.18 shows a more complex container system that collects data from GPS equipment, temperature, humidity, tampering, explosive, and biological contamination sensors. This complex system collects data from all sensors and transmits all

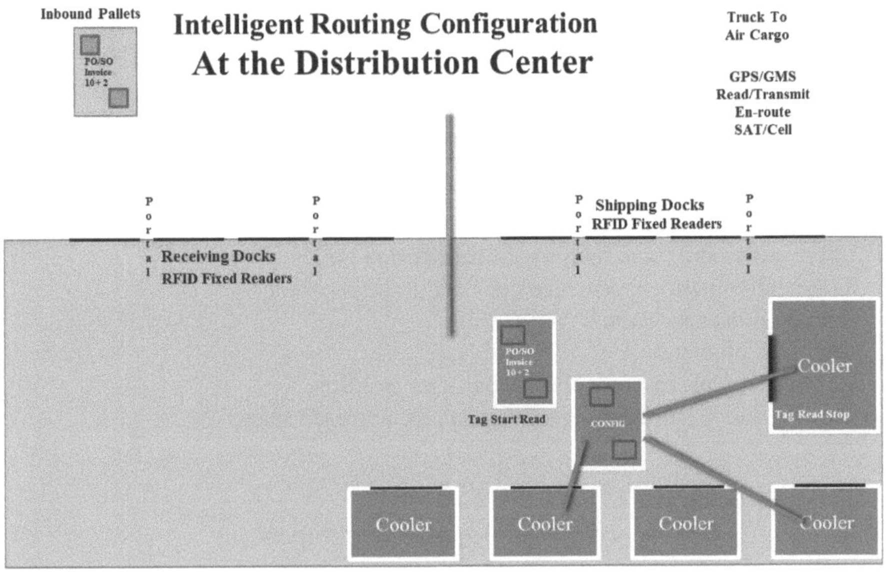

FIGURE 9.17

Intelligent food routing configuration at the distribution center.

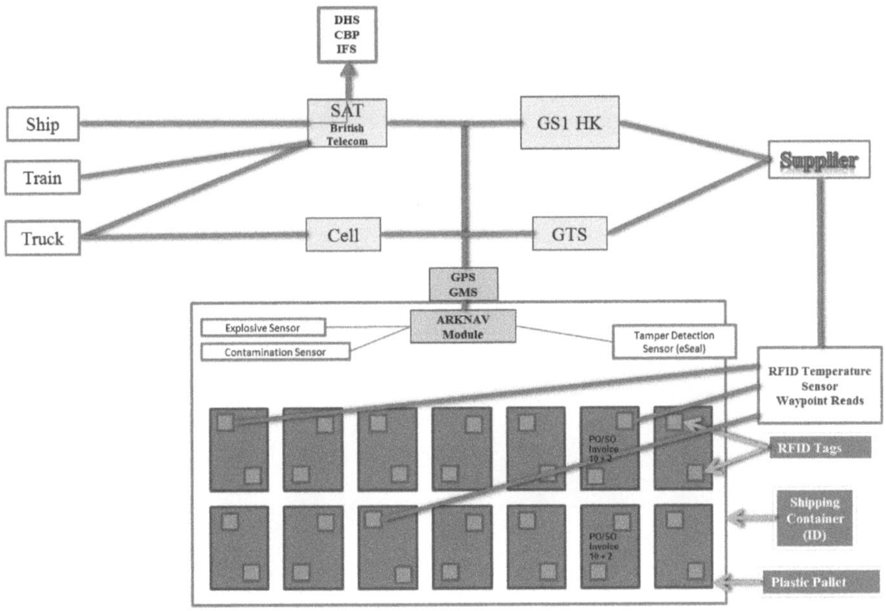

FIGURE 9.18

Intelligent food routing systems applied to shipping containers.

data into a reader that transmits all data into a device that sends all data to satellites. The transmitted data is then available to shippers, carriers, and receivers as well as CBP and DHS officials concerned with shipments entering and exiting countries.

A basic temperature monitoring system is shown in six steps in Figs. 9.19–9.24. Such systems as those depicted in Figs. 9.19–9.24 have several advantages including:

- Preventing food safety and quality problems
- End-to-end seamless monitoring in a real time mode
- Improved security and integrity of transported goods
- Traceability platform provides track and trace capability
- Reduced cost and waste
- Improved efficiency
- Consumers can see product traceability in real time
- Improved food safety and quality result in increased sales

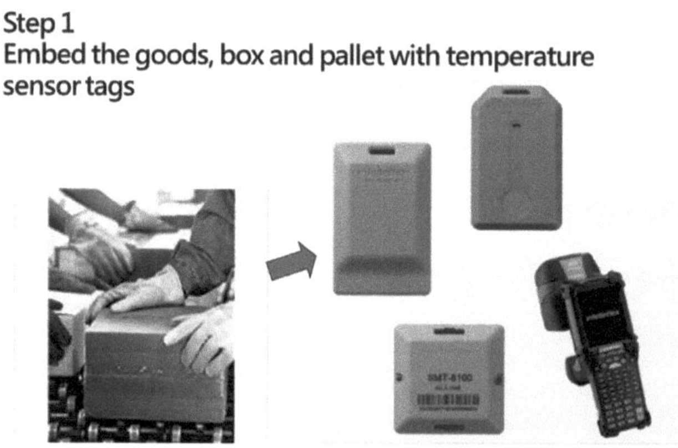

FIGURE 9.19

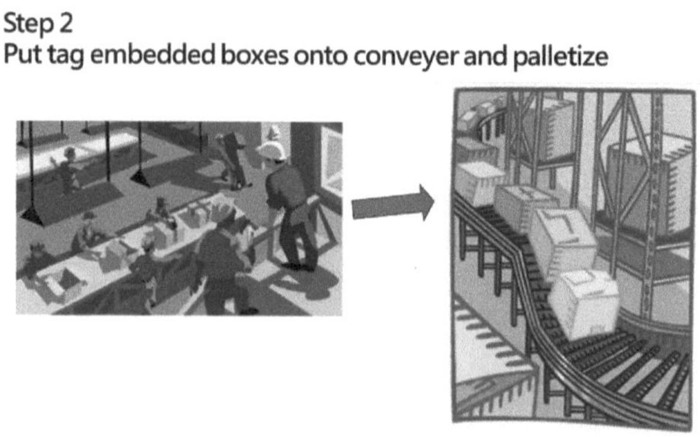

FIGURE 9.20

Step 3
Place pallet embedded with tags tags onto storage shelf with inventory address

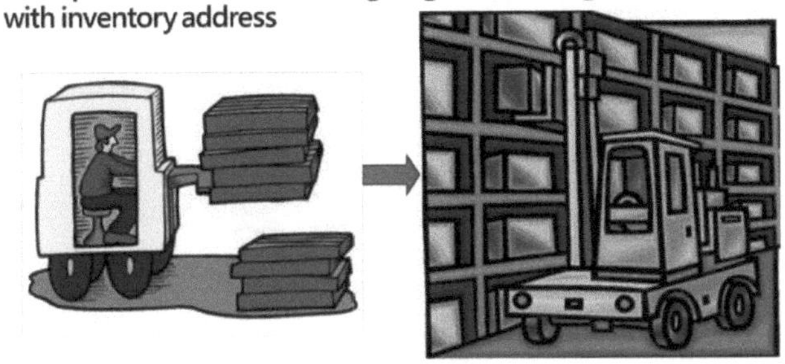

FIGURE 9.21

Step 4
When delivery is not in refrigerated trucks, temperature control insulated containers can be employed to monitor the integrity of product.

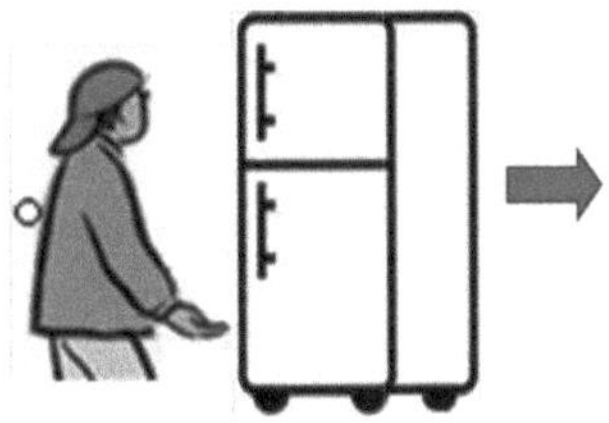

FIGURE 9.22

Step 5
Once insulated container is on the truck, use a fleet tracking solution to monitor safety and freshness of goods

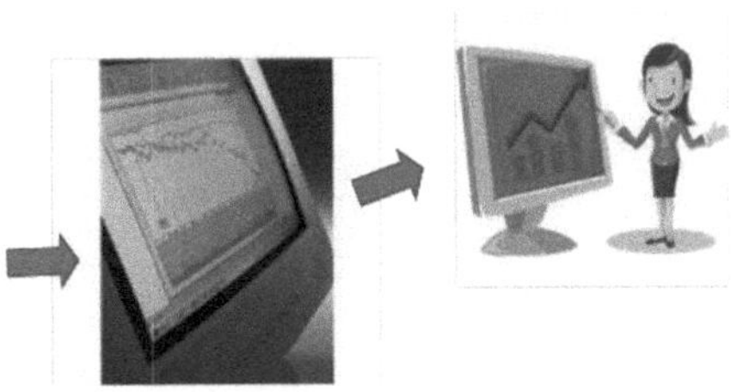

FIGURE 9.23

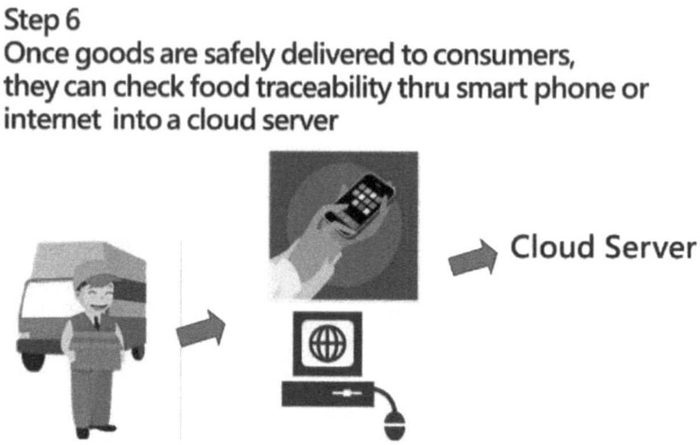
Step 6
Once goods are safely delivered to consumers, they can check food traceability thru smart phone or internet into a cloud server
Cloud Server

FIGURE 9.24

The capabilities offered by today's cell phone–enabled tagging and monitoring systems provide the supply chain with facility and reefer monitoring designed to assure that food is properly temperature maintained during production, through transportation to distribution, during distribution, and transportation from distribution into retail outlets. Fig. 9.25 shows suppliers such as bakeries, processors, or packers that have installed facility level temperature monitors throughout the facility. Data is transmitted using what are known as Zigbee technology from point to point throughout the facility until it becomes stored in a computer tied to higher level networking systems. Distributors and reefers are similarly outfitted with temperature monitors. Reefer temperature data is collected during transit and automatically downloaded into facility computer upon arrival at unload locations.

The advantages offered by Zigbee systems are that they are capable of being calibrated (environmental monitoring accuracy), extremely easy to install (no technical assistance needed), and designed for harsh environments where temperatures ranges are excessive.

Of equal importance is the capability of such systems to a centralized system for sharing among all supply chain participants such as shown in Fig. 9.26 where data from suppliers, supplier-to-distribution reefer transportation, distribution center, distribution center-to-store transportation, and store-level monitoring data is available for analysis and preventive action by FIT teams.

By expanding the Zigbee system even further to cover multiple regional distribution networks, all data from all regions can be accessed, analyzed, and preventive actions taken by corporate-level teams assigned to managing members of regional supply chains as shown in Fig. 9.27.

Some companies such as Chipotle are (or should be) concerned with capturing temperature monitoring data as soon as possible from harvest sites. The process that involves harvest through some level of packaging and the placement of harvest cases or packages onto pallets is known at the grower pallet loop (Fig. 9.28). In many instances, GPS-enabled mobile barcode printing and tagging systems are utilized to

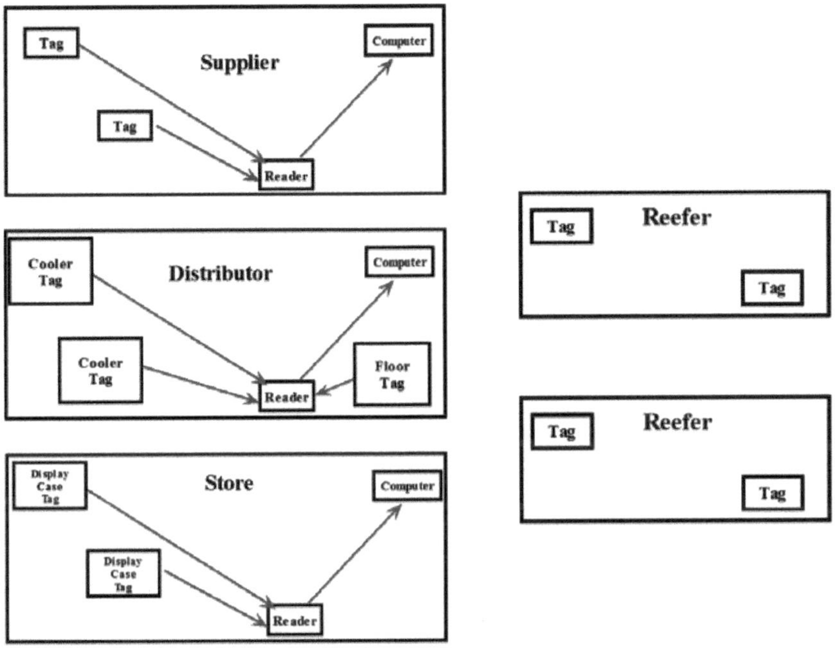

FIGURE 9.25

Supply chain Zigbee monitoring systems.

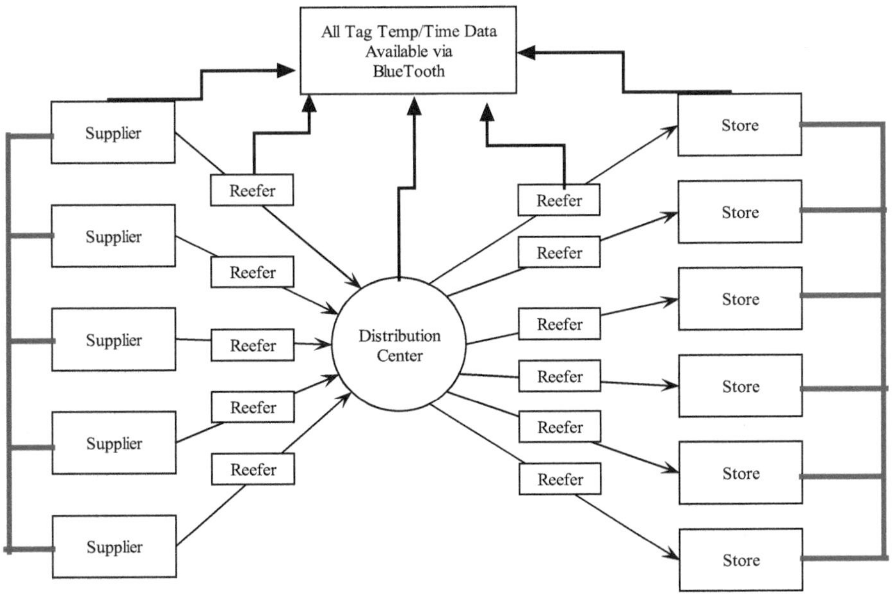

FIGURE 9.26

Collecting and sharing supply chain data from suppliers to store outlets.

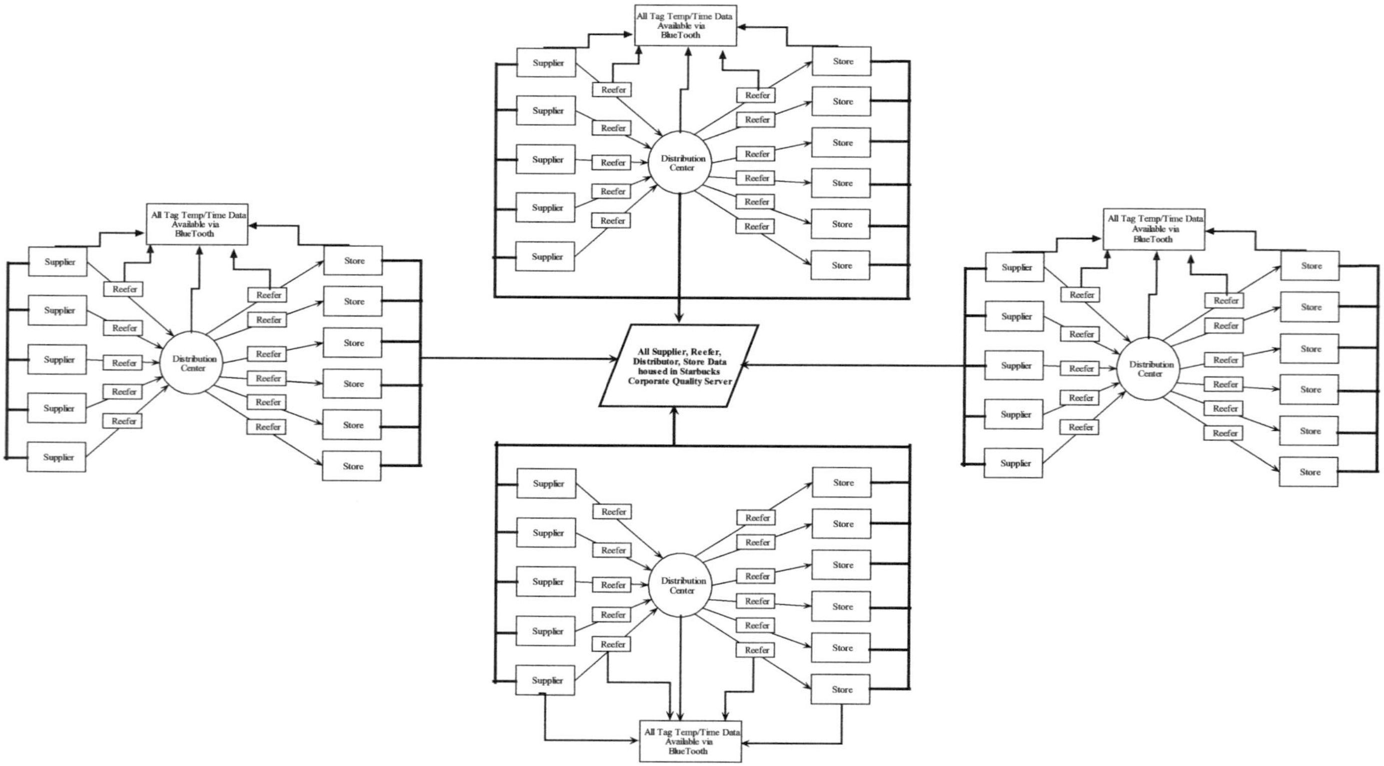

FIGURE 9.27

Corporate monitoring, reporting, and preventive action systems.

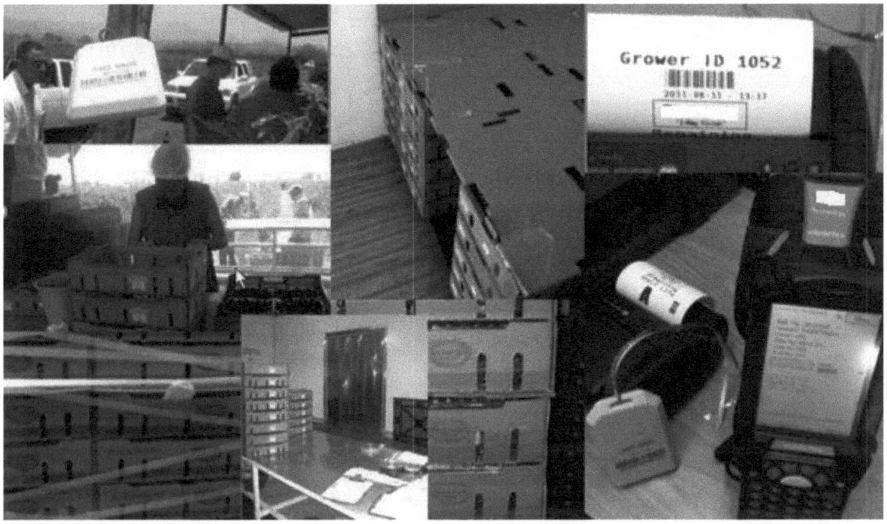

FIGURE 9.28

Capturing data from the grower pallet loop.

immediately lable cases when they are filled. In this manner, the exact field harvest location is automatically recorded. In the event of a recall when a particular case or food is identified as hazardous, the exact location where it was harvested can be checked for the hazard under question.

In many instances and at many farms and packing houses, pallets of produce or fruit may be harvested at different times and from different locations. There are also differences in how precool systems are able to properly cool product that is in the middle of cases or pallets when these cases and pallets are insulated by other cases and pallets (thus "protecting" them from being cooled according to procedural requirements). These missteps result in pallets with different shelf lives being loaded in the same shipment. Such scenarios represent mismanagement of inventory from a food quality and food safety perspective. Recall that warmer temperatures help bacteria to grow.

In the top row of Fig. 9.29, pallets of mixed shelf lives have been randomly loaded into a container. The numbers on each colored section show the remaining shelf life in days for each set of cases load on the pallet. For instance, 15+ indicates that these cases have at least 15 days of saleable shelf life remaining based on industry temperature control standards. Unfortunately, truck trailers and containers tend to be unloaded from the rear at the first stop which is usually the closest stop requiring shorter remaining shelf life because the produce has not had to travel very far between loading and unloading. The illustration shows that long shelf life cases will be unloaded at points where shorter shelf life shipments will fulfill receiver requirements.

Mixed loads like those shown in Fig. 9.29 (top) are the result of a lack of appropriate precool or improper time to temperature measurements and record keeping before or during inventory storage.

The bottom row in Fig. 9.29 shows that the company has been careful to monitor temperatures and shelf lives, thus allowing the company to deliver short shelf life pallets to closer destinations and to deliver longer shelf life pallets to distances further away where transportation times are longer.

Another preventive temperature control issue commonly occurs from the front of the trailer (near the reefer) to the rear of the trailer. Fig. 9.30 shows the result of research that indicates the reefer (and pallet) temperatures in the middle of the truck are generally maintained at a higher temperature than the areas closest to and furthest away from the reefer.

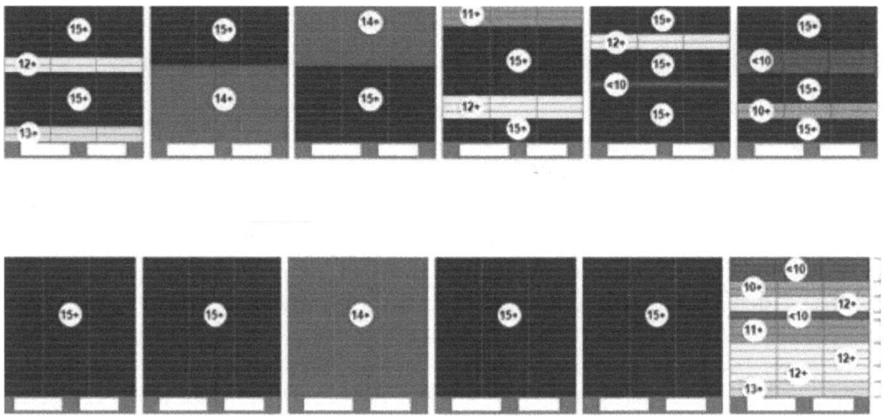

FIGURE 9.29

Mixed and sorted shelf life loading.

Reprinted with permission from Intelleflex, Corporation.

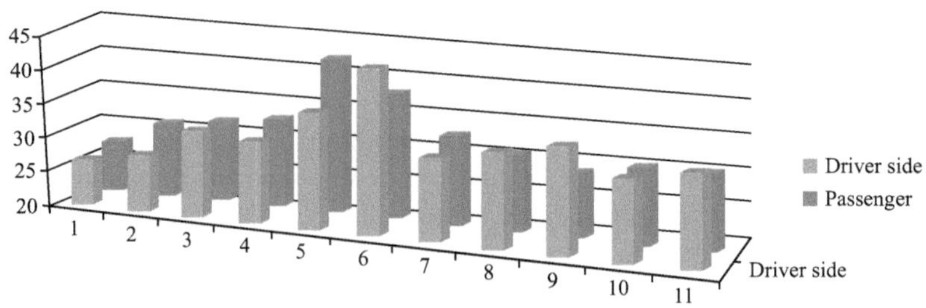

FIGURE 9.30

Front-to-rear temperature monitoring results.

Reprinted with permission from Intelleflex, Corporation.

Transoceanic container shipments represent another type of temperature management scenario. In Fig. 9.31, a shipment of avocados is picked up from a California farm, transported to downtown Los Angeles, California then to the Port of Los Angeles.

Fig. 9.32 shows the long journey by ship from the Port of Los Angeles to Honolulu, Hawaii where the pallet was delivered to a distribution center.

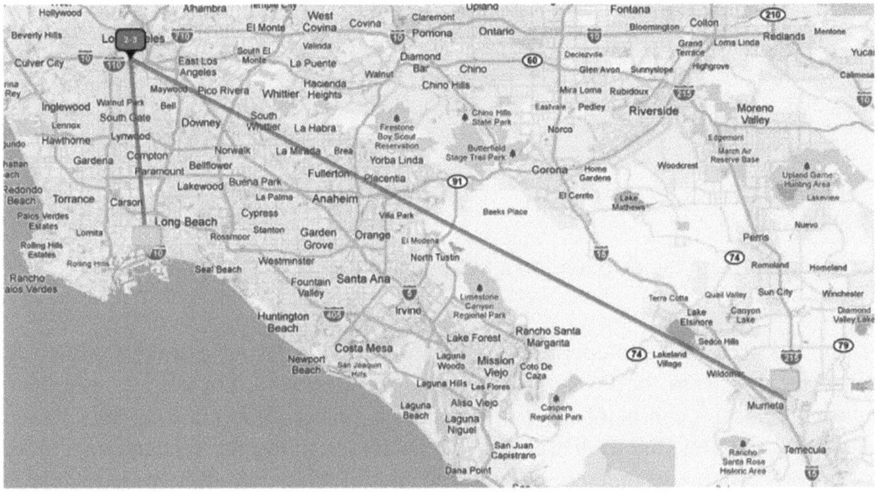

FIGURE 9.31

California pallet routing.

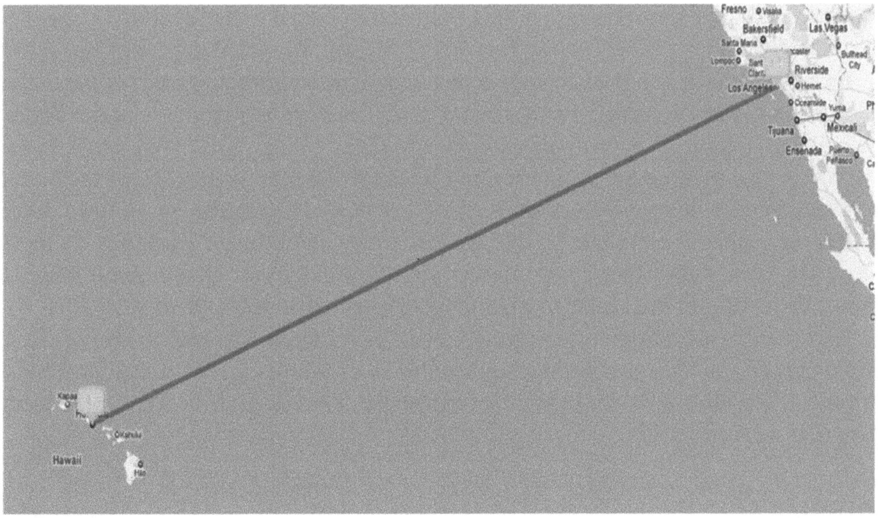

FIGURE 9.32

Trans-pacific routing.

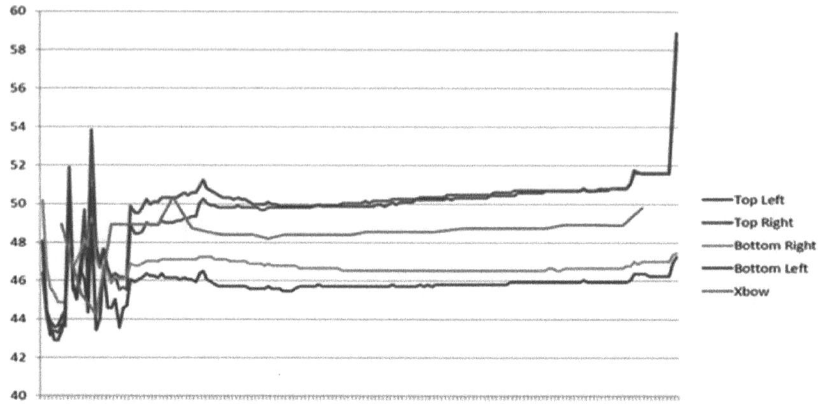

FIGURE 9.33

Monitoring container temperatures on a trans-pacific voyage.

Fig. 9.33 shows the temperature monitoring profiles for several days while food moved by ship from the Post of Los Angeles to Honolulu. On the left side of the data trend chart, it can be observed that pallet temperature monitoring tags showed erratic temperatures due to distribution center loading after the container sat on the loading dock for an extended period of time and for temperatures recorded while the container sat on the Port of Los Angeles ship loading dock.

Five temperature monitoring tags were placed randomly on five different pallets. Two tags were placed at the bottom the pallets, two on top and one was placed in the middle of the pallets.

Notice how the monitoring tag data flattened out during the several voyage days across the Pacific.

From the date in Fig. 9.33, it can be seen that temperatures at the top of the pallets recorded container temperatures at least 5°F higher than temperatures at the bottom the pallets.

Notice also that the temperature trend lines for the tags at the tops of the pallets show an increase in temperature as the freighter moves across the ocean from cooler California waters and climate to the warmer water and climate Hawaiian temperatures. The data shows that even relatively modest external climate conditions can impact the ability of the reefer to maintain compliance temperatures.

European wine shipping in reefer containers from Europe to Hong Kong (Fig. 9.34) shows a pattern similar to that shown above for the California to Hawaii Shipment. Recall that wine, especially expensive wine, should be kept at temperatures not to exceed 75°F.

EQUIPMENT

Although traceability equipment is sold with and without temperature or other sensor-enabled equipment and at a vast range of prices, traceability and monitoring

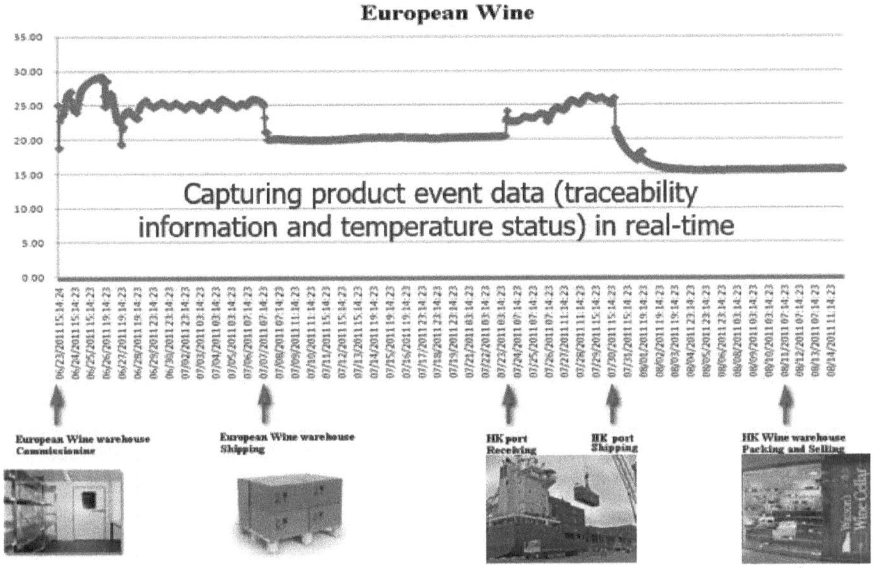

FIGURE 9.34

Wine trans-oceanic temperature monitoring profile.

preventive control requirements should be established based on the circumstances surround the product needs and process capabilities.

Fig. 9.35 shows high endurance barcode equipment that is available from many suppliers. The equipment is water and drop resistant and made for relatively harsh environments such as might be encountered in processing, loading, and unloading operations.

As the need to incorporate temperature monitoring increases because of food safety and legal requirements, other types of equipment are becoming more popular. Fig. 9.36 shows a number of temperature monitoring tags and devices on common use for both process audits and for continuous monitoring. The blue temperature sensor-enabled tags on the left can be used only one or two times, usually for audit purposes, and cost about \$50 U.S. each, whereas the green tags are battery operated (also about \$50 U.S. each) and can be used for continuous monitoring for up to several months on different loads. Both of these types of tags dump data into data upload points at receiving docks.

On the right side of the picture is a fully rechargeable temperature/GPS/date/time/humidity monitoring device with full software support showing all the ILC mentioned above in the section on traceability. This \$500 device can be used indefinitely. Database access to monitoring results cost about \$50 per year. Don't lose this one. Make sure you have a good return system in place.

Of course, the simplest type of device that can be used to monitor GPS for any load, anywhere, is shown in Fig. 9.37. At a cost of about \$150 in small quantities,

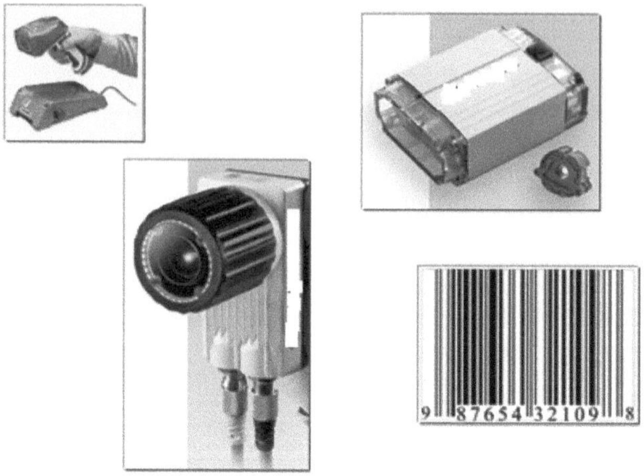

FIGURE 9.35

High impact barcode readers.

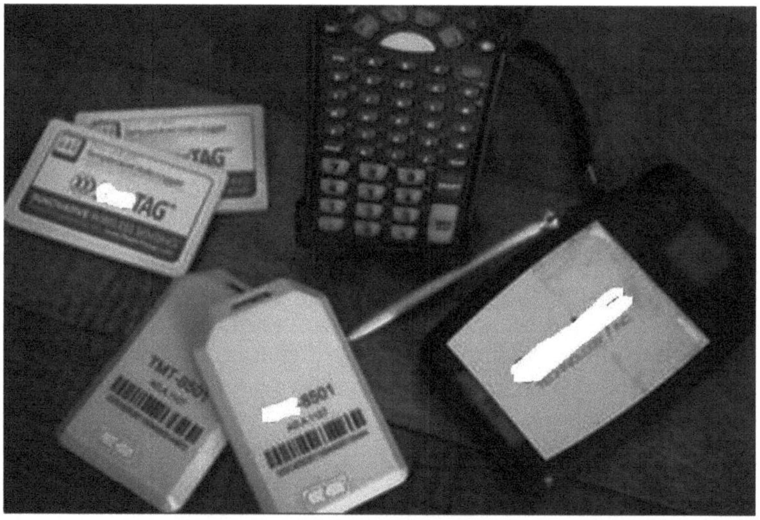

FIGURE 9.36

Different temperature monitoring options.

other technologies have surpassed its usefulness due to the added sensor-enabled features available at a similar or lower price.

Fig. 9.38 shows a temperature/GPS RFID system installed on the front interior wall of a reefer. The reader/sender is and antennas are clearly shown. The antenna picks up temperature data from RFID tagged pallets and transfers the data to the

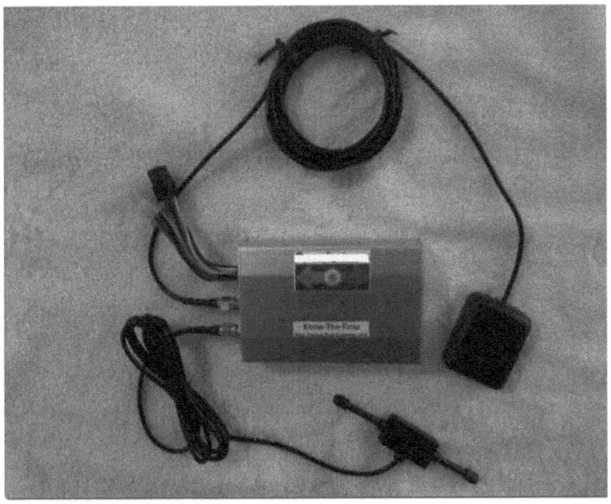

FIGURE 9.37

Basic GPS monitoring device.

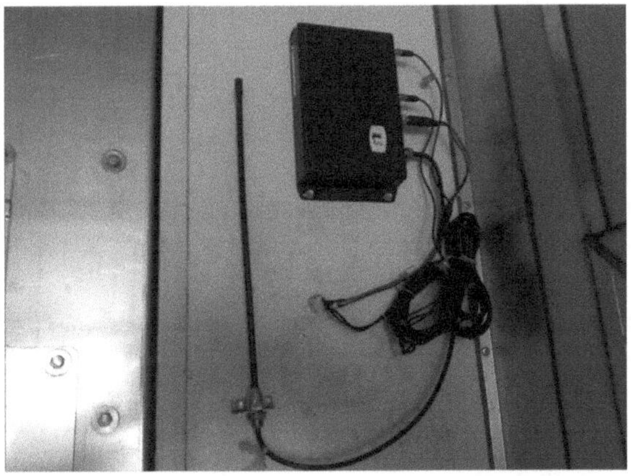

FIGURE 9.38

RFID/GPS/temperature rental system.

reader/sender device. Wires exit the reefer wall through a hole and are attached to a cell phone receiver/transmitter and to the reefer battery (to power the unit). The system rents for about $35 per month thus reducing the need to establish a capital asset fund. All data is uploaded to the cloud where reports are available.

- While today's technology marketplace is fraught with wireless devices, wireless temperature/GPS monitoring systems clearly offer the best advantages at the most reasonable prices. Additionally, such devices are
- Quickly installed—No techies are needed

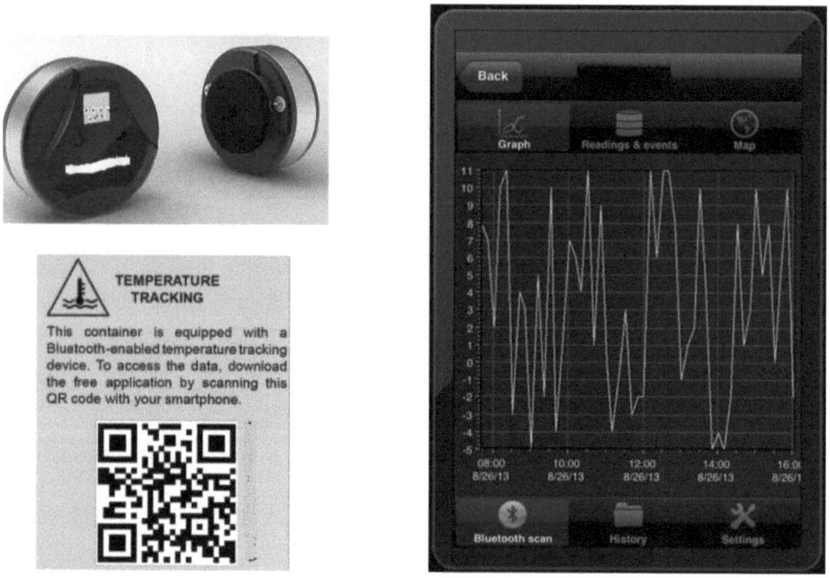

FIGURE 9.39

The hockey puck.

- Offer wireless tracking using cell phones and tablets
- Free Apps are included
- Can be used to monitor storage facilities, cooling equipment and packages in transit anywhere around the world
- Allow for data sharing via the clout
- Allow for viewing route details on full color maps
- Provide different read distance ranges
- Are federal communications commission (FCC), federal aviation administration (FAA), and Bluetooth certified
- Allow remote configuration
- Provide alerts and notification for out-of-control conditions
- Record times and temperatures according to local requirement
- Are often approved for use in many countries

For example, the small round device in Fig. 9.39 is one of the more advanced temperature/GPS monitoring devices to enter the Bluetooth marketplace. This hockey puck is about 2 in in diameter and is easily attached to reefer walls or pallets (for those needing pallet temperature monitoring). A free downloadable App is used to talk, configure, and read from the device. Data, routing, and many other bits of information are available to shippers, carriers, and receivers, whereas food is on route or in storage. The outer silver ring on the hockey puck captures ambient data without case interference. It is battery operated. The battery can be easily changed after a 1 to 2-year activity period. The device can be calibrated for an additional cost. Local software must be installed to talk to a cloud data repository. Full analysis and reports are available.

ADVANCED CONTAINER ID SYSTEM (CID): COMPLIANCE WITH FDA FSMA RULES

Designed specifically for keeping shipping container and truck trailers in full compliance with the new FDA FSMA rules on the sanitary transportation of human and animal foods, the container ID (CID) system collects data from GPS, temperatures, load/unload operations, wash operations and allows drivers to register container or reefer problems. By loading a temperature tag or two into the shipping compartment, temperatures are collected at intervals set by the user. The data is stored in the tag until uploaded into a cell phone or tablet containing a free downloadable App where the data is then transmitted by cell phone technology to cloud servers to comply with FSMA record keeping requirements. Fleet and container-level wash, temperature, load, and other analyses are available using a low cost ($25/year) system (Fig. 9.40).

The tag is RFID enabled which allows users to establish unique container identification numbers on the basis of GS1 international standards. Regardless of where the container or truck are in the world, it is internationally registered under this number and all load, wash, unload, temperature, GPS, and other data are matched to that unique ID number.

Once the free App is downloaded into the cell phone or tablet, a data entry screen is shown that allows the user to select where and how the container or trailer was sanitized, shipper and load information, and information that allows recording of reefer critical failures and container maintenance problems. All data is uploaded by cell phone technology (anywhere/anytime) to the container cloud data system.

Temperature profiles and GPS routing (Fig. 9.41) for any particular route can be accessed by shipper, receivers, and carriers using cell phones or tablets when permissions are granted.

Fig. 9.42 shows the data upload functions that appear on the cell phone or tablet.

Once the carrier maintenance (wash/test) button is clicked, the carrier maintenance (wash/test) screen (Fig. 9.43) appears that allows, by touch screen, all data

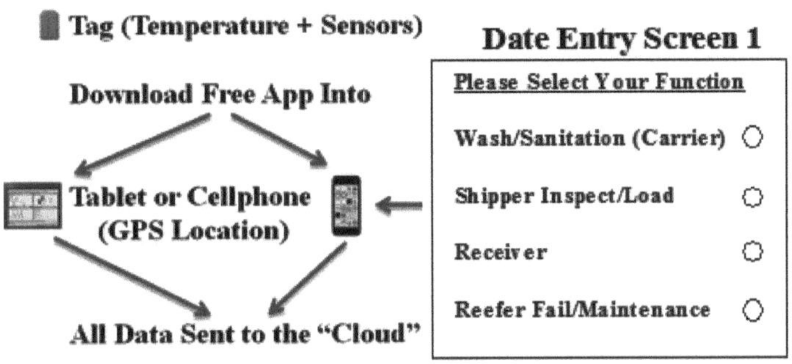

FIGURE 9.40

Meeting FDA requirements at the container carrier level with the CID system.

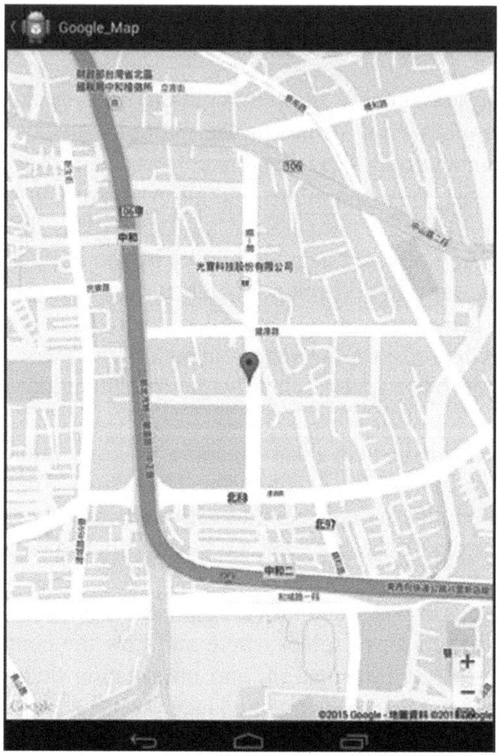

FIGURE 9.41

CID cell phone GPS route map.

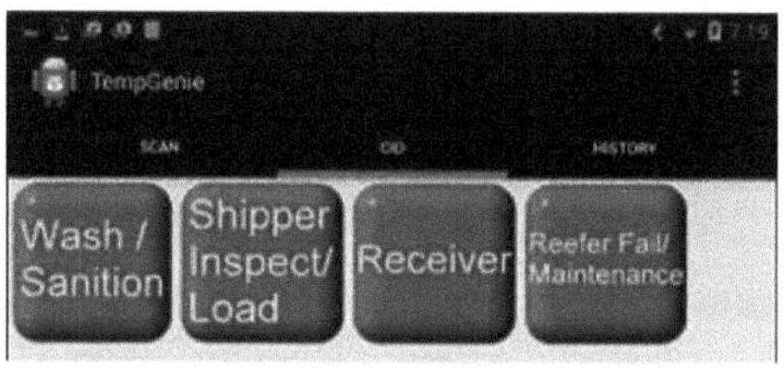

FIGURE 9.42

CID service data upload screen options.

to be uploaded concerning wash requirements, temperatures, wash environmental monitoring test results, and other details.

When the container or trailer are loaded, the Shipper Load Data Entry Screen allows load personnel to click on and upload details concerning what load was loaded and under what conditions. Inspection initials are required to record who

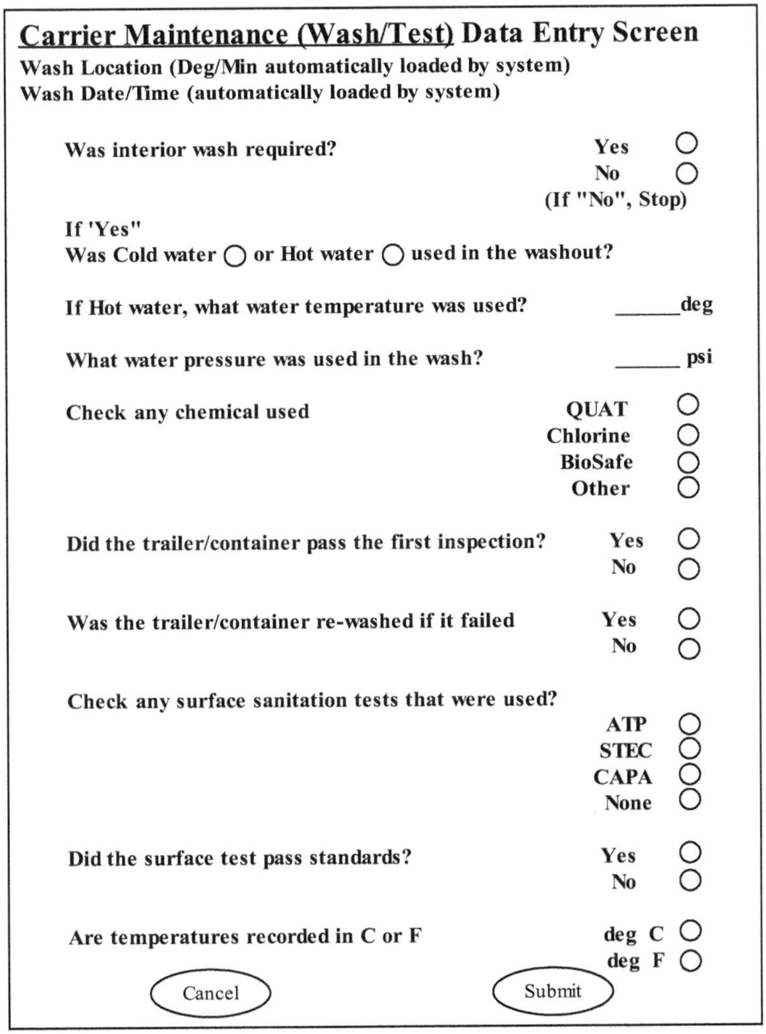

Carrier Maintenance (Wash/Test) Data Entry Screen

Wash Location (Deg/Min automatically loaded by system)
Wash Date/Time (automatically loaded by system)

Was interior wash required? Yes ○ No ○ (If "No", Stop)

If 'Yes"
Was Cold water ○ or Hot water ○ used in the washout?

If Hot water, what water temperature was used? ______deg

What water pressure was used in the wash? ______ psi

Check any chemical used QUAT ○ Chlorine ○ BioSafe ○ Other ○

Did the trailer/container pass the first inspection? Yes ○ No ○

Was the trailer/container re-washed if it failed Yes ○ No ○

Check any surface sanitation tests that were used? ATP ○ STEC ○ CAPA ○ None ○

Did the surface test pass standards? Yes ○ No ○

Are temperatures recorded in C or F deg C ○ deg F ○

Cancel Submit

FIGURE 9.43

CID carrier wash/test documentation record.

was in charge of the load operation. Load date/times and locations are automatically uploaded (Fig. 9.44).

A third screen is available at the unload operation that includes checking temperatures and security systems for the container (Fig. 9.45).

According to the FDA FSMA rules on the sanitary transportation of human and animal foods, any failure to keep transported perishables at specified temperatures or in a sanitary condition should be recorded. Furthermore, such failures should be corrected so as to prevent recurrence. Fig. 9.46 shows the clickable screen used to

Shipper Load Data Entry Screen

A1 Load Location (Deg/Min automatically loaded by system)
A2 Date/Time (automatically loaded by system)

Enter the Initials for your Name X X X

Is this Unit refrigerated? Yes ○ No ○

Did the container pass sanitation inspection? Yes ○ No ○

This food is for human consumption ○
This food is for animal consumption ○

Is the food perishable? Yes ○ No ○

Please check the shipment contents
Produce ○
Seafood ○
Dairy ○
Meat ○
Poultry ○
Fish ○
Frozen ○
Bulk ○
Other ○

Check here if non-Food is included in this shipment ○

Is Special Handling Required? Yes ○ No ○

If yes,
What type of Special Handling? Halal ○ Kosher ○ Other ○

Did you place the security tag/lock on the container? Yes ○ No ○

Are temperatures recorded in deg C ○ deg F ○

What is the pre-load temperature set at? _______deg

What is the upper limit for in-transit temperature? _______deg

What is the lower limit for in-transit temperature? _______deg

Cancel Submit

FIGURE 9.44

CID recording load required data.

record either critical reefer failure codes or to record needed container maintenance. The system records the time/date and location of the failure as well.

The CID system data uploads are stored and analyzed to provide shippers, carriers, and receivers with multiple carrier management capabilities at both the single container (FIT teams at local sites) and fleet (CC teams at corporate). A sample of the

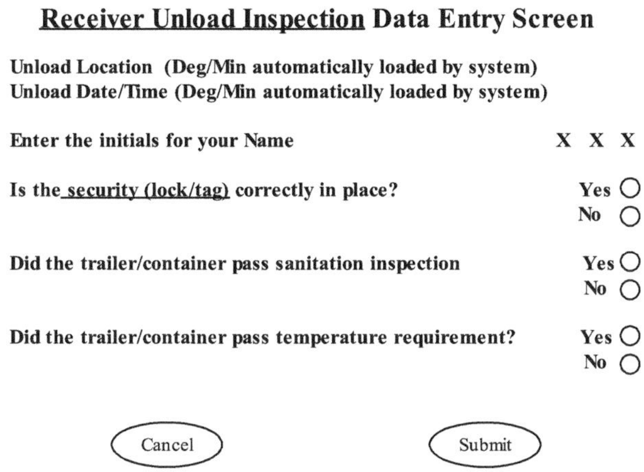

FIGURE 9.45

CID shipment receiver data entry screen.

type of reports is shown in Fig. 9.47. Both food safety and quality control personnel will find the analyses and trends useful to drive preventive action activities.

Record keeping for container and trailer loads covers sanitation and temperature monitoring and controls. Sanitation and temperature controls are critical components for any food transportation operation. Data collection systems need to be established, maintained, and made available to CC and FIT teams for purposes of analysis and their abilities to determine and improve processes that can be considered valid in terms of their abilities to control and eliminate hazards through many types of processes.

PACKAGING

Like the other topics in this chapter, assuring that packaging is food safety and food quality perfect is primarily a problem that comes under the needed planning control of CC teams. Once the packaging supply chain is qualified and certified, procedures are written to keep it clean and people are trained, in general, packaging issues come under the protection of FIT teams as work to continually measure and solve assignable causes.

When you sit down to eat lunch or dinner today, like us, most people will check their plate and utensils for cleanliness. Once food is cleaned, processed, and ready for transport, the packaging that carries the food through the supply chain should be sanitized and should protect the food from adulteration. Clean food should be moved in sanitary packaging. No food industry member should package or transport clean food in uncontrolled dirty packages, trailers, or containers.

Packaging demands a new way of thinking. Packaging is a food contact surface and must comply with packaging & food contact substances (FCSs) laws. In the United States, "The term 'food contact substance' (FCS) is defined in Section 409(h)(6) of the Federal Food, Drug, and Cosmetic Act as 'any substance intended for use

Container/Reefer Maintenance Data Entry Screen

Maintenance Location (Deg/Min automatically loaded by system)
Maintenance Date/Time (automatically loaded by system)

Enter the Initials of the person performing maintenance X X X

Container/Trailer Maintenance/Repair Record

- 1 Door
  - 2 Gaskets
  - 3 Retaining Strips
- 4 Chute
- 5 Seal
- 6 Floor
- 7 Roof
- 8 Wall Panel
- 9 Ducting
- 10 Rails
- 11 Drains
- 12 Cross Members
- 13 Insulation
- 14 Electrical Circuitry
- 15 Lock
- 16 Other

Take Immediate Action Alarm Codes

- 10 HIGH DISCHARGE PRESSURE (OR TEMP)
- 12 SENSOR OR DIGITAL INPUT SHUTDOWN
- 23 COOLING CYCLE FAULT
- 24 HEATING CYCLE FAULT
- 27 VAPOR MOTOR RPM HIGH (CR)
- 32 REFRIGERATION CAPACITY LOW
- 35 CHECK RUN RELAY CIRCUIT
- 36 ELECTRIC MOTOR FAILED TO RUN
- 38 ELECTRIC PHASE REVERSED
- 44 CHECK FUEL SYSTEM
- 47 REMOTE SENSOR SHUTDOWN
- 48 CHECK BELTS OR CLUTCH
- 60 CHECK BOOST CIRCUIT
- 62 AMMETER OUT CALIBRATION
- 63 ENGINE OR VAPOR MOTOR STOPPED
- 66 LOW ENGINE OIL LEVEL
- 75 CONTROLLER RAM FAILURE
- 76 CONTROLLER EPROM FAILURE
- 77 CONTROLLER EPROM CHECKSUM FAILURE
- 78 DATA LOG EPROM FAILURE
- 82 HIGH COMPRESSOR TEMP SHUTDOWN
- 90 ELECTRIC OVERLOAD
- 91 CHECK ELECTRIC READY INPUT
- 93 LOW COMPRESSOR SUCTION PRESSURE
- 97 FAILED REMOTE RETURN AIR SENSOR
- 99 HIGH COMPRESSOR PRESSURE RATIO
- 101 CONTROLLING ON EVAP COIL OUTLET TEMP
- 102 LOW EVAPORATOR COIL TEMPERATURE
- 114 MULTIPLE ALARMS- CAN NOT RUN

Cancel　　Submit

FIGURE 9.46

CID reefer and container maintenance record-keeping component.

Percent of Containers Washed and Tested for Sanitation
Compare to Process Control Procedural Requirements

Analysis of Contamination Trends
Which chemicals are used for different load contents
Comparison of ATP/STEC test results to appropriate chemical use
Which load locations are in compliance/pass unload condition requirements?

Analysis of Temperature Monitoring and Sanitation Trends
Adulterants plus out of control temperature (bacterial growth)= recallable loads

Comparison of Pass Conditions at Load and Pass Conditions at Unload
Load Condition should equal Unload Condition 100%

Comparison of Security Seals set at Load and Security Seals Still Set at Receiving

Number still set at Unload/Receiving = Percent seals received as set
Number set at Load/Shipping

FIGURE 9.47

CID sample of individual container and fleet records and reports.

as a component of materials used in manufacturing, packing, packaging, transporting, or holding food if such use is not intended to have any technical effect in such food.' Examples of FCSs include polymers (plastic packaging materials), pigments and antioxidants used in polymers, can coatings, adhesives, materials used during the manufacture of paper and paperboard, slimicides and biocides (antimicrobial agents), and sealants for lids and caps."

Further "The term "safe," as it refers to food additives and ingredients (including food contact substances), is defined in 21 *CFR* 170.3(i) as a "reasonable certainty in the minds of competent scientists that a substance is not harmful under the intended conditions of use."

In general, "Food packages shall be in a good condition and protect the integrity of the contents so that the food is not exposed to adulteration or potential contaminants from the packaging or from external sources [7]."

Packaging is a product and putting clean food in dirty, poorly designed or poorly manufactured packaging does not promote preventive food safety control. Cleanliness, cleanability, and sanitation controls must be considered for:

- Package design
  - Marketing communications
  - Graphic design
  - Point of sale display
- Security
  - Tamper resistance
  - Tamper evident

  - Package pilferage
  - Retail loss prevention

- Convenience
  - Distribution
  - Handling
  - Stacking
  - Display
  - Sale
  - Opening, reclosing, use, and reuse

- Physical protection
  - Shock
  - Vibration
  - Compression
  - Temperature

- Barrier protection
  - Oxygen, water vapor, dust, etc.
  - Permeation
  - Desiccants and oxygen absorbers
  - Modified atmospheres
  - Controlled atmospheres
  - Clean
  - Fresh
  - Safe for the intended use
  - Shelf life

- Disposal
- Transportation
  - Pallets
  - Containment or agglomeration (cross contamination)
  - Liquids
  - Powers
  - Granular materials
  - Information transmission
  - Labels
  - Recycling
  - Disposal
  - Instructions for use
  - Required by governments
  - Marketing
  - Labels
  - Use by marketers
  - Portion control
  - Bulk
  - Single serving

Some basic examples of food packaging covered by current laws include but are not limited to:

- Beverage—Bottled and aseptic
- Paper
- Bags
- Bakery
- Cans
- Boxes
- Flexible packaging (bagged spinach)
- Wrappers
- Aseptic processing
- Plastic trays

As an example paperboard containers and boxes include:

- Containers, food, sanitary: Except folding
- Cups, paper: Except those made from pressed or molded pulp
- Dishes, paper: Except those made from pressed or molded pulp
- Drinking cups, paper except those made from pressed or molded
- Drinking straws, except glass or plastics
- Food containers, nonfolding paperboard, sanitary
- Food containers, sanitary: Except folding
- Frozen food containers, nonfolding paperboard
- Ice cream containers, nonfolding paperboard
- Milk cartons, paperboard
- Plates, paper: Except those made from pressed or molded pulp
- Soda straws, except glass, or plastics
- Spoons, paper: Except those made from pressed or molded pulp
- Utensils, paper: Except those made from pressed or molded

In the United States, the total domestic demand for nonfolding food containers equaled \$3.5 billion, whereas \$131.0 million of product was imported with exports worth \$313.4 million. That's just nonfolding food containers such as paperboard beverage cartons, round and nested food containers, paper cups for hot or cold drinks, stamped plates, dishes, spoons, and similar products.

Several variables are critical to consider when working on issues and a plan to protect both the packaging and food—Temperatures, humidity, sanitation (and testing for sanitation), process monitoring, verification, and validation of preventive controls and package traceability.

Packaging must be controlled at the supplier, producer, packer, processor, in-transit, at the store, or restaurant. Equipment and tools used to produce packaging must be controlled and be, themselves, appropriately sanitized. Generally, packaging suppliers can create or incorporate hazards to food. CODEX and Current good manufacturing practices (CGMP) preventive controls must be established at packaging suppliers for all foods. Such controls should cover:

Personnel: Head covers, gloves, face masks, smocks, shoe covers, employee health/wash/jewelry/tobacco, handling

Facility: Clean rooms, floors, walls, lighting (no glass), ceilings, water, stainless steel, hepa-filtering (air cleanliness) systems, sanitation

Implies sanitary process controls throughout the packaging supplier, farm, packer, distributor, manufacturing, filling, transportation, loading/unloading, distribution, receiving, and shelf display operations.

QUALIFYING AND CERTIFYING THE PACKAGING SUPPLY CHAIN

If a couple of basic concerns are investigated by the CC planning team, the team can begin by considering whether or not the packaging supplier is food safety certified and has validated their food safety plans and operates under a Hazard Analysis Critical Control Point (HACCP), Hazard Analysis and Risk-Based Preventive Controls (HARPC), or other preventive controls system. One could begin by assessing their own and their supplier's employee training and procedures such as:

- Employee health requirements
- Personal cleanliness and hygienic practices
- Hand washing and hand washing facilities
- Clothing
- Jewelry
- Handling
- Hand sanitizing
- Tasting, eating, and drinking
- Clean fingernails
- Restrictions on tobacco use

Fig. 9.48 is a shot of an onion packaging line at a food distribution operation. Notice the aprons, gloves, stainless steel line surfaces (stabilizable and testable), and head covers.

Meanwhile, at an apple packing plant (Fig. 9.49), the apples are packed in plastic bags on a conveyor system prior to being placed in shipping cases and loaded onto pallets. The shipping case storage and pallets show no protection from environmental contaminants, no gloves or aprons in spite of food safety requirements.

The CC team should review all internal and packaging supplier packaging operations, packaging materials, and personnel with regards to how closely the packaging operations comply with basic preventive control concepts.

LABELING

In general, labeling is considered a critical aspect of the packaging operation. The FDA guidance for industry: A food labeling guide, general food labeling requirements lists the following basic requirements:

- General
  - Name of food
  - Juices

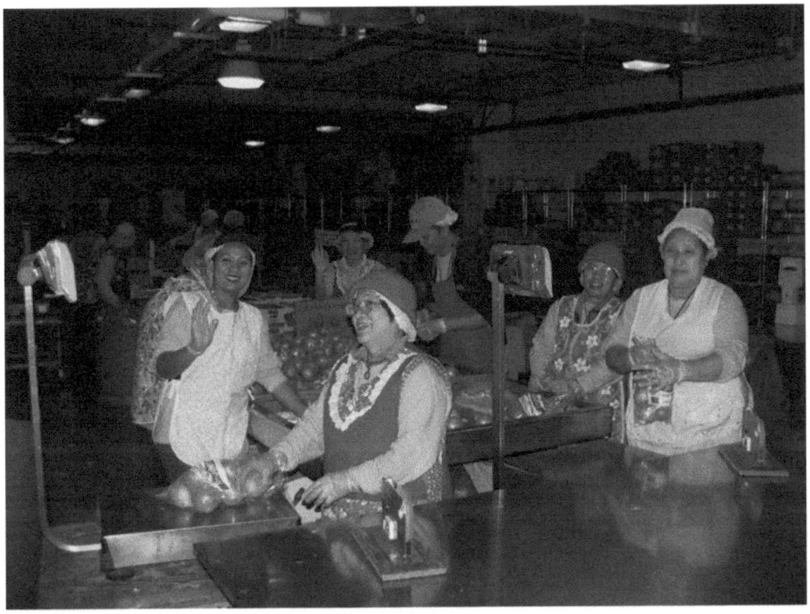

FIGURE 9.48

Onion packing line.

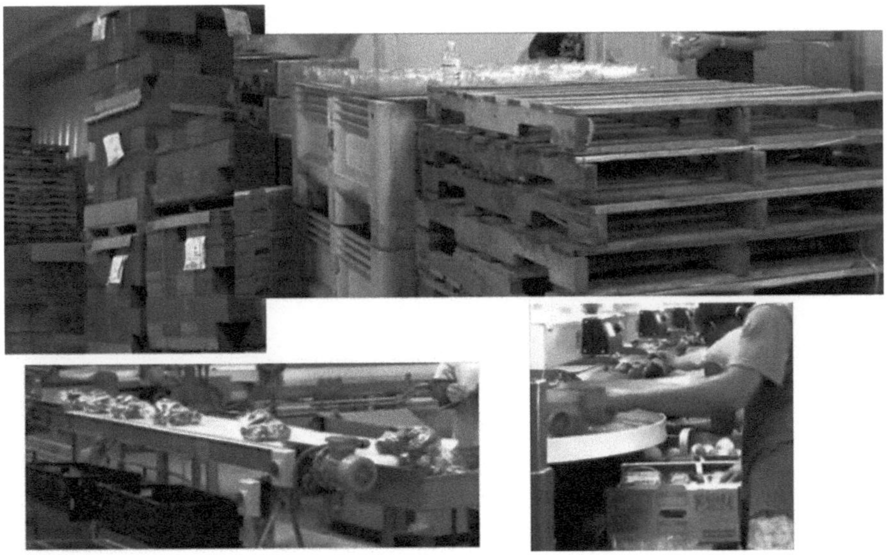

FIGURE 9.49

Apple packaging operations.

  - Net quantity of contents statements
  - Ingredient lists
  - Nutrition labeling
  - Colors
  - Food allergen labeling
  - Nutrient declaration
  - Products with separately packaged ingredients
- Label formats/graphics
  - General
  - Specific label formats
  - Trans fat labeling
  - Miscellaneous
  - Serving size
  - Exemptions/special labeling provisions
- Claims
  - Nutrient content claims
  - Health claims
  - Qualified health claims
  - Structure/function claims [8]

EXPERT COMPOSITIONAL REVIEWS

As most companies that purchase packaging do not have the internal expertise to perform the many tests that should be applied to packaging, it is suggested by the American Society for Testing and Materials (ASTM) that an expert compositional review should be conducted [9].

On the ASTM website, they recommend "Evaluation and testing of the physical, mechanical, and chemical properties of various pulp, paper, and paperboard materials that are processed primarily to make containers, shipping boxes and parcels, and other packaging and labeling products.

These standards help to identify characteristics such as

- chemical content
- acidity or alkalinity
- tensile breaking strength
- peel adhesion
- water, oil, and tear resistance among others

Also, these paper and packaging standards help papermaking plants, packaging and shipping companies, and other producers and end-users of paper materials and products in the proper processing and assessment procedures to ensure their quality towards efficient commercial use."

For a quick review, CFR—Code of Federal Regulations, Title 21 addresses adhesives, and laminate structures and recommends analysis of each for use in packaging dry snacks, aqueous and fatty foods, microwaveable products, fresh frozen, frozen, dry foods, nonfoam fresh cut produce, hot-filled condiments, jams, jellies, sauces, boil-in bag products, foods containing oil or fatty components, and the temperature ranges under which each can or should not be used [10].

PACKAGING EQUIPMENT

As preventive controls apply to suppliers, packaging suppliers must be qualified and certified by companies purchasing packaging from them. There are quite a number of issues for the purchasing company to review when qualifying suppliers of packaging and packaging equipment used by packaging suppliers. Some of these types of equipment are listed for review:

- Auto-coders (label and date verification)
- Vacuum packaging
- Capping, over-capping, lidding, closing, seaming, and sealing
- Carton makers
- Case and tray forming, packing, unpacking, closing and sealing check weight
- Cleaning, sterilizing, cooling, and drying
- Conveying, accumulating, and related
- Feeding, orienting, placing, and related
- Filling machines: Handling liquid and powdered products
- Package filling and closing
- Form, fill, and seal
- Inspect, detect, and heck weight
- Labeling
- Palletizing/de-palletizing
- Product identification: Labeling, marking, etc.
- Tracking
- Wrapping machines
- Converting machines
- Others

In addition to assure that the supplier's equipment is appropriate, sanitize able and operating in a clean environment, and to successfully provide an initial assessment of potential, the product's end user's needs, design, manufacturing conditions, and filling requirements must be considered.

Preventive controls would require that the packaging supplier undergo a complete CGMP assessment, and it is recommended that operational areas and equipment used in the production environment should be color coded to prevent cross-contamination throughout the process. A typical packaging operation and facility are shown in Fig. 9.50

The food packaging operation itself, from incoming through any required package wash, into storage, movement into the packaging operation and into labeling must all be controlled to prevent cross contamination.

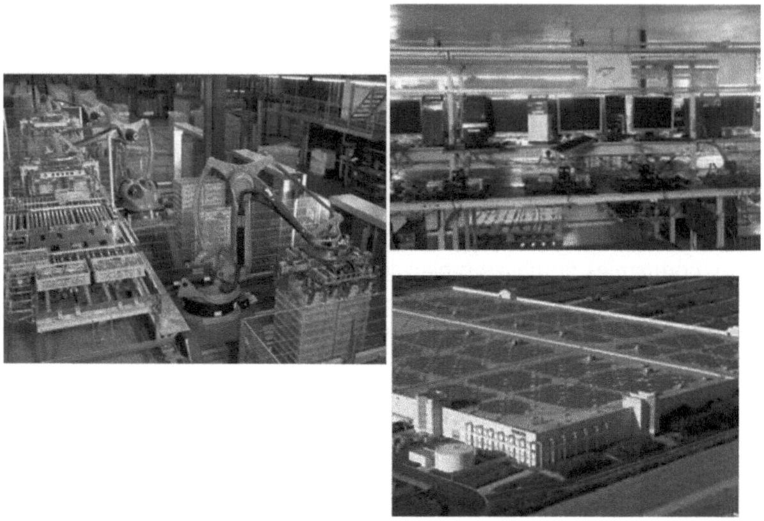

FIGURE 9.50

Automated packaging manufacturing lines.

A simple example of a U.S. state-level set of regulations comes from the Illinois Sanitary Food Preparation Act where packaging is clearly identified as basic to any food safety regulations.

> *Sec. 1. That every building, room, basement, enclosure or premises, occupied, used or maintained as a bakery, confectionery, cannery, packing house, slaughter house, creamery, cheese factory, restaurant, hotel, grocery, meat market, or as a factory, shop, warehouse, any public or place or manufacturing establishment used for the preparation, manufacture, packing, storage, sale or distribution of any food as defined by statute, which is intended for sale, shall be properly and adequately lighted, drained, plumbed and ventilated, and shall be conducted with strict regard to the influence of such conditions upon the health of the operatives, employees, clerks, or other persons therein employed, and the purity and wholesomeness of the food therein produced, prepared, manufactured, packed, stored, sold or distributed [11].*

In some cases, however, laws can be highly questionable as in the case of using a carbon monoxide treatment during store-level packaging operations (Fig. 9.51). Carbon monoxide is used in store-level packaging to preserve the color of meats and other products, whereas carbon monoxide treatment is generally regarded as safe (GRAS) by the FDA, food safety experts question the fact that such equipment and the process were tested by the equipment manufacturers prior to being certified as GRAS. Questions of the interactions between the Styrofoam cases, the wrapping and the meat remain as do questions regarding which comes first:

Food Appearance?
Or
Food Safety?

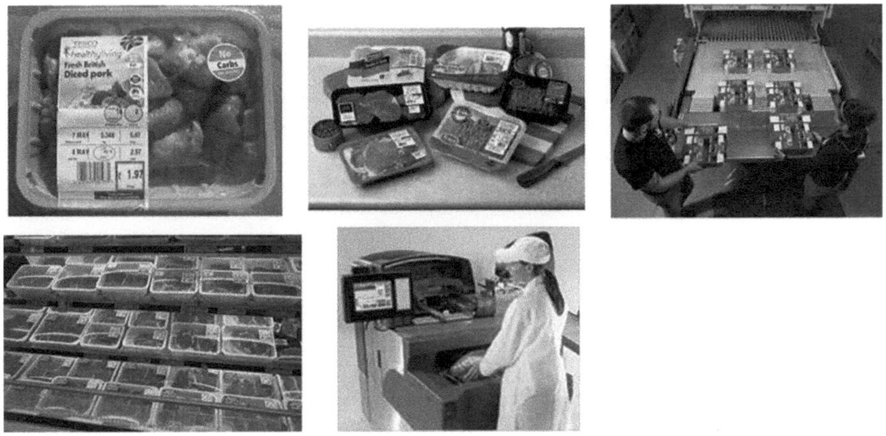

FIGURE 9.51

Packaging using carbon monoxide.

Regardless of where it comes from or how it ends up, food packaging is a critical issue when it comes to food safety and quality. All food supply companies either employ or handle food packaging in some way. As food packaging represents a contact surface, any company's ability to apply preventive control requirements needs to be addressed, documented, and defended in light of preventive control rules.

FOOD FRAUD

In Europe, probably the most notorious example of food fraud came when horsemeat was fraudulently shipped into unsuspecting food supply chains under beef labels. Ikea meatballs, Burger King hamburger patties, cottage pies, and frozen lasagna were a few of the products impacted by the 2013 European horsemeat scandal. In the United Kingdom (UK) where horses are viewed as pets, people were somewhat horrified to find that they had been fooled into thinking that horsemeat was ground beef. In some countries, horsemeat is a normal product. It has the same amount of protein as beef, less fat, and poses no threat to human health (Fig. 9.52).

What's the problem with selling horsemeat labeled as beef? Horsemeat doesn't pose any real public health threat. Horse reportedly has the same amount of protein as beef and less fat, horsemeat is cheaper than beef, and in some countries, horsemeat is a totally acceptable thing to eat (not everyone thinks of them as pets).

While selling horsemeat identified as beef might seem to be blatant example, the perpetrators apparently penetrated many supply chains and impacted many companies and consumers.

Food safety and quality systems designed to prevent food fraud should under go validation planning and implementation regardless of industry or governmental requirements.

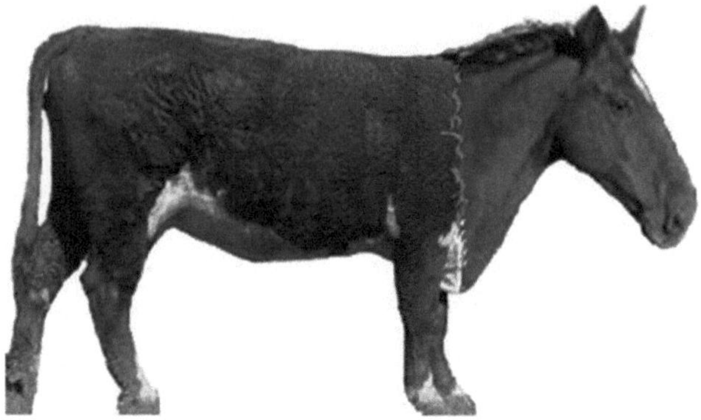

FIGURE 9.52

A new species?

In 2008, most people will remember the melamine dilution of dairy products that came out of China, which caused 290,000 infant illnesses, 860 hospitalizations and at least 6 deaths and cost the industry an estimated $3 billion when it was discovered. For those children, the impact may last throughout their entire lives. In the melamine case, the demand for milk far outstripped the supply, watering down the milk was a way to increase the product, reduce costs and profits, and tests were fooled because melamine with its high nitrogen content was added to the watered down milk to artificially inflate the protein content. The side effect caused kidney stones and fatalities.

In one case, the guardian (European Union (E.U.)) reported that "Fake-food scandal revealed as tests show third of products mislabeled". The article highlighted cheese substitution with noncheese products, meat emulsion (pink slime), adding water to frozen prawns to increase weights, adulteration of ground beef with substituted pork or poultry, putting glucose powder in withdrawn prescription drugs at higher than the normal dose, additives in fruit juices, ham made from poultry meat, brining processes to add pink colors, excessive salt in sausages, water in seafood to increase weights, and counterfeit vodka. More importantly, many of the samples came from fast-food restaurants, stores, restaurants, and wholesalers.

Is anything to be trusted [12]?

There are many ways to commit food fraud and get away with it. Most of these are just not labeled as food fraud either because there is a lack of legal definition for food fraud or because most people are focused on intentional substitution. Consider these few examples:

- Adding ice and water to products to increase weight and volume
- Adding extra salt
- Blended coffees
- Flame retardants in juices

- Meat emulsion or "pink slime" (no label identification)
- False vitamin claims
- Drugs in food
- False and misleading labels

Food fraud impacts just about all foods in the supply chain. Just a few examples that have been highlighted in the news include:

- Melamine
- Fish
- Horsemeat
- Olive oil
- Coffee
- Milk
- Juices
- Honey
- GMO products
- Alcoholic beverages
- Cheese

For example, consider the following open-door opportunities food suppliers have to commit food fraud or to walk on the thin line between current definitions of food fraud that rely on concepts associated with intentional substitution:

- Label "Sell by," "Best Used by," Expiration," and "Use by" dates
- No label identification for the use of modified atmosphere packaging (MAP)
- Weight fraud
- Organic, natural, and "Locally Grown" misidentification
- Bottled water from the tap sold as "Spring" or other nice sounding sources
- Vitamins and herbal supplements
- Theft and resale (see section: Food Cargo Theft)
- Transshipment fraud
- Knowingly packing in a dirty environment using dirty packaging

In many countries, there is no legal definition of food fraud. More importantly, food fraud is most often defined as the intentional substitution of one ingredient for another. But, that's the tip of the iceberg. There are hundreds of incidents where laws cover different aspects of food fraud but companies simply choose not to obey those laws.

It is not known how widespread food fraud is in the United States or worldwide. It is also assumed that those who commit food fraud want to avoid detection. If you review the sample lists above and consider that just about any food can include salt or water in unknown quantities, be transshipped, have a false label that includes a false expiration date, include Genetically Modified Organisms (GMO) food sources (no identification of GMO is required in the United States), could include extra salt to make it taste better, includes illegal or unidentified drugs, packed in a dirty environment, and has substituted ingredients, you can begin to get an idea of how complex the problem really is and how inadequate any definition that focuses on intentional substitution really is.

Meanwhile, in the United States, the FDA FSMA rule for Focused Mitigation Strategies to Protect Food against Intentional Adulteration is just that: Focused on intentional adulteration. That rule would require the largest food businesses to have a written food defense plan that addresses significant vulnerabilities in a food operation. Although not included in the United States preventive control rules, a "food defense plan" clearly refers to prevention and the requirement for U.S. companies to implement preventive controls. The rule focuses on manufacturing, processing, packing, and holding and requires that companies:

1. Prepare and implement a written food defense plan
2. Identify and implement focused mitigation strategies at each actionable process step to prevent adulteration at each step
3. Establish procedures
4. Corrective action plan
5. Verify that monitoring is being conducted
6. Train personnel
7. Keep records

Cable news network (CNN) U.S. reported "Unprecedented verdict: Peanut executive guilty in deadly salmonella outbreak" on September 19, 2014. Participants in the fraud (economically motivated adulteration) were charged and found guilty on multiple counts. The owner, his brother, and the quality control manager were convicted, fined, and sentenced to prison for knowingly shipping salmonella-contaminated peanut products that ended up in many food processing plants and hundreds of products. The plant manager was told that samples of the product contained *Salmonella*, and the owner replied "Just ship it," resulting in some 714 illnesses and 9 deaths [13].

Interestingly, the question of whether or not food fraud is a food safety issue remains debated. The FDA definition is as follows:

> *"Fraudulent, intentional substitution or addition of a substance in a product for the purpose of increasing the apparent value of the product or reducing the cost of its production, i.e., for economic gain." However, in the U.S., no single federal agency and no single U.S. law or statute directly addresses food fraud or economically motivated adulteration of food and food ingredients [14,15].*

Current good manufacturing practices (CGMP) require that manufacturers are responsible to determine that representations or claims about their product are substantiated and nor misleading or false. Further, final rules require that food and ingredients must be consistently manufactured to assure purity, composition, strength, and identity.

CGMP requirements include design and construction of the physical plant, establishing quality control procedures, testing manufactured product and supplements, maintaining records, handling complaints, training of processing and supervisory personnel, segregation of food allergens during storage and handling, validated cleaning procedures for food contact equipment, prevention of cross-contact during processing, product label reviews, label storage and control and a stringent supplier control program for ingredients and labels. Further, the rules require a written environmental pathogen control plan and written sanitation procedures.

In the meantime, the grocery manufacturers association (GMA) published the 2010 "Consumer Product Fraud: Deterrence and Detection" and estimated that fraud could be costing the international food industry between $10 billion and $15 billion annually and affected nearly 10% of all commercial foods. They further estimate annual lost sales between 2% and 15% [16].

The GMA reported that the organization was concerned over increasing product recalls, contamination incidents, the significance of economic and health consequences, media coverage, growing consumer advocacy, and government scrutiny.

The GMA recommends a number of preventive control strategies:

- Establish an intelligence sharing clearinghouse
- Improve shared audit programs
- Create basic ingredient standards
- Develop shared library of ingredient reference samples
- Partner with academia to forecast risk
- Improve product safety and quality
- Implement traceability
- Audit suppliers
- Establish deterrence strategies
- Deploy a holistic program throughout the organization (TQCM)
- Establish partnerships with federal and state governments
- Establish an integrated food safety system (IFSS)
- Establish IFSS from the business side
- Integrate federal, state, and local government IFSS data into business IFSS
- Invest in new low cost/high turnaround test technologies

The E.U. provides a definition of food fraud: "Food fraud is a collective term used to encompass the deliberate and intentional substitution, addition, tampering, or misrepresentation of food, food ingredients, or food packaging; or false or misleading statements made about a product for economic gain".

Within E.U. rules food traceability, labeling and food fraud prevention are required. The food fraud prevention scenario from the E.U. includes:

- RASFF (rapid alert system for food and feed)
- Testing program
- Horse passport (verification of horse slaughter)
- Origin labeling
- Official controls, implementation, and penalties [17]

Although it is very difficult to test every ingredient for potential food fraud, in an article published by Food Online, the United Kingdom "government promises proactive solutions in food laboratories, along with improved supply-chain audits, to curb the uprising trend of food fraud [18]."

To illustrate how far companies will go to commit food fraud and how complex their efforts can become, Bloomberg Business week reported in an article entitled "The Honey Trap" how a German company was buying honey in China, shipping it in 50-gal drums to India, Malaysia, Indonesia, South Korea, Russia, Mongolia, Thailand, Taiwan, and the Philippines to avoid US tariffs on honey imported from China. The article reported that the scam was worth around $80 million and was the largest scam in the history of the United States.

Although honey can be tested for pollen content and the type of pollen in the honey traced back to regional origins, farms in the United States were part of the scam and participants were prosecuted as part of an undercover operation [19].

In the meantime, Walmart sponsored a food fraud prevention online course for people in China. In June 2014, Walmart Facts and News reported, "Walmart has agreed to sponsor the translation of a Food Fraud Prevention online course to the Mandarin language. The course was developed by Dr. John Spink, Professor at Michigan State University (MSU) and Director of the University's Food Fraud Initiative. Dr. Spink, a recognized expert in this area joined Walmart in their efforts to help customers, regulators, suppliers, and retailers increase public awareness of food fraud prevention in China and prevent food fraud through the joint efforts in the market."

Further, Frank Yiannas, Vice President of Food Safety for Walmart, said, "At Walmart, we take the issue of food fraud very seriously. Because prevention of food fraud is a shared responsibility and education is a key to deterrence, Walmart is delighted to be able to help Michigan State University make the course more broadly available to regulatory officials, industry professionals, consumers and other stakeholders in China."

While food fraud remains relatively unencumbered by a lack of legal definition and leadership in most countries as well as inadequate detection and enforcement capabilities, Science Time reported, "Chinese consumers are outraged after Walmarts sell donkey meat that is adulterated with cheap fox. But China is hardly the only country grappling with fraudulent meat."

DNA testing of product that was supposed to be donkey meat intended for snacking contained other sources of meat including fox, mink, and rat meat [20].

DETECTION TESTING TECHNOLOGIES

Although the world tends to focus on the ingredient substitution issue, one must remember that testing for any potential substitute in all types of food is complex, expensive, and impossible. Today's detection technology world contains at least the following capabilities:

- high-performance liquid chromatography;
- standards for infrared spectroscopy;
- gas chromatography;
- isotope ratio mass spectrometry (horse/pork);

- hyphenated mass spectrometry methods;
- near infrared spectroscopy;
- polymerase chain reaction (PCR);
- capillary electrophoresis;
- enzyme-linked immuno-sorbent assay;
- thin-layer chromatography;
- site-specific natural isotope fractionation;
- mid-infrared spectroscopy;
- Raman spectroscopy;
- nuclear magnetic resonance spectroscopy;
- high-performance anion exchange chromatography;
- resonance spectroscopy;
- high-performance anion exchange chromatography; and
- differential scanning calorimetry.

The problem is that most companies, even if they knew what to test for, probably do not have the ability or money to either establish their own lab or to pay for such expensive analyses thereby leaving even substitute testing undone.

Take a simple example: A pizza. How many small pizza vendors are there in the United States, many of whom are independent of the control required by large corporate entities. How many ingredients go into a pizza sauce, toppings and dough? Maybe dozens that could require some type of testing if their vendors did not fulfill testing requirements for every known substitute in every ingredient.

The choice of analytical test development and methods are primarily determined by preexisting knowledge of the potential adulterant. That means that until an illegal substitute causes a problem, no one tests for the substituted ingredient. Further, perhaps there is no known test for the substitute. There is simply no way of knowing who could put what into what to save money or change the appearance of a product. In short, the food industry is constantly lagging in detection test technology. Testing for ingredient substitutes is not a preventive strategy. It is a reaction to a cause.

For insight into other potential problems related to testing for substitute ingredients and for food fraud in general, here are a few more common product types to consider:

Vitamins and Herbal supplements
Bottled water
Organic produce

RECOMMENDED PREVENTIVE VALIDATION STRATEGIES

1. Establish chain of custody as a standardized food supply chain traceability requirement. Make sure incoming products can be traced back to original sources using competent case, pallet, and container-level traceability strategies and systems. Chain of custody means that the formalization of the traceability system is a legally required system requirement.

2. Take responsibility for potential food fraud in the company product line. Identify fraud as a potential hazard and establish a control plan.
3. Get some training for food safety and quality personnel, establish goals and objectives related to food fraud, establish CC teams to handle the overall planning and management and FIT teams to monitor, measure, analyze, look for causes, and take action on findings.
4. Establish preventive purchasing practices that will identify, qualify, certify, and buy only from suppliers capable of certification under supplier preventive control rules.
5. Know your supply chain. Vicarious liability practices under new preventive control rules mean you are partially responsible for purchasing fraudulent ingredients because you approved them as suppliers.
6. Establish a system of distributed authority. Make it clear to all employees that food fraud is a potential food safety and quality threat, and they have the authority and responsibility to help with potential problems. Invest in preventive approaches by establishing a system of continuous improvement. Dump the "If it ain't broke, don't fix it!" attitude and recognize food fraud for what it is. Companies are either in support of food fraud or against it as demonstrated by their determination to establish fraud prevention systems.
7. Hire honest people. Fraud is not only the intentional or unintentional substitution of one ingredient for another. Many common business practices that can be attacked by CC teams are indeed intentional if the participants know that the functioning system is in some way supporting the fraudulent delivery of products to consumers.
8. Proactively cooperate with the competition. Help each other to identify and attack potential food fraud as a means of saving the supply chain from recall disasters.
9. Help prosecute and publicize those found guilty of providing the supply chain with fraudulently grown, manufactured, packed, transported, or otherwise injecting fraudulent foods into the supply chain [21].
10. Validate the preventive food fraud plan.

There are quite a number of resources available to help identify potential food fraud issues. Here are a few to investigate:

- Rapid alert system for food and feed (RASFF) [22]
- New Adulterant Screen software [23]
- International experts
  - Dr. Chris Elliot, director of the Institute for global Food Security at Queen's University Belfast, Northern Ireland
  - Liz Moran is the president of the Association of Public Analysts in the UK
  - Dr. John Spink (Michigan State University (MSU), Food Fraud Initiative)
  - Dr. Douglas C. Moyer is an associate Professor and public health instructor for the University of Michigan
- Better Seafood Board (BSB) [24]
- Barfblog lists examples of food fraud practices [25]

The US Pharmacopeial Food Fraud Database [26]

- Food Fraudster [27]
- UK Food Standards Agency "Reporting Food Fraud" [28]
- European Commission Official Controls and Enforcement [29]
- National Center for Food Protection and Defense: Food Fraud Resources [30]
- RASFF [31]

FOOD FRAUD CONFUSION REIGNS

Food fraud and the potential for food fraud come from many more directions than mere substitution of one product or ingredient for another. And food fraud is practiced at many levels from the restaurant waitress telling customers that tilapia is cod to the blatant replacement of beef with horse meat and the use of contaminated packing materials to save money. Though food fraud has been around since time began and is costing billions of dollars each year on a world-wide basis, the drive to bring things under some semblance of control is in its infancy.

The entire supply chain is called to task to begin to work on assessments and plans focused on risk reduction and preventive planning and to work collectively to establish a chain of custody system.

FOOD CARGO THEFT

Companies that do not prepare and implement preventive theft control plans leave food safety and quality at the options of thieves, fences, and buyers needing to keep costs low. The food supply chain is a food security and food safety issue. It represents a relatively easy and vulnerable target that is tied to the complexity of food systems. Cargo is involved with smuggling and provides a potential for terrorism.

Food cargo theft is a critical aspect of food safety and quality and needs to come under the preventive control umbrella requiring CC team planning and FIT team oversight.

Overall, an estimated $30 billion in cargo is stolen annually.

- In California, violent gangs such as Ms-13—El Salvador
- In Canada, the Chinese Triad crime organization
- Mexico warring drug cartels
- United States organized cargo theft rings is being funneled back to terrorist organizations such as Al Qaeda and Hezbollah
- Trucks and trailers are unattended
- Warehouses used to temporarily store the freight are burglarized
- Hijackers hook up their recently acquired stolen tractor to the loaded trailer and drive away
- Fences (people who knowingly buy stolen property to resell) dispose of stolen goods [32]

Here are some details:

- Food and drink loads remained the hottest targets.
- Average loss per incident = $600,000.
- Products with the same batch numbers must be recalled and destroyed.
- Recovery, replacement, increases in insurance premiums, reputation loss.
- Thefts by deceptive pickup—Thieves fraudulently posing as drivers to receive loads from shippers—Accounted for 14 thefts in the quarter.
- Incidents involving theft of trailer/container accounted for the vast majority of thefts.
- Seventy-one, 31%, of the thefts tend to occur in California. Florida had 30 thefts reported, and Illinois and Texas each had 28. Georgia saw 15, and New Jersey had 9.
- Unsecured parking once again topped the list of locations where theft was most likely to occur, accounting for 113 reported incidents, primarily at truck stops.
- Thefts of trailers and containers accounted for 75% of all reported incidents.
- Hottest days for theft: Friday and Saturday.
- On holidays, there is increased activity on roads and decreased activity around warehouses when shipments are more likely to be left alone for long periods of time [33].

What foods tend to be stolen?

- Beer and wine
- Eggs
- Chocolate
- Walnuts
- Kentucky bourbon
- Hamburger patties
- Soup
- Nutella
- Cheese
- Chicken wings
- Maple syrup
- Frito-Lay
- Kellogg's products
- Crisco
- Green giant canned corn
- Frozen foods
- The product your company ships

CargoNet reports a food and beverage breakdown by subtype.

1. Non-alcoholic beverages
2. Meat products
3. Alcoholic beverages

4. Produce
5. Seafood products
6. Candy and gum
7. Baking and cooking ingredients
8. Condiments and spices
9. Snack product
10. Frozen foods
11. Dairy product
12. Beans and seeds
13. Animal food
14. Baby products
15. Bakery products

Some companies refuse to report stolen food cargos because recalls can impact all products of the same type, the recovered product is likely to be unusable, the victim company will suffer a loss of reputation and a negative public perception. Furthermore, competitors are quick to take advantage of the slack control stolen goods represent, and the cost of insurance policies will surely go up.

The federal and state governments have established inconsistent laws regarding food cargo theft. Many victim companies lose direct and related sales and are unable to receive replacement shipments. Raised trucking rates and food prices are passed on to consumers.

Some things contribute to food cargo theft that may or may not be under the control of victim companies. These include:

- Poor reporting
- Mandatory reporting
- Specific cargo theft statutes
- Weak prosecution and aggressive district attorneys
- Bail strategies for criminals
- As well as fiscal and personal constraints on the part of the victim [34]

CargoNet reports the following theft locations in order of highest-to-lowest for the period June 1, 2012 through June 1, 2014:

1. Warehouse/Distribution center
2. Unreported location
3. Parking lot
4. Truck stop
5. Secured yard
6. Unsecured yard
7. Carrier/terminal lot
8. Side of road
9. Other
10. On route (hijacking)

CargoNet also reports theft by state ranked high-to-low below:

1. California
2. Florida
3. Texas
4. Illinois
5. Georgia
6. New Jersey
7. Michigan
8. Pennsylvania
9. Indiana
10. North Carolina [35]

VALIDATING PREVENTIVE FOOD THEFT SYSTEM COMPONENTS

Preventive control provides companies the potential to halt thefts through improved hiring practices (background checks), training, and technology requiring some up-front investment.

A basic preventive strategy includes some key approaches and CC team upgrades to theft control practices including:

- Risk assessment—Where, when, how are you exposed?
- GAP analysis—Where is your preventive system today?
- Training—Upgrade your personnel
- Audits & certification—Internal or external to determine system status

The following proven approaches need to be considered:

- Technology—Trackers, geo-fences, alarms, immobilization
- Locks, air brake valve locks, glad hand locks (locking the trailer's airline), seals to alert intrusion
- Staying alert
- Be on information distribution channels
- Response planning
- Knowledge of the supply chain
- Basic safety practices
- Screen employees (inside theft)—Background checks
- Site controls—Cameras, gates, guards, know the driver
- Training employees

Test Your System, set improvement goals and track improvements.

Document all improvement cycles using the solution tracking sheet (STS) A food theft preventive approach links security management to many other aspects of the business management, can serve to reinforce food security management, and can be measured and improved. In some cases, surveillance (cameras, etc.), reward money, and GPS locaters as well as watching for tips from law enforcement, insurance companies, and concerned citizens are important.

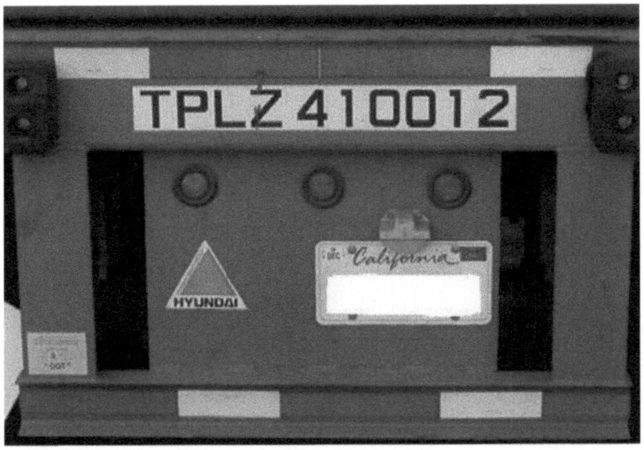

FIGURE 9.53

Owner applied number and unusual markings.

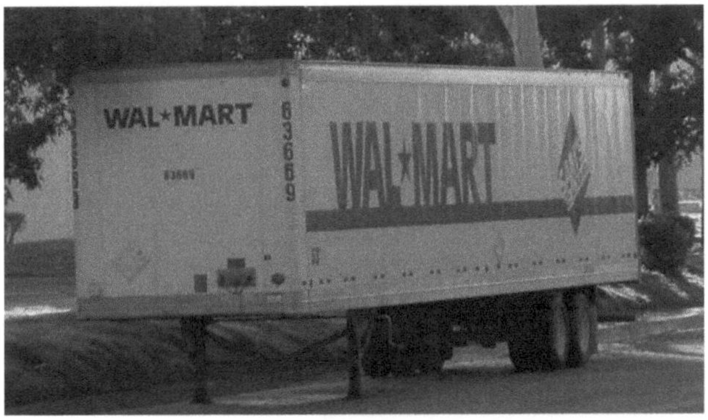

FIGURE 9.54

Unattended trailer.

If theft does occur, it is important to be able to report as many specifics about the theft as possible, immediately report theft to local State police or the sheriff's department. Tractors and trailers should have owner applied (or international) numbers for the tractor (Fig. 9.53), trailer and containers. Carriers should think about unusual markings such as roof numbers for easy identification from the air. Reporting requires a grand theft report along with the bill of lading and a statement from the driver and reporting party.

Fig. 9.54 shows an easy target.

Theft of trailers is accomplished by what is known as bob-tailing. The thief rives a tractor without a trailer attached, hooks up to the unattended trailer by coupling the tractor truck to the trailer and driving off. The tractor is often also stolen. Once stolen, the trailer, tractor, and goods are sold to a fence.

In some cases, cargo is unloaded or the ignition removed to take the trailer contents or the tractor (Fig. 9.55).

Other strategies include breaking the tractor window or disconnecting the satellite navigation system (Fig. 9.56).

Easy targets include outside storage of product and open doors (Fig. 9.57).

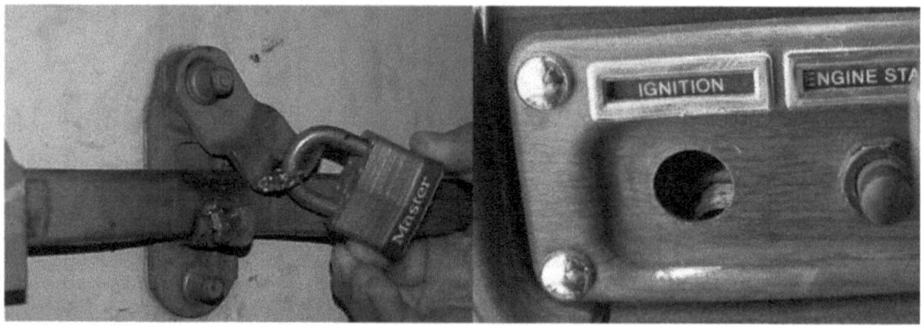

FIGURE 9.55

Welding cut used to open trailer and removed ignition.

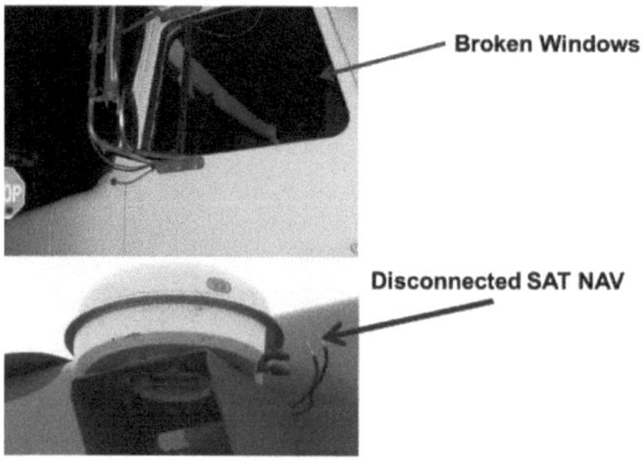

FIGURE 9.56

Broken window and disconnected SAT NAV system.

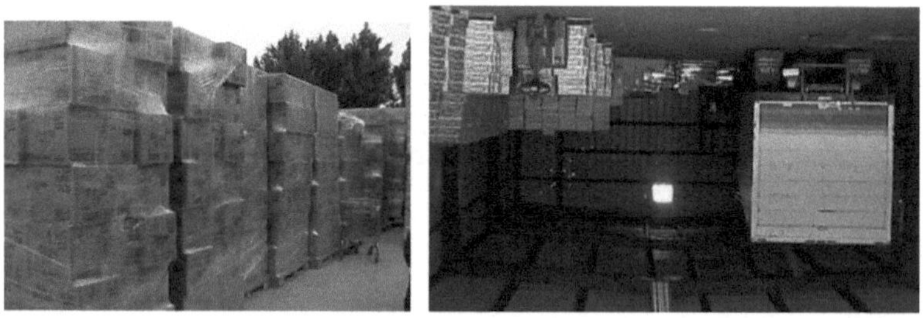

FIGURE 9.57

Easy targets.

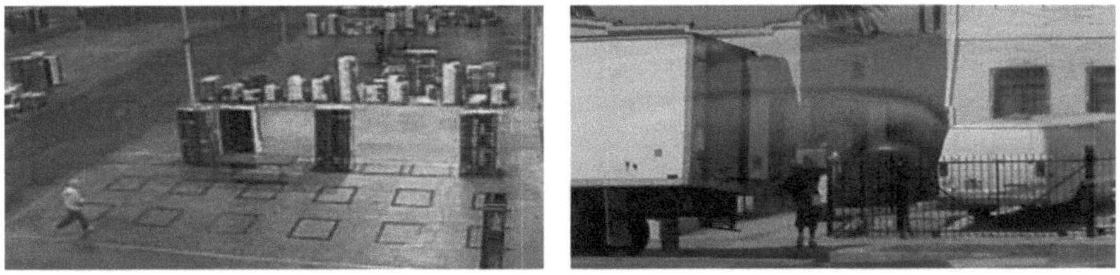

FIGURE 9.58

Distribution center theft.

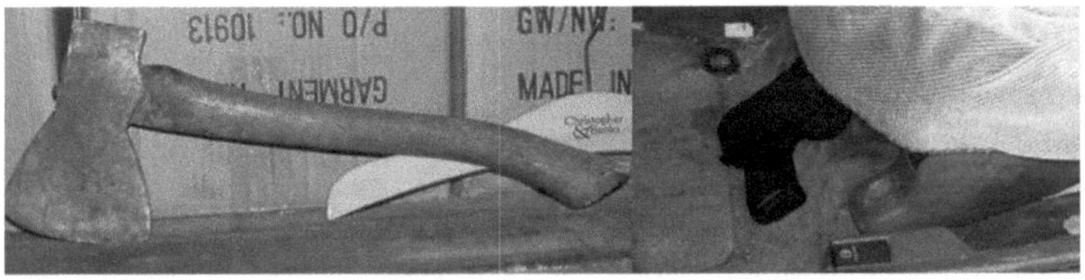

FIGURE 9.59

Cargo theft weaponry.

Cameras can prevent distribution center theft (Fig. 9.58).

Some warnings from anti-theft professionals are important for cargo theft witnesses.

Cargo theft is often a violent crime with violent criminals so witness safety should be a primary concern. Hardened criminals will not let your live impede their freedom (Fig. 9.59).

THE U.S. FBI ON CARGO THEFT

The FBI defines cargo theft as "The criminal taking of any cargo including, but not limited to, goods, chattels, money, or baggage that constitutes, in whole or in part, a commercial shipment of freight moving in commerce, from any pipeline system, railroad car, motor truck, or other vehicle, or from any tank or storage facility, station house, platform, or depot, or from any vessel or wharf, or from any aircraft, air terminal, airport, aircraft terminal or air navigation facility, or from any intermodal container, intermodal chassis, trailer, container freight station, warehouse, freight distribution facility, or freight consolidation facility.

For purposes of this definition, cargo shall be deemed as moving in commerce at all points between the point of origin and the final destination, regardless of any temporary stop while awaiting transshipment or otherwise."

They provide a Cargo Theft User Manual (2013)—Uniform Crime Reporting Program that is free to download and use [36].

The FDA also has some prevention and response that are basically in line with preventive control rules. They state “When a theft occurs, FDA is committed to work with the affected firm to minimize the public health risks and ensure an appropriate public health response.

The agency has developed streamlined procedures to rapidly respond to reports of theft and ensure consistency as we work with firms that have experienced a cargo or warehouse theft [37].”

In that document, they state that information about stolen products, a risk assessment and an action plan are recommended. They also push for taking preventive measures, planning, and establishing an appropriate public health response covering recalls for related product in the supply chain. They require details for stolen food products including:

- Finished product (prescription, over the counter (OTC), infant formula), samples, bulk product, API, etc.)
- Description of product stolen (capsules, injectables, powders, etc.)
- Quantity of each product stolen
- Description of packaging/containers
- Lot number(s) and national drug code (NDC) number(s)
- Storage/handling requirements for the product(s)
- Tampering protections in packaging

Other publications have likewise chimed in on cargo theft. Food Logistics magazine (http://foodlogistics.com) published an article in September 2011 highlighting “Eight Ways to Prevent Cargo Theft” focused on their clients. In that article, they recommend reconciling inventories through frequent audits, firing dishonest employees, providing background checks, using cameras and security systems, aligning the company with enforcement organizations, training personnel to catch suspicious activities and strangers, establishing safe vehicle parking habits and establishing vehicle and trailer alarms, locks, and other security devices [38].

As some theft involves drive-aways by unauthorized drivers (under the noses of gate guards and dispatchers), details about drivers and demanding commercial driver licenses (CDLs) from drivers as well as recording trailer numbers prior to trailer pick-ups are recommended.

What happens to stolen trucks and trailers? Here is a list:

- Cargo sold cheaply to any buyer
- Buyers reserve the right to purchase stolen trucks and trailers
- Shopping lists of trucks/trailers and cargos
- Used for replacement parts
- Altering the vehicle identification number (VIN)
- Sold for scrap
- Purchasing cheap stolen trucks/trailers—No maintenance, tires, etc.
- When they wear out, get another stolen one

Some thieves are caught. Truckinginfo.com published an article in March 2014 entitled "Three convicted in $1 Million Truck, Trailer and Cargo Theft Conspiracy." The perpetrators were indicted by the US federal government. They stole cargo in Missouri, Kansas, Florida, Oklahoma, Nebraska, and Arkansas. They stole meat, chicken, beer, sausage, and Nike shoes and sold the product. They collaborated with each other to pay for stolen product and vehicles [39].

Some resources for those companies desiring more information about preventive planning and current events involving food cargo theft can be found at:

http://www.freightwatchintl.com
http://cargonet.com
http://www.tracersystems.us (U.S. food and drug administration (USFDA) food related alerts, missing/overdue drivers, stolen cargo)
http://www.tsa.gov (Transportation Security Administration)
http://www.dhs.gov (Department of Homeland Security (DHS)
http://www.RLA.org

The Reverse Logistics Association (RLA) provides some issues for reverse logistics control of stolen food freight including help with:

- Planning
- Recouping cash loss
- Recall handling
- Regulatory compliance
- Salvage
- Package recycling
- Liability
- Notification of supply chain partners
- Information capture
- Quality and safety of the food
- Facilitation product handling and labeling
- Management of consumer notifications
- Return for reconditioning
- Disposal and disposal costs (bacteria laden, environmental protection association (EPA)

Some security systems currently available to carriers and shippers include these options:

- Alarms
- Trailer and auto lock systems (remotes)
- Software
- Cameras
- Truck security starter disarmers
- Tracker systems

- Ignition cut out switch
- Fuel cut out switch
- Steering wheel lock
- Transmission lock
- Wheel lock/boot
- Lockable fuel cap and wheel nuts

Jammers are a problem when used by thieves. They are illegal devices that interrupt and block signals put out by GPS tracking devices in phones and other wireless devices.

The illegal use of jammers should be reported to the FCC at the Jammer Tip Line (Phone 1-8555-55NOJAM).

To sum up, food shippers working to establish preventive food theft controls need to be aware of fake phone numbers, fake contacts, fake CDLs and identification cards, fake dispatchers, and fake liability insurance.

Basic start-up steps include:

1. Analyze your current exposure
2. Plan to improve
3. Train your people
4. Know how to respond and report
5. Have an action plan in the event of theft
6. Validate the plan

There are a few books carriers might consider purchasing including

Cargo Theft Prevention: A Handbook for Logistics Security by Louis A. Tyska and Lawrence J. Fennelly
Contraband, Organized Crime and the Threat to the Transportation and Supply Chain Function by Mario Possama
Transportation and Cargo Security: Threats and Solutions by Kathleen M. Sweet
Securing Global Transportation Networks: A Total Security Management Approach by Luke Ritter, J. Michael Barrett, and Rosalyn Wilson

Food theft can occur at any time, in any place. The number one cargo theft throughout the world is food. There are multiple agencies established to provide assistance in planning and prevention that can be contacted for more information. Food theft is a preventable food safety and food quality issue that impacts a company's bottom line. Food theft can destroy a small company while larger companies may not want the notoriety associated with the lack of preventive controls and may choose to hide the theft in order not to have unwanted publicity or increased insurance costs.

REFERENCES

[1] USDA Current Recalls and Alerts. http://www.fsis.usda.gov/wps/portal/fsis/topics/recalls-and-public-health-alerts/current-recalls-and-alerts; August, 2016.

[2] US FDA Animal and Veterinary Recalls Archive. http://www.fda.gov/animalveterinary/safetyhealth/recallswithdrawals/ucm393160.htm; August, 2016.

[3] US FDA Industry Guidance: Information on Recalls of FDA Regulated Products. http://www.fda.gov/Safety/Recalls/IndustryGuidance/default.htm; February, 2016.
[4] US FDA Safety. http://www.fda.gov/Safety/Recalls/ucm165546.htm; August, 2016.
[5] Responding to a Food Recall: Procedures for Recalls of USDA Foods. http://www.fns.usda.gov/sites/default/files/Responding_Food_Recall_FNS_Final_May_30_2014.pdf; August, 2016.
[6] The Food Recall Manual. http://edis.ifas.ufl.edu/pdffiles/fs/fs10800.pdf; August, 2016.
[7] US FDA Regulatory Report: Assessing the Safety of Food Contact Substances. http://www.fda.gov/Food/IngredientsPackagingLabeling/PackagingFCS/ucm064166.htm; August, 2016.
[8] US Department of Health and Human Services: A Food Labeling Guide. http://www.fda.gov/downloads/Food/GuidanceRegulation/UCM265446.pdf; August, 2016.
[9] ASTM International: Paper Standards and Packaging Standards. https://www.astm.org/Standards/paper-and-packaging-standards.html; August, 2016.
[10] US FDA CFR – Code of Federal Regulations Title 21. https://www.accessdata.fda.gov/scripts/cdrh/cfdocs/cfcfr/CFRSearch.cfm?fr=177.1390; August, 2016.
[11] Illinois Compiled Statutes. http://www.ilga.gov/legislation/ilcs/ilcs3.asp?ActID=1584&ChapAct=410; August, 2016.
[12] theguardian, Fake-food scandal revealed as tests show third of products mislabeled. http://www.theguardian.com/world/2014/feb/07/fake-food-scandal-revealed-tests-products-mislabelled; February, 2014.
[13] Unprecedented verdict: Peanut executive guilty in deadly salmonella outbreak. http://us.cnn.com/2014/09/19/us/peanut-butter-salmonella-trial/index.html?sr=sharebar_linkedin; August, 2016.
[14] R. Johnson, Food Fraud and "Economically Motivated Adulteration" of Food and Food Ingredients, Congressional Research Service. http://fas.org/sgp/crs/misc/R43358.pdf; January 10, 2014.
[15] ibid.
[16] Consumer Product Fraud: Deterrence and Detection. http://www.gmaonline.org/downloads/wygwam/consumerproductfraud.pdf; August, 2016.
[17] European Parliament 2013 Report on the food crisis, fraud in the food chain and the control thereof. http://www.europarl.europa.eu/sides/getDoc.do?type=REPORT&reference=A7-2013-0434&language=EN; August, 2016.
[18] FoodOnline 8 Actions to Stop Food Fraud. http://www.foodonline.com/doc/actions-to-stop-food-fraud-0001?utm_source=linkedin&utm_medium=social&utm_content=Oktopost-linkedin-group&utm_campaign=Oktopost-2014-09+General+Campaign; August, 2016.
[19] Bloomberg, Honey Sting Leads to U.S. Charges of Smuggling From China. http://www.bloomberg.com/news/articles/2013-02-20/u-s-probe-nets-largest-honey-smuggling-scheme-in-history; April, 2016.
[20] Time, Waiter, There's Fox in My Donkey Meat: The Global Scandal of Food Fraud. http://science.time.com/2014/01/02/china-fake-meat-food-fraud-scandal/; August, 2016.
[21] John M. Ryan, Food Fraud, Elsevier Academic Press, London, 2015,
[22] https://webgate.ec.europa.eu/rasffwindow/portal/?event=SearchForm&cleanSearch=1; July, 2015.
[23] Food Safety and Quality. http://www.perkinelmer.com/industries/food-beverage-nutraceuticals/food-fraud.xhtml; July, 2015.

[24] US FDA FDA DNA Testing at Wholesale Level to Evaluate Proper Labeling of Seafood Species. http://www.fda.gov/Food/GuidanceRegulation/GuidanceDocuments RegulatoryInformation/Seafood/ucm419982.htm; August, 2015.
[25] Food fraud Rudolph edition: Alaska restaurant labels New Zealand venison as native reindeer. http://barfblog.com/tags/food-fraud/; July, 2015.
[26] USP Food Fraud Database. https://www.foodfraud.org; August, 2016.
[27] http://nfpcportal.com/FQTools/FoodFraudster/tabid/329/Default.aspx; April 15, 2015.
[28] https://www.food.gov.uk/enforcement/the-national-food-crime-unit/foodfraud; August 3, 2015.
[29] http://ec.europa.eu/food/safety/official_controls/food_fraud/index_en.htm; August 4, 2015.
[30] http://www.foodfraudresources.com/publications/; August 1, 2015.
[31] https://webgate.ec.europa.eu/rasffwindow/portal/?event=SearchForm&cleanSearch=1; July 27, 2015.
[32] http://www.freightwatchintl.com/; December 15, 2015.
[33] http://www.landlinemag.com/Story.aspx?StoryID=27597#.VDap4haqzAw; August 22, 2016.
[34] http://www.aapa-ports.org/files/SeminarPresentations/06_Security_Huerta.pdf; August 22, 2016.
[35] CargoNet.com; June 12, 2014.
[36] http://www.fbi.gov/about-us/cjis/ucr/cargo-theft-user-manual; August 22, 2016.
[37] http://www.fda.gov/ICECI/CriminalInvestigations/ucm209979.htm; August 22, 2016.
[38] http://www.foodlogistics.com/article/10365265/eight-ways-to-prevent-cargo-theft; August 22, 2016.
[39] http://www.truckinginfo.com/channel/fleet-management/news/story/2014/03/three-convicted-in-1-million-truck-trailer-and-cargo-theft-conspiracy.aspx; August 22, 2016.

CHAPTER

Step-by-step implementation of your valid food safety and quality preventive control system

10

If you have not caught on yet, there is a critical and basic perspective personnel in any company must come to grips with if effective and validated preventive control food safety and quality systems are to be established by food suppliers. Yes, there are a million details, or so it seems. And where or how to start can be, at the very least, confusing.

NOT A PROBLEM

There are two parts to this chapter. The first part covers a general system implementation process to help guide implementers, whereas the second part provides guidance in defining system details.

START SOMEWHERE!

Throughout this book, there has been a strong emphasis on separating common causes from assignable causes and the need to separate responsibilities for each class of causes in mind and in action. Common causes are system causes and they are the responsibility of management and are addressable through the activation of CC teams. As the Chipotle case study demonstrates, a failure on the part of management to recognize and act upon responsibilities under their control can lead to mismanagement, huge financial losses, and even, perhaps, jail time. Functional improvement teams (FITs) take on the responsibilities within their sphere of control and are given authority and responsibility to attack functional problems using the solution tracking sheet (STS) and statistical process control (SPC) tools discussed in Chapter 4, Developing a Preventive Controls Plan: Food Safety and Quality.

Food safety and quality are not issues to ignore or assume that the "problem" is caused by governmental laws and will go away with a change in those people elected to manage the government. Product and, now, personal liabilities are involved. As a result of the passage of the food safety modernization Act (FSMA) in the United States as an example, regardless of corporate protection, management is now held to

Validating Preventive Food Safety and Quality Controls. DOI: http://dx.doi.org/10.1016/B978-0-12-810994-6.00010-9

a different set of standards and can be prosecuted for the impact of noncompliance on consumers and the public. Regardless of enforcement activities, companies wishing to protect their own financial longevity and stability should have a vested interest in avoiding system failures that result in external failure costs such as those associated with recalls, loss of reputation and lawsuits.

The U.S. FSMA perspective on preventive controls is incomplete when trying to avoid such losses. A validation system designed to preventively control threats to food safety and quality goes far beyond FSMA regulations or any preventive control qualified individual (PCQI) training you will receive.

Recall that validation requires that your company proves that products and processes have been established that bring potential hazards under control and keep them under control. The validation stream includes process design, pilot processing, volume processing, and controls through to the customer. Teams, the solution tracking sheet (STS), and statistical process control (SPC) are primary tools available to focus efforts on hazard reduction.

In addition to the Team STS/SPC approach outlined here, remember that related research, mathematical modeling and even sampling can be used as validation tools.

Regardless of FDA FSMA preventive control rules and the omissions included in them, many food safety aspects must be controlled in order to prevent illness and deaths. Many tools are available to assure valid supplier and transportation controls are in place and to work on food fraud and theft issues.

Up to this point, the chapters in this book covered the following general validation topics:

1. Laws causes and costs
2. Teams and teamwork
3. Environmental monitoring and sampling
4. Solution tracking sheet and SPC
5. Cross contamination
6. Supplier controls
7. Cycle time analysis
8. Critical issues you cannot ignore
   a. Recall
   b. Traceability
   c. Temperature monitoring
   d. Packaging
   e. Food fraud
   f. Food cargo theft

Fig. 10.1 depicts a flowchart that can be used to serve as guidance to one of many sequences you might consider following as you begin your journey to full compliance with both customer and food and drug administration (FDA) FSMA requirements. In each box on the flowchart are the numbers that are discussed in the paragraphs below.

All food safety and quality planning starts with a company policy that is the responsibility of the chief executive officer (CEO) and upper management (1). This policy must be communicated to all company employees.

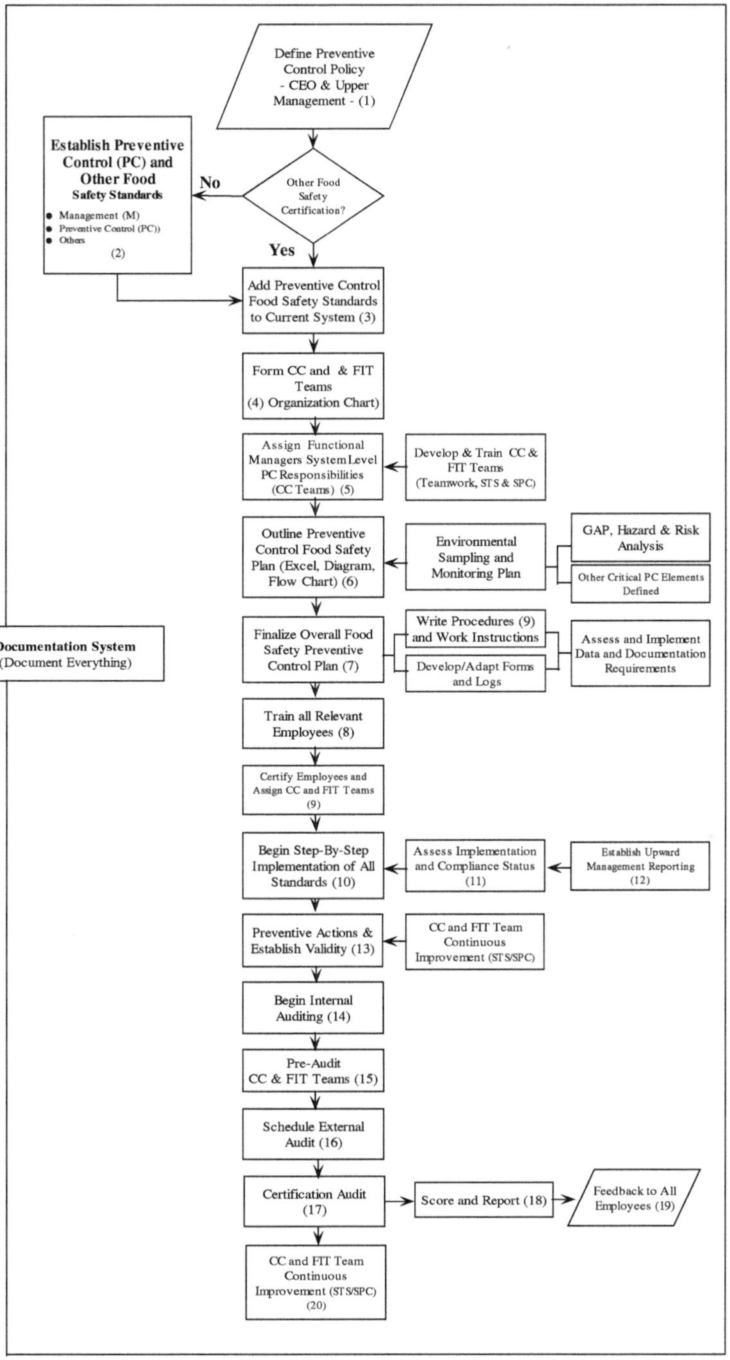

FIGURE 10.1

Implementation flowchart.

Each company must develop, adapt, or copy a set of food safety and quality standards that include, but are not limited to, management, preventive controls, and others that apply to the organization (2). These standards are critical to guiding the development of the overall plan.

Most companies already have some type of food safety plan and, generally speaking, are undergoing food safety audits by their internal audit teams and third-party auditors. The new company preventive control standards and requirements must be merged into the company current food safety plan. The company that might be hired to conduct third-party audits should be consulted to assure that any changes they might have made to their own set of standards and audit activities have been upgraded to meet current legal requirements such as those provided by the FDA under FSMA (3).

The company must clearly understand and organize management and hourly workers into common cause (CC) and functional improvement (FIT) teams and begin to assign priorities and responsibilities for each set of system (CC teams) and process requirements (FIT teams) to tackle both common system and assignable causes (4). Team and individual assignments should be specified on lower-level organizational chart. If there is a single individual in charge of organizing and overseeing the entire preventive control system, that responsibility and the person in charge should be delineated on the upper-level organizational chart. Showing the specific person responsible for preventive controls and food safety in general is a common audit requirement.

FIT and CC teams need to undergo initial training. Remember that a trained and certified individual must be assigned to oversee the initial planning and must approve any changes to the plan. These teams and the system validation person should show up on the organizational chart (5).

The steps leading into item 6 that calls for teams to outline the preventive controls plan using FIT and CC team input to Excel, diagrams, and flow charts, good agricultural practices (GAP), hazard and risk analysis, environmental monitoring, and other critical components (see chapter: Cycle Time Analysis in Preventive Food Safety and Quality Control Practices) are included to get a visual understanding of what each company must work on.

Inputs to step 7 call for an assessment and implementation of data and documentation requirements, writing procedures and work instructions, and developing or adapting the data collection system (forms, logs, software, etc.). All of that should then be added to the initial plan developed under item 6 in Fig. 10.1.

Step 8 calls for the training of all employees whose responsibilities impact food safety and planning. The training needs to be documented and documents recorded in each person's human resource (HR) file. The process diagram, flowchart, and Excel spreadsheet data should be used in the training to add a component of visualization for employees. Some companies require each employee to pass a test for such certification.

With certification training in the rear view mirror, final assignment of members of CC and FIT teams to activities prioritized by team member discussions can be completed to get the teams up and running (step 9). Do not forget to have someone trained as an overall team/program facilitator.

Implementation of teams, teamwork, and the plan begin in step 10 with support from support and reviews from management (step 12) and assessment and compliance reviews (step 11).

Assuming that a few months have gone by, step 13 calls for CC and FIT teams to demonstrate (probably through quarterly reviews) continuous improvement through STS and SPC presentations.

There is a basic and classic SPC reference book you can download for free that was developed by a now defunct company named Western Electric. The book provides readers with many different types of SPC applications that are beyond the scope of this book. [2]

With the system up and running and some number of teams operational, the internal audit team can begin to review the system (step 14). Step 14 is normally activated prior to organizing CC and FIT team representatives whose responsibility is now to assure that the system is ready for a third-party audit (step 15). In other words, do the internal auditing before the external audit is called for and scheduled.

Schedule and complete the audit (step16), review scoring and the final report (step 18), and provide feedback to all employees (step 19).

With that all compete, management is expected to review the system on a continuous basis and teams are expected to demonstrate their control over causes using objective data and analyses such as can be supplied by use of STS and SPC results (step 20).

REFERENCES

[1] Developing food safety and quality plans: an aquaponics process control example. Food Safety Magazine 2012: http://www.foodsafetymagazine.com/enewsletter/developing-food-safety-and-quality-plans-an-aquaponics-process-control-example/.

[2] Statistical Quality Control. http://www.contesolutions.com/Western_Electric_SQC_Handbook.pdf; October, 2016.

CHAPTER 11

Case study Chipotle: Common cause failures

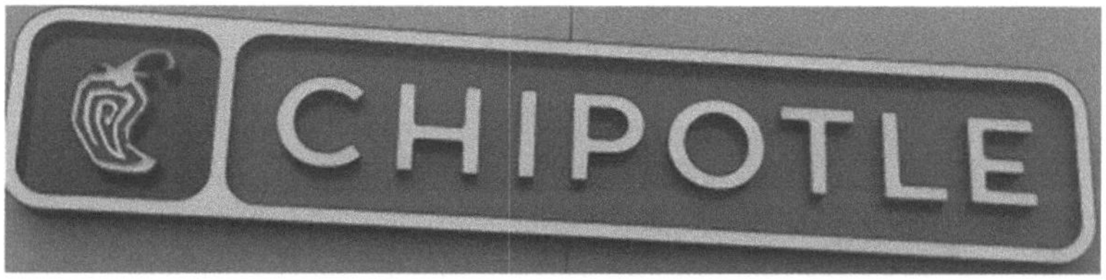

Take, for instance, one of the costlier outbreaks involving *Escherichia coli* 026 (Shiga toxin producing). Chipotle had lost billions in value, and, even after months of diligent work on the part of company employees. It has not been able to determine a cause. However, Chipotle is a great example of what ails the overall food industry and company reacts by promising the best food safety system in the world.

The Chipotle case demonstrates a classic misunderstanding of the difference between common causes (CCs) and assignable causes and the results of the failures that result from not recognizing and planning for those differences.

While Chipotle is considered a retail operation and therefore exempt from the preventive control rules and exempt from validation requirements, the case illustrates the fact that when retailers are exempt and get out of control, the entire food supply chain is impacted.

GREAT REASONS TO ESTABLISH PREVENTIVE CONTROLS: DOLLARS, DEATHS, AND ILLNESS

In August 2015, a Simi Valley, California Chipotle restaurant outbreak was blamed for sickening 243 people with Norovirus. In December 2015, a second restaurant in Boston, Massachusetts sickened 143, also from Norovirus. In August 2015, *Salmonella* somehow invaded tomatoes in Minnesota and Wisconsin sickening 64 people, then *E. coli* hit another 60 people in California, Delaware, Illinois, Kansas, Maryland, Minnesota, New York, Ohio Oklahoma, Oregon, and Washington states. The outbreaks have continued through March 2016.

The cost of such outbreaks can be catastrophic to even the best of companies. In 1993, outbreaks at Jack in the Box saw their stock value plunge 22% due to an

Validating Preventive Food Safety and Quality Controls. DOI: http://dx.doi.org/10.1016/B978-0-12-810994-6.00011-0

E. coli (0157:H7) outbreak that saw over 170 people impacted with four children dying from complications. Finger pointing and lawsuits regarding whom was responsible ensued between Jack in the Box, Vons, and eight meat suppliers with Jack in the Box finally accepting a $58.5 million from these suppliers.

From a food safety perspective, and in addition to the large financial losses supply chain members suffered, Wikipedia reports many food safety related results as shown below.

As a direct result of the outbreak:

- *E. coli* O157:H7 was upgraded to become a reportable disease at all state health departments
- the Food and Drug Administration (FDA) increased the recommended internal temperature for cooked hamburgers from 140°F (60°C) to 155°F (68°C)
- the United States Department of Agriculture (USDA)'s Food Safety and Inspection Service (FSIS) introduced safe food-handling labels for packaged raw meat and poultry retailed in supermarkets, alongside an educational campaign alerting consumers to the risks associated with undercooked hamburgers. The labels and the educational campaign came with criticism and objection from the industry [1]
- the FSIS introduced testing for *E. coli* O157:H7 in ground meat
- the USDA reclassified *E. coli* O157:H7 as an adulterant in ground beef
- the USDA introduced the Pathogen Reduction and Hazard Analysis and Critical Control Point (PR/HACCP) program
- the national cattlemen's beef association (NCBA) created a task force to fund research into the reduction of *E. coli* O157:H7 in cattle and slaughterhouses
- Jack in the Box completely overhauled and restructured their corporate operations around food safety priorities, setting new standards across the entire fast food industry.
- Parents of victims formed STOP Foodborne Illness (formerly Safe Tables Our Priority, or S.T.O.P.), a national nonprofit organization dedicated 'to prevent Americans from becoming ill and dying from foodborne illness' by advocating for sound public policy, building public awareness, and assisting those impacted by foodborne illness.
- Parents of the victims played key roles in spreading awareness and advocating for change—speaking directly to President Bill Clinton, meeting with Vice President Al Gore, testifying before the Clinton Healthcare Task Force, working with the Secretary of Agriculture, and discussing food safety issues with lawmakers in Washington, D.C.
- Some parents, including Darin Detwiler (who lost his son, Riley, to *E. coli* and hemolytic-uremic syndrome during the outbreak), later served as regulatory policy advisors to the USDA for meat and poultry inspection [1].

Chipotle stock peaked in October 2105 at around $750 per share (Fig. 11.1). After the March 2016, Norovirus outbreak, the stock was selling at about $455 per share. This represents a 39.3% loss to those invested in the company's stock. Estimates at the end of 2015 were that Chipotle's total net income fell some 44% and net sales fell 15% which translates into $53 million [2].

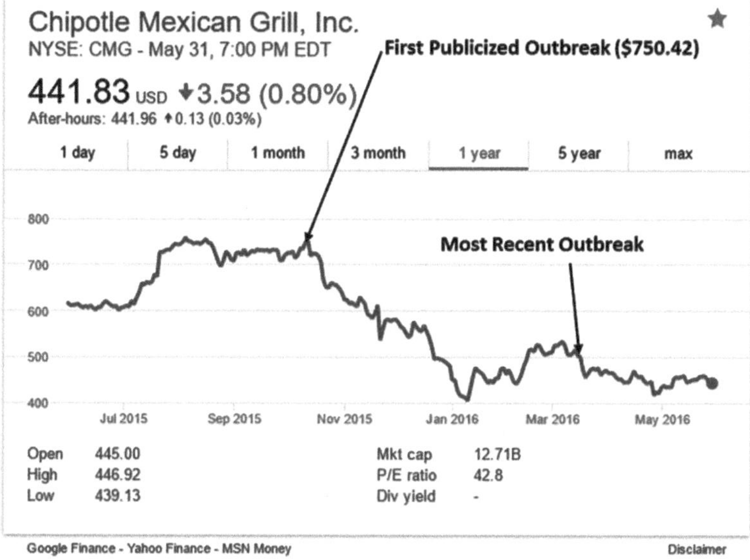

FIGURE 11.1

Chipotle stock trend [3].

Chipotle had no food safety officer prior to the first outbreak but hired one 4 months later.

Taking a bit closer look at the Chipotle multistate outbreak involving *E. coli*, the FDA, and the CDC issued this information:

- "Confirming that all microbial testing performed by the company did not yield *E. coli* (more than 2500 tests of Chipotle's food, restaurant surfaces, and equipment all showed no *E. coli*)
- Confirming that no employees in these restaurants were sickened from this incident
- Expanded testing of fresh produce, raw meat, and dairy items prior to restocking restaurants
- Implementing additional safety procedures, and audits, in all of its 2000 restaurants to ensure that robust food safety standards are in place
- Working closely with federal, state, and local government agencies to ensure that robust food safety standards are in place
- Replacing all ingredients in the closed restaurants
- Conducted additional deep cleaning and sanitization in all of its closed restaurants (will conduct deep cleaning and sanitization additionally in all restaurants nationwide)

The FDA conducted trace backs of multiple widely distributed ingredients. Trace back can be difficult with Mexican-style foods given they are often complex dishes containing multiple ingredients. No product of interest was identified. Even without a definitive item to follow, the FDA traced back to their origins some widely distributed ingredients in an effort to identify a source for the outbreak. Unfortunately, the distribution path did not lead to an ingredient of interest.

The FDA also conducted investigations of some suppliers, but did not find any evidence that those suppliers were the source of the outbreak. Ultimately, no food item has been identified as causing the outbreak, and by the same token, no food has been ruled out as a cause [4]."

Chipotle is a great case study from a system point of view. The reaction from the company in media included live interviews and as many apologies and assurances as could be publicly delivered in as short a time possible. Regardless of Chipotle's many problems, the crowds continue to enjoy Chipotle lunches (Fig. 11.2).

From the Chipotle chief executive officer (CEO) comes this statement:

The fact that anyone has become ill eating at Chipotle is completely unacceptable to me and I am deeply sorry. As a result, we are committed to becoming known as the leader in food safety, just as we are known for using the very best ingredients in a fast food setting. I want to share with our customers' specifics about some of the significant steps we are taking to be sure all of the food we serve is as safe as it can be [5].

Will Chipotle become "the leader in food safety?" Here is an outline of their plan from their website. This list is what Chipotle calls "Our Food Safety Procedures."

1. At the Company Suppliers
   New supplier guidelines that include "high-resolution" testing methods. Samples are taken and tested, sometimes in the field before harvest and again after wash and pack operations. The company say they take statistically random samples from each field using a "Z" pattern.
2. In Central Kitchens
   Tomatoes, for example, are washed, diced, rinsed, tested and passed or failed based on a "zero defects" sampling plan. Zero defects means that if any tested piece fails, the batch is scrapped.
3. In the Restaurants
   Marinate chicken and steak only at night to prevent cross contamination of fresh ingredients.

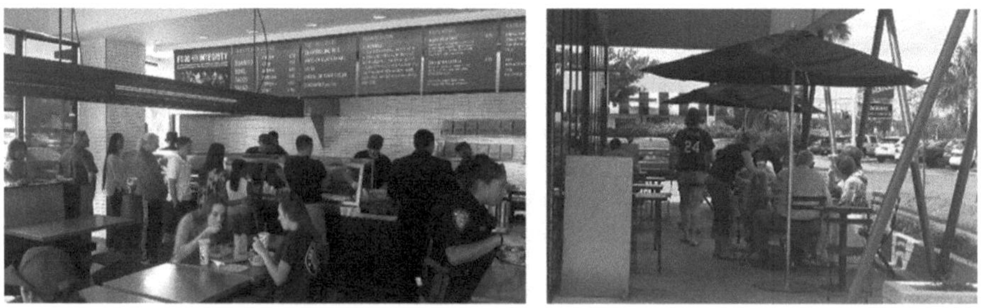

FIGURE 11.2

Photos of local Chipotle restaurant (March 2016).

Produce blanching (or submerging in boiling water for 5 seconds) for lemons, limes, jalapenos, onions, and avocados to eliminate surface bacteria. Surface bacteria can be carried into the product when a knife blade passes through the contaminated surface into the inner product thus carrying the contamination into the protected part of the product.

Higher frequency disinfecting and sanitizing food contact surfaces (table tops, etc.) during operating hours and restaurant-wide cleaning at closing time.

Field leaders trained in food safety to perform weekly inspections with annual inspections by Chipotle corporate staff food safety team members, health experts, and government health officials.

4. At the Employee Level
Food Safety training and evaluation, paid sick leave to prevent employees coming to work when ill, a reward system for restaurants achieving high marks on food safety and assigning the duty senior manager as the "food safety owner" to assure that procedures are followed.
5. A 10-million dollar find established for local grower support to provide them with food safety training, grants to help pay for new costs, and new partnerships with companies employing new technologies. Chipotle calls this the "Local Grower Support Initiative" [6].

It is interesting to note that nowhere in the Chipotle website discussion is there any mention of prevention or the food safety modernization act (FSMA). What is also interesting is that Chipotle has recognized at some aspect of their supply chain beginning with farms then processing of raw produce followed by some in-restaurant blanching of a few commodities, heightened restaurant sanitation with audits and inspections, employee wellness, training, financial assistance, and the development of new greenhouse and technology partnerships.

Recognizing the fact that many growers cannot meet Chipotle's food safety standards, the company allocated the $10 million in funds to support the food safety effort.

The significant question that must be raised from Chipotle's list is whether or not the planned system is comprehensive enough to be considered a preventive system? In early February 2016, a 90-minute all employees meeting was broadcast live via the web to announce a new food safety system that was planned to descend on retail outlet operations. Daily "Food Safety Notes", "Crew Confidence Sheets" (requiring pre shift meetings covering a variety of procedures), "Food Safety Rollout Checklists", standards, "Food Safety Evaluation" forms, "Field Leader Observation Guides", and other documents were distributed over the next few months. All hourly and salaried managers were scheduled to complete ServSafe Food Manager certification training and compliance testing no later than March 31, 2016.

Daily Food Safety notes cover such items as dishwashing, allergens, sick time policies, food from nonChipotle approved sources, Chipotle ingredients, new recipes, general operational cleanliness, employee and customer vomit controls, flies and pests, hot holding (temperature controls), sick policies, and others.

Field leader evaluations designed to rate restaurant compliance cover dumpster areas, dining rooms, restrooms, drink stations, appearance, and taste of food ingredients (tortillas, rice, beans, fajita mix, barbacoa, chicken, steak, carnitas, sofritas, salsa, sour cream, cheese, guacamole, lettuce, chips), station set-up, take-out lines, dish and chemical controls, crew standards, storage and walk-ins, grills, kitchen management, accounting/office, safety/licensing, security, compliance/training, and service management. Most of the field leader's guide covers normal operational quality concerns rather than food safety issues.

The Chipotle food safety evaluations cover general food safety (and operational) audit issues such as employee health, personal cleanliness, hygienic practices, eating, drinking, tobacco use, contamination prevention, hand washing, use of approved food sources, utensil storage, food contact surfaces, self-service item use, ware washing, storage and use of wiping cloths, time/temperature controls, reheating, cooling, cold and hot holding, records maintenance, date marking/disposition, thawing chemicals, hazard analysis critical control point (HACCP), and pest controls. Each food safety evaluation included a cover sheet that appropriately identified the evaluated site, the manager, the auditor and contact information.

EXTENDING THE COST OF EXTERNAL FAILURES: CHIPOTLE NEWS ITEMS

Chipotle dumped the centralized kitchen concept because products arriving at retail stores were not fresh enough. The centralized kitchen was established to better control food safety of product coming from farms. Chipotle reportedly shifted gears and began to eliminate small produce suppliers and replace them with large scale farming operations.

References to food safety disappear from the Chipotle.com website.

In this book, the discussion of the potential external failures (costs associated with the most expensive aspect of a lack of food safety and quality control) reveals that the lack of preventive controls can be financially devastating to a company. Often external failure costs do not include the costs of lawsuits that may follow on the heels of outbreaks when such costs should be included.

In March, 2016, 24/7 Wallst published an article detailing multiple lawsuits from investors and employees. The lawsuits cover sexual harassment, failure to pay workers overtime, hiring practices, gender discrimination, failure to pay overtime, wrongful termination, retaliation, and discrimination [7].

Other lawsuits include false genetically modified organisms (GMO) claims, securities class action, attempted coverup of the outbreaks, and even allowing a kitchen manager to work for 2 days while sick with gastrointestinal symptoms [8–11].

Such external failure costs resulting from high profile outbreaks similar to the Chipotle fiasco are yet to be determine but will surely amount to millions of dollars.

News reports tend to follow a story as long as the public tunes in, and the Chipotle saga has become a never-ending shark feeding fest.

Spring the early summer of 2016, Chipotle dumped the centralized kitchen concept because products arriving at retail stores were not fresh enough. The centralized kitchen was established to better control food safety of product coming from farms. Chipotle reportedly shifted gears and began to eliminate small produce suppliers and replace them with large scale farming operations.

References to food safety disappear from the Chipotle.com website.

In May 2016, Chipotle announced that it would enter the burger market (a $73 billion market) by announcing it would start a new burger chain named "Better Burger." Within hours, the Chipotle stock value dropped [12].

American broadcasting company (ABC) News reports that "Hundreds of Chipotle restaurants aren't serving pork after the national chain suspended a supplier for violating its standards [13]."

The New York Times reports that "Chipotle Mexican Grill closed its more than 2000 restaurants for four hours on Monday to hold a "virtual" town hall meeting with its employees about steps it said it was taking to improve food safety and regain consumers' trust [14]."

Chipotle ramps up restaurant manager training requiring all managers to undergo food safety training with a company known as ServSafe. According to ServSafe, "The ServSafe online training program provides food safety training, exams, and educational materials to foodservice managers. Students can earn the ServSafe Food Protection Manager Certification, accredited by the American National Standards Institute-Conference for Food Protection." Chipotle paid ServSafe $100 per manager for training and $35 per manager for certification testing.

NBC News reports on June 8, 2016 that Chipotle offered part-time workers improved benefits including sick pay, paid vacation, and tuition reimbursement [15].

Food Safety News reports that "Federal officials slapped down claims by Chipotle Mexican Grill's corporate lawyers that the public didn't need to know details about E. outbreaks that sickened at least 60 people across 14 states in late 2015" [16].

Chicago Tribune reports on July 18, 2016 that "Mark Crumpacker, 53, the chain's chief creative and development officer, appeared in New York state court last week on misdemeanor charges that he bought cocaine on seven occasions since January, according to prosecutors. He's accused of being one of 18 'repeat customers' of a cocaine-delivery service who were indicted Thursday along with three ringleaders."

"Crumpacker's alleged drug purchases coincide with some of the company's worst days of 2016, with Chipotle struggling to bounce back from a string of *E. coli* and norovirus outbreaks. Crumpacker, whose compensation was $4.28 million last year, led the marketing effort to restore the company's image [17]."

In July 2016, Chipotle's chief creative officer was arrested in New York for criminal possession of cocaine, a controlled substance. He was placed on administrative leave.

Grub Street published a report regarding an employee who was terminated for complaining about wages and beginning a break policy petition. The case went to court. The judge required Chipotle to rehire the employee and repay lost wages [18].

Will Chipotle's stock ever recover? As of late August, 2016, the Chipotle stock continues to decline (Fig. 11.3).

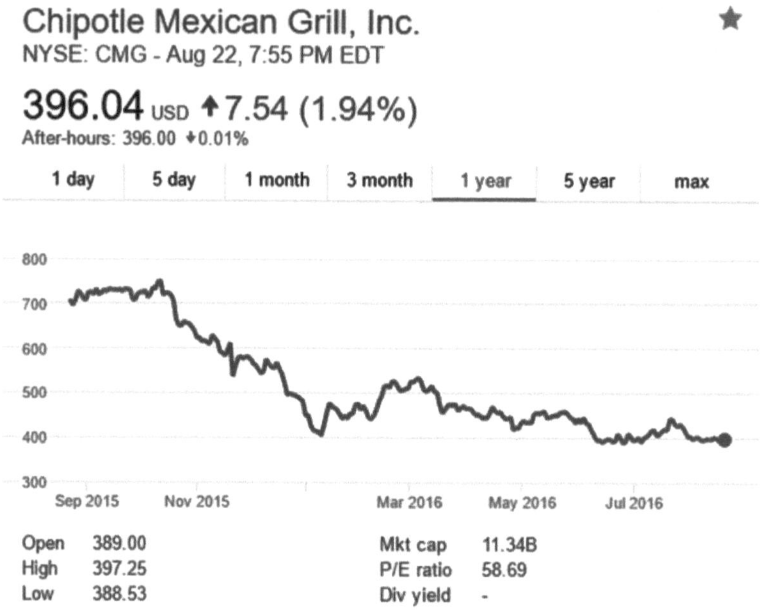

FIGURE 11.3

Chipotle stock trend late August 2016 [19].

Chipotle drops the centralized food preparation operations due to a decline in food quality. This reversal is a shift away from food safety and a shift back to appearance and taste (date unknown).

Steve Ells, the Chipotle founder, chairman and Co-Chief Executive Officer placed a full page announcement in the USA Today (Page 5A) on September 21, 2016 that attempted to update the public regarding Chipotle's food safety advancements. In that announcement, Ells listed eight advancements made by the company.

1. Supplier Interventions (increased food safety steps at suppliers)
2. Advanced Technology ("high pressure")
3. Farmer Support & Training (providing funding and training)
4. Enhanced Restaurant Procedures (new food safety procedures)
5. Food Safety Certification (managers and field leaders)
6. Restaurant Inspections (increased in number and intensity)
7. Ingredient Traceability (electronic tracking)
8. Advisory Council (independent industry experts)

CASE STUDY QUESTIONS

1. Outline a basic CC team list of priorities for Chipotle's management staff.
2. Given a perspective of preventive controls, describe how you would plan to bring food safety into Chipotle's processes.

a. Where would you start?
b. What priorities would you set?
c. How would you change the priorities apparently established by Chipotle management?

3. Under subpart G of the supplier preventive control rules and concepts of vicarious liability, is Chipotle liable for buying product from small, local, fresh farms?
4. Name 3 critical incidents that occurred between January 2016 and July 2016 that might have caused set-backs for the overall food safety improvement effort.
5. Why did Chipotle offer improved benefits to part-time workers in June 2015?
6. What preventive control might Chipotle have enforced when it fired the pork supplier?
7. Do you think Chipotle turned to unapproved suppliers due to some type of shortage in deliveries from approved suppliers? Does the shortage of an ingredient cause other supply chain members to buy from unapproved suppliers when a shortage hits?
8. Do you think the arrest of Chipotle's chief creative and development officer impacted the business?
9. Under FSMA, the law eliminated small farms from having to comply with new regulations. Congressional arguments went back and forth over the idea that small farms were still farms and could easily contaminate the food supply chain. Others claimed that small farms would be unable to comply with FSMA rules due to costs and the lack of small farm expertise. Early on, Chipotle established a $10 million fund to help their small farm suppliers upgrade food safety systems.

   Should Chipotle have eliminated the small farms?

   Is there another strategy Chipotle could have followed that would have allowed the company to continue with the small farm, locally grown, freshness concept while protecting food safety?
10. Do you think Chipotle has the food safety and quality preventive controls in place well enough to begin a Better Burger chain?
11. Discuss the potential issues and costs of external failures resulting from the Chipotle story.
12. Google "Chipotle Food Safety", update and discuss changes Chipotle has made since the publication of this book.

REFERENCES

[1] 1993_Jack_in_the_Box_E._coli_outbreak. https://en.wikipedia.org/wiki/1993_Jack_in_the_Box_E._coli_outbreak; March, 2016.

[2] Here's How Many People Stopped Eating at Chipotle During Their E. Coli Outbreak. http://gizmodo.com/the-cost-of-chipotles-e-coli-outbreak-measured-in-bur-1756830015; March, 2016.

[3] Chipotle Mexican Grill, Inc. https://www.google.com/webhp?sourceid=chrome-instant&rlz=1C1CHZL_enUS683US683&ion=1&espv=2&ie=UTF-8#q=chipotle%20stock; June, 2016.

[4] FDA Investigates Multistate Outbreak of E. coli 026 Infections Linked to Chipotle Mexican Grill Restaurants. http://www.fda.gov/Food/RecallsOutbreaksEmergencies/Outbreaks/ucm470410.htm; March, 2016.
[5] Our Food Safety Advancements: A letter from Chiptle Founder Steve Ells. http://chipotle.com/founderletter; March, 2016.
[6] Chipotle Local Grower Support Initiative. http://chipotle.com/localgrowersupport; March, 2016.
[7] Former Chipotle Employees Go After Company in Court. http://247wallst.com/services/2016/03/23/former-chipotle-employees-go-after-company-in-court/; August, 2016.
[8] Judge Green Lights Lawsuit Against Chipotle Over GMO Claims. http://www.eater.com/2016/4/21/11481534/chipotle-gmo-lawsuit; August, 2016.
[9] Chipotle Mexican Grill Inc., The Rosen Law Firm. http://www.rosenlegal.com/cases-809.html; August, 2016.
[10] Chipotle Tried to Cover Up Foodborne Illness Outbreak, Lawsuit Claims. https://thinkprogress.org/chipotle-tried-to-cover-up-foodborne-illness-outbreak-lawsuit-claims-b4429e866634#.eimglmgyl; August, 2016.
[11] Robertson & Associates, LLP Files Class Action Against Chipotle Mexican Grill, Inc. Alleging Norovirus Outbreak Sickened Hundreds. http://www.businesswire.com/news/home/20160119006866/en/Robertson-Associates-LLP-Files-Class-Action-Chipotle; August, 2016.
[12] Chipotle's new burger chain. https://www.washingtonpost.com/news/wonk/wp/2016/04/01/why-chipotle-is-thinking-about-opening-up-a-burger-chain-and-what-it-might-look-it/; August, 2016.
[13] Chipotle: Why Hundreds of Restaurants Don't Have Pork on the Menu. http://abcnews.go.com/Business/chipotle-hundreds-restaurants-pork-menu/story?id=28217932; July, 2016.
[14] Chipotle Meeting Outlines Food Safety to Workers and Message for Public, New York Times. http://www.nytimes.com/2016/02/09/business/chipotle-meeting-outlines-food-safety-to-workers-and-message-for-public.html?rref=collection%2Ftimestopic%2FChipotle%20Mexican%20Grill%20Inc.&action=click&contentCollection=business®ion=stream&module=stream_unit&version=latest&contentPlacement=4&pgtype=collection&_r=0; July, 2016.
[15] Chipotle to Offer Part-Time Workers Paid Vacation, Sick Pay, Tuition Reimbursement. http://abcnews.go.com/Business/chipotle-offer-part-time-workers-paid-vacation-sick/story?id=31619921; July, 2016.
[16] CDC to Chipotle: Public has a right to know about outbreaks, Food Safety News. http://www.foodsafetynews.com/2016/05/cdc-to-chipotle-public-has-a-right-to-know-about-outbreaks/#.V4-ebbiANBc; July, 2016.
[17] Chipotle executive's alleged cocaine buys line up with company's worst days, Chicago Tribune. http://www.chicagotribune.com/business/ct-chipotle-executive-cocaine-20160718-story.html; July, 2016.
[18] Chipotle Broke the Law by Firing Employee Who Circulated Petition. http://www.grubstreet.com/2016/08/chipotle-broke-the-law-by-making-an-employee-delete-tweets.html; August, 2016.
[19] Chipotle Mexican Grill, Inc. NYSE https://www.google.com/?ion=1&espv=2#q=chipotle%20stock; August, 2016.

Index

Note: Page numbers followed by "*f*" and "*t*" refer to figures and tables, respectively.

D

E

F

Kolibri 360 GmbH
Ferdinand-Jühlke-Straße 7
99095 Erfurt, Deutschland
produktsicherheit@kolibri360.de